From the eleventh century to the Black Death in 1348 Europe was economically vigorous and expanding, especially in Mediterranean societies. In this world of growing wealth new educational institutions were founded, the universities; and it was in these that a new form of medicine came to be taught and which widely influenced medical care throughout Europe. The knowledge of the university medical practitioner, both physician and surgeon, was built on translations of Greek and Arabic texts, together with personal experience of medical practice.

The essays in this collection focus on the practical aspects of medieval medicine, and among other issues they explore how far this new learned medicine percolated through to the popular level; how the learned medical men understood and coped with plague; the theory and practice of medical astrology, and of bleeding (phlebotomy) for the cure and prevention of illness. Several essays deal with the development and interrelations of the nascent medical profession, and of Christian, Muslim and Jewish practitioners one to another. Special emphasis is given to the practice of surgery and to innovation in surgical technique, to the development of surgical treatises which made learned surgery more widely available, and to the role of royal surgeons. The problems of recovering knowledge of a large proportion of medical care – that given by women – are also explored.

This collection forms a companion volume to *The medical renaissance of the sixteenth century* (1985, edited by Andrew Wear, Roger French and I. M. Lonie), *The medical revolution of the seventeenth century* (1989, edited by Roger French and Andrew Wear), *The medical enlightenment of the eighteenth century* (1990, edited by Andrew Cunningham and Roger French), and *The laboratory revolution in medicine* (1992, edited by Andrew Cunningham and Perry Williams).

Practical medicine from Salerno
to the Black Death

Practical medicine from Salerno to the Black Death

EDITED BY
LUIS GARCÍA-BALLESTER,
ROGER FRENCH, JON ARRIZABALAGA
AND ANDREW CUNNINGHAM

Consejo Superior de Investigaciones Científicas, Barcelona
and
Wellcome Unit for the History of Medicine,
Cambridge University

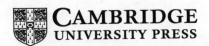
CAMBRIDGE
UNIVERSITY PRESS

616.0094
P881

AG01 '94

Published by the Press Syndicate of the University of Cambridge
The Pitt Building, Trumpington Street, Cambridge CB2 IRP
40 West 20th Street, New York, NY 10011–4211, USA
10 Stamford Road, Oakleigh, Melbourne 3166, Australia

First published 1994

Printed in Great Britain at the University Press, Cambridge

A catalogue record for this book is available from the British Library

Library of Congress cataloguing in publication data

Practical medicine from Salerno to the Black Death / edited by
Luis García-Ballester et al.
　　p.　　cm.
　ISBN 0 521 43101 8 (hc)
　　1. Medicine, Medieval – History. 1. García-Ballester, Luis.
[DNLM: 1. History of Medicine, Medieval – congresses. WZ 54 P895]
R141.P7　1994
616'.0094'0902 – dc20
DNLM / DLC　92–49013　CIP

ISBN 0 521 43101 8 hardback

94-0090

CE

Contents

Illustrations and tables

TABLE

Contributors and editors

Jole Agrimi, Department of Philosophy, University of Pavia, Italy

Jon Arrizabalaga, Consejo Superior de Investigaciones Científicas, Barcelona, Spain

Chiara Crisciani, Department of Philosophy, University of Pavia, Italy

Andrew Cunningham, Wellcome Unit for the History of Medicine, University of Cambridge, UK

Roger French, Wellcome Unit for the History of Medicine, University of Cambridge, UK

Luis García-Ballester, Consejo Superior de Investigaciones Científicas, Barcelona, Spain

Pedro Gil-Sotres, University of La Laguna, Canary Islands, Spain

Monica H. Green, The Institute for Advanced Study, Princeton, New Jersey, USA

Danielle Jacquart, Directeur de Recherche au CNRS, Paris, France

Peter Murray Jones, King's College, Cambridge, UK

Michael R. McVaugh, The University of North Carolina at Chapel Hill, USA

Cornelius O'Boyle, University of Notre Dame, Indiana, USA

Nancy Siraisi, Hunter College of the City University of New York, USA

Acknowledgements

The present volume arises from the conference on 'Practitioners and medical practice in the Latin Mediterranean, 1100–1350' (Barcelona, April 1989), organized by the Department of the History of Science of the CSIC in Barcelona and the Wellcome Unit for the History of Medicine of the University of Cambridge, and would not have been possible without the enthusiastic collaboration of all those attending, both the contributors of papers and those who took part in the ensuing discussions. The conference was made possible thanks to the generous help of the Dirección General de Investigación Científica y Técnica of the Spanish Ministry of Education and Science. We are also grateful for the financial assistance of CSIC (Madrid), CIRIT of the Generalitat de Catalonia, the Subdirección General de Cooperación Internacional of the Spanish Ministry of Education and the Wellcome Trust (London). The stimulating atmosphere of discussion was further encouraged by the warm welcome offered by the President and staff of the Institut d'Estudis Catalans, on the premises of which in the former Hospital de Sant Pau i de la Santa Creu the conference took place. Our thanks also go to the management and staff of the CSIC's residence for research-workers in Barcelona for their hospitality; to Maribel Sevillano and Elena Orriols, secretaries of the Department of the History of Science in Barcelona; to Fernando Salmón, Montserrat Cabré and Lluís Cifuentes, at the time Ph.D. students at the CSIC.

The final text of this book owes much to the suggestions of two anonymous referees of Cambridge University Press.

Note on names

In the vexed matter of the appropriate form of medieval names, we have mainly followed the usages in Nancy Siraisi, *Taddeo Alderotti and his Pupils: Two Generations of Italian Medical Learning* (Princeton, 1981), and Michael R. McVaugh and Nancy Siraisi (eds.), *Renaissance Medical Learning: Evolution of a Tradition* (*Osiris*, 2nd series, 6 (1990)). Alternative versions of names are given in the index.

It has been impossible to achieve consistency throughout the volume in the spelling and accenting of Peninsula place names, and we have generally opted for forms most familiar to the English-language reader.

Introduction: Practical medicine from Salerno to the Black Death

LUIS GARCÍA-BALLESTER

This book brings together the majority of the papers presented at a conference held in Barcelona in April 1989. The principal aim of the meeting was to assemble a group of scholars working in the field of medieval medicine in order to discuss to what extent medicine based on natural philosophy reached medieval medical practitioners, both physicians and surgeons. It was felt that it was important to restrict discussion to a significant geographical area and a well-defined period of time. The geographical area chosen was the Christian lands of the western Mediterranean, since this question could be most appropriately investigated there, and the period selected was from the twelfth century until the mid fourteenth century.

The reasons for these chronological limits are quite simple. We took as our starting point the fact that in the twelfth century a remarkable development took place in the southern part of Latin Christendom (the south of Italy, Sicily, and especially Salerno), an event that was to be of considerable influence in the intellectual history of European medicine. This was the basing of medical practice on the 'natural' part of philosophy, in particular on Aristotle's philosophy, which gave rise to a new form of medicine and a new way of perceiving medical training. Naturally, this did not happen by chance, and for this reason it is of great interest to enquire about its origins and why it developed in this particular area. The other event, providing our closing date, also came to be considered as remarkable in many ways, and this was the so-called 'Black Death' of 1348. It was remarkable not because it was the only such plague, nor even the first one, but because it marked a turning point even in the perceptions of the very people of the later Middle Ages themselves. Moreover, it coincided with the moment when the first process we are concerned with (the developing relationship between medicine and 'natural' philosophy) had reached a level of maturity in both intellectual and social terms. Its intellectual maturity was attained in the context of the introduction of medicine into universities in the course of the thirteenth century, while the extent of its social maturity can be demonstrated through the wide geographical distribution by this date of physicians or surgeons who based their practice on this new form of medical Galenism. It thus seemed reasonable to enquire to what extent, if any, there was a response from university medical circles and the new professionals in the field of medicine to the extraordinary phenomenon of the Black Death, and whether there was any communication over this issue between society and the medical world (with its Galenic paradigm). Such, then, were the chronological justifications.

We wanted to enquire, by means of new and directed research, whether the scholastic medicine that was being developed by scholars inside the universities was seen as merely an intellectual phenomenon, of concern only to a minority, or whether it was seen also as something that could be applied to the daily life of the new society that was being shaped in these southern parts of Latin Christendom at this period. We also wished to investigate whether university institutions were able to develop routes by which they might offer intellectual resources for the benefit of the health of citizens and cures for their illnesses, and not just for the minority of *beati possidentes* of the time (such as members of royal families, members of the civil and ecclesiastical nobility, and the new rich of the period). In short, what sort of contacts (if any) were established between the world of medicine based on the natural part of philosophy on the one hand, and society on the other – for such an interaction, if it in fact took place, must have worked in both directions.

Recent research has drawn attention to the existence of some intellectual products developed by the universities, and which were welcomed and applied by society in the area of medical practice. First there was the introduction and diffusion in the Latin West of Roman Law, which spread from northern Italy around the western Mediterranean from the late twelfth century onwards, and then at a faster rate in the following two centuries. The new physicians and surgeons learned how to make use of the new legal opportunities and of the conceptual world offered by the scholastic reception of Roman Law, for example, the concept of *salarium*, to conform with and adapt to the new social and economic order. In turn, town councils, institutions which were characteristic of the new social order in northern Italy in the early thirteenth century, were able to create a market for these new professionals, and did not hesitate to hire well-trained physicians to attend the medical needs of their citizenry, and not only the poorest members.[1] Secondly, there was the promotion of the university model of the medical professional as the only acceptable one in the field of professional practice. This was well established by the first decade of the

---

[1] See, Vivian Nutton, 'Continuity or rediscovery. The city physician in classical antiquity and mediaeval Italy', in A. W. Russell (ed.), *The town and state physician in Europe from the Middle Ages to the Enlightenment* (Wolfenbüttel, 1981), and bibliography therein. On the diffusion of Roman Law throughout the present-day French Midi and Catalonia, see André Gouron, *La science du droit dans le Midi de la France au moyen age* (London, Variorum Reprints, 1984).

fourteenth century. For instance, a development of this kind took place in the first third of the fourteenth century in the lands of the Kingdom of Valencia (Crown of Aragon), which had been won for Christendom shortly before (1240–5).[2] The urban bourgeoisie played a leading role in both these kinds of development.

There has been considerable recent interest in the development of medieval medicine. One area of interest has been that of medical and dietetic prescriptions and therapeutic indications. The editors of a recent volume[3] on this pay special attention in their lengthy introduction to the relevant 'Fachliteratur', the professional technical medical literature. Although it had a complex relationship with medical texts in Latin and it deeply influenced the world of medical practice, this form of medical literature was often produced and used by anonymous practitioners mainly of non-academic origin, who did not spurn expressions derived from common speech. This extraordinarily popular kind of medical writing was professional in nature, full of technical expressions, and it made interesting contributions to lexical issues in various European languages. It allows us to draw closer to the real world of medical practice, of which it was a product and to which, at the same time, it served as a stimulus. It might almost be dubbed 'underground literature', and on occasions was indeed on the very frontier between academic knowledge and uneducated empiricism: for it drew upon the complex intellectual and technical medical world intro- duced into Europe by means of Latin translations of the writings of Greek or Arab doctors in the university sphere, while it simultaneously reflected local healing traditions. Both Anglo-Saxon[4] and German[5] scholarship has paid due attention to this field.

Moreover, medieval medicine is presently also being studied from the broad perspective of an intellectual and social 'renaissance' spanning the period from the twelfth to the sixteenth centuries.[6] Some of us are also engaged in studying medical learning and its social penetration into the complex society of the fourteenth-century Crown of Aragon, where three cultures lived alongside one another (Jews, Muslims and Christians), with different models for understanding and practising the social task that

---

[2] Luis García-Ballester, Michael R. McVaugh, and Augustin Rubio-Vela, *Medical licensing and learning in fourteenth-century Valencia, Transactions of the American Philosophical Society*, 79, part 6 (Philadelphia, 1989).

[3] Gerhard Baader and Gundolf Keil (eds.), 'Einleitung' to *Medizin im mittelalterlichen Abendland* (Darmstadt, 1982), pp. 1–44, especially from p. 25 onwards.

[4] Tony Hunt, *Popular medicine in thirteenth century England. Introduction and texts* (Cambridge, 1990).

[5] See, amongst others, Gundolf Keil, 'Das Arzneibuch Ortolfs von Baierland', *Sudhoffs Archiv*, 43 (1959), 20–60; Keil, 'Der Kodex Kohlhauer. Ein iatromathematisch-hauswirt- schaftliches Arzneibuch aus dem mittelalterlichen Oberfranken', *Sudhoffs Archiv*, 64 (1980), 130–50; and also Gundolf Keil (ed.), *Fachprosa-Studien* (Berlin, 1981).

[6] Michael R. McVaugh and Nancy Siraisi (eds.), *Renaissance medical learning. Evolution of a tradition* (*Osiris*, 2nd series, 6 (1990)), esp. 7–160.

medicine represented and still represents.[7] Recently too, the relationship between Arabic medicine and the Latin West has been reconsidered using a wider knowledge of the Arabic sources and greater familiarity with the Latin manuscripts.[8] Meanwhile, such a thorny subject as twelfth-century medicine in Salerno has recently been dealt with from a new standpoint.[9] All these explorations have strengthened our interest in enquiring what role medical learning had for the practice of physicians and surgeons over this reasonably short and coherent period.

THE SOCIAL DIFFUSION OF UNIVERSITY MEDICINE

Studies of the historical sociology of theology have demonstrated how efficient later medieval preaching was in spreading from the university world of scholasticism specific theological ideas and a particular vision of the world and man.[10] Recent studies on the social expansion of knowledge in the Latin West in the thirteenth and fourteenth centuries[11] similarly reveal the diffusion of written knowledge within society through the network of grammar schools that spread across southern Europe in these centuries.[12]

The world of the liberal arts thus had a well-established and institutional-ized channel of social diffusion as well as offering a wide and interesting range of job opportunities. This diffusion of the liberal arts was assisted by the so-called 'scientific encyclopedias' of Vincent of Beauvais, Bartholo-maeus Anglicus, Thomas of Cantimpré, Albert the Great, and Juan Gil de Zamora, all dating from the thirteenth century.[13] (By the mid thirteenth

---

[7] See note 2 above.

[8] Danielle Jacquart and Françoise Micheau, *La médecine arabe et l'occident médiéval* (Paris, 1990).

[9] Piero Morpurgo, *Filosofia della natura nella schola salernitana del secolo XII* (Bologna, 1990).

[10] See the lucid study of the role of preaching in thirteenth- and fourteenth-century Latin Europe, in Fernando Rodríguez Reboiras and Abraham Soria Flores (eds.), *Raimundi Lulli Opera latina, Summa sermonum in civitate Maioricensi ... composita*, vol. xv (Turnhout, 1987).

[11] Peter Denley, 'Governments and schools in late medieval Italy', in T. Dean and C. Wickham, *City and countryside in late medieval and Renaissance Italy* (London and Ronceverte, 1990), pp. 93–107: 'The clear acceleration of state sponsorship of education in the fourteenth and fifteenth centuries is very much in tune with the findings of historians who are looking at state provision for medicine, public health and other aspects of civic government in the period' (p. 98). See also Nutton, 'Continuity or rediscovery', pp. 32–3.

[12] Michael R. McVaugh and Luis García-Ballester, in their current work about practitioners and medical practice in the fourteenth-century Crown of Aragon, have found a lot of evidence in the Catalonian notarial records on the spread of grammar schools in small and large towns and the role in this played by university people trained in the faculty of arts; for an example, see the contracts between the municipal council of the town of Manresa (Catalonia) and Bonanatus, *magister in artibus*, 'magister scholarium gramatice' (Arxiu Historic Municipal, Manual de Consells, 1365–73, fols. 59, 18 June 1367 and 137r–v, 13 September 1369).

[13] Recent research has stressed the role played by members of the mendicant orders educated in Paris in the diffusion of Avicenna's *Canon*: see Nancy Siraisi, 'The medical learning of

century the liberal arts had largely been transformed into natural philosophy, with medical doctrine and material forming a substantial part of it). Scholastic society was thus capable of building routes of communication along which there flowed currents of ideas and values between university circles and the rest of society, and was also capable of creating suitable (or at least acceptable) conditions for a labour market attractive enough for university graduates.

It is reasonable to think that a similar phenomenon took place also in the medical world. Was scholastic medicine indeed perceived by lay society as a suitable technical means for the analysis of illness and capable of creating a medical system which could face up to the problems presented by illness, both in normal social conditions and in extraordinary situations? A full answer to all these questions that underlie the concept of this present book would require a reinterpretation of the medical manuscript sources, in the light of the new approaches of the social and intellectual history of medicine. However, the medical sources, of whatever nature, would not suffice for a complete answer, and it would be necessary to use both civil and ecclesiastical archive sources and other forms of lay or non-professional literary evidence (chronicles, accounts, sermons, all types of written material) to enable us to identify the daily activity of the new type of healer who emerged from the university lecture halls, and of those non-university healers who in one way or another were associated with the values of university medicine. Furthermore, if it were possible, our aim should be not only to detect their presence and activity, but also to assess the social impact of this new type of healer in terms of the perceptions of people of the time. A full account along these lines lies beyond the scope of this book, but it is in some way present within it.

Medical practice in this period was not limited to the activities of the professional, whether physician or surgeon, emerging from the academic world equipped with the intellectual tools provided by natural philosophy. In these years such medical practitioners were a novelty, and, of course, given their numbers, they were unable to provide medical attention to the whole population of Europe: we need only consider, on the basis of the limited data available, the ratio of inhabitants to university physicians even in the most privileged regions of southern Europe at this period.[14] So, what relationship existed between this academic form of medicine (that of the physicians and surgeons) and that of those other physicians, surgeons and

---

Albertus Magnus', in J. A. Weisheipl (ed.), *Albertus Magnus and the sciences* (Toronto, 1980), pp. 379–404, on pp. 392–3; D. Jacquart and C. Thomasset, 'Albert le Grand et les problèmes de la sexualité', *History and Philosophy of the Life Sciences*, 3 (1981), 73–93.

[14] M. R. McVaugh and L. García-Ballester, work in progress quoted in note 12. For Barcelona city and Valencia city (1325–34), the approximate ratio was between two and six physicians per 10,000 inhabitants. These figures have been established from the names of the physicians (*phisici*), which appear in the notarial records, and from the population as estimated by historians of demography (20,000–25,000 inhabitants).

barbers without direct access to academic circles, but who fulfilled an important role in providing a socially respectable form of medicine (for they were certainly not considered to be 'quacks')? Practitioners belonging to this latter category lacked any form of access to the academic world either because of their religion (Jewish or Muslim) or their sex, even though they lived alongside the dominant Christian group, or belonged to it. Many of these practitioners, for socio-economic and cultural reasons, did not consider academic medicine to be something necessary for proper professional activity. Moreover, in their opinion, the route towards proper medical practice did not need to pass through a faculty of medicine, in spite of the fact that this professional model, generated by these same institutions, became the norm, at least in the minds of those who ruled society and dictated its laws,[15] and even though this scholastic model, and the new professional who emerged from it, continued to hold a certain fascination, at least for Jewish physicians.[16]

THE APPEARANCE OF A NETWORK OF MEDICAL CARE

Another feature of medicine in southern Europe in the twelfth to the fourteenth centuries was that the type of medical practitioner moulded in the Galenic paradigm and shaped by scholasticism often formed part of an incipient network of medical care and attention.[17] In effect the professional physician or surgeon placed himself at the service of a medical system – a true network of medical care – that took shape over this period, and spread rapidly all around the western Mediterranean. By means of this system, civil society (basically the city councils) endeavoured to provide medical care of its citizens through the hiring of technically trained medical professionals.[18] University physicians answered this demand, and one could suggest that they did so with a certain degree of prestige, judging by their generous salaries.[19] The existence of such a network, the extent and density of which can be measured in many regions of Italy from the mid thirteenth

---

[15] Pearl Kibre, 'The faculty of medicine at Paris, charlatanism and unlicensed medical practices in the later Middle Ages', *Bulletin of the History of Medicine*, 27 (1953), 1–20, at 8–11.

[16] Luis García-Ballester, Lola Ferre, and Eduard Feliu, 'Jewish appreciation of fourteenth-century scholastic medicine' in McVaugh and Siraisi (eds.), *Renaissance medical learning*, 85–117 (*Osiris*, 2nd series, 6 (1990), 85–117).

[17] L. García-Ballester and M. R. McVaugh, work in progress quoted in note 12 above. The documentary evidence deals with the fourteenth-century (1280–1400) territories of Catalonia, Valencia, Aragon and Majorca.

[18] See documents published by Michael R. McVaugh, 'Bernat de Berriacho (fl. 1301–43) and the *ordinacio* of Bishop Ponç de Gualba', *Arxiu de Textos Catalans Antics*, 9 (1990), 251–4.

[19] Luis García-Ballester, 'Medical ethics in transition in thirteenth–fourteenth century Latin medicine: new problems on physician–patient relationship, and the doctors' fee', in A. Wear and R. French (eds.), *Medical ethics: historical aspects* (Amsterdam, 1993).

century onwards,[20] and in the lands of the Crown of Aragon from the closing years of the same century,[21] is in our view the great novelty in the field of the historical sociology of European medicine. This new development was closely related to the one already mentioned in the intellectual field: the basing of medical practice on natural philosophy. Nevertheless, the information available does not allow us to establish a causal relationship between the two phenomena.

Under normal conditions, such professionals provided a reasonably satisfactory response to the problems that illness produced for the inhabitants of towns and cities and also of villages, and to the health requirements of a society that had reached a high degree of complexity as a consequence of the process of urbanization and the dynamic growth resulting from intense commercial activity. By supporting this new type of physician, the new bourgeois group (merchants, artisans, liberal professionals, *rentiers*) together with the nobility and the Church itself, provided him with the backing of their own social position and prestige. It is obvious that this could not have been achieved if the physician was not satisfying the expectations about health and illness that society as a whole and individuals within it had of him. It is impossible to conceive the increasing spread of learned practitioners, both physicians and surgeons, as anything other than a consequence of the effectiveness of their presence and as a demonstration of a positive response to their work by those who had it in their power to make decisions in this medieval European society. It goes without saying that this efficacy must be measured in accordance with the criteria of the society of that time. In fact, the new university bodies, through the geographical spread of university-trained practitioners, demonstrated that the conversion of medicine into a *scientia* was perceived as socially beneficial. Civil authorities came to establish a link between the desire for health (*spes salutis*) and the presence of professionally suitable physicians and surgeons (that is, those educated in the medical *scientia*).[22] The evidence that we currently possess about France, Italy and the east of the Iberian Peninsula (the former Crown of Aragon) seems to confirm this view.[23] This does not mean that the practice of these professional physicians and surgeons was totally free from criticism, or even from cruel caricatures or violent rejection, but at no time did lay society question the model of the practitioner who had been produced by the university. However, it was to

[20] See Nutton 'Continuity or rediscovery'.

[21] See note 17 above.

[22] 'Ut provisiones medicorum phisice et cirurgie et apothecariorum ... ut per eorum providenciam et scienciam medicine Nos [the king] et nostri subditi preserventur a noxis et habere possimus absque periculo spem salutis', Arxiu de la Corona d'Aragó, C., reg. 1145, fol. 24v (12 February 1354).

[23] See Danielle Jacquart, *Le milieu médical en France du XIIème au XVème siècle*, Hautes études médiévales et modernes, 46 (Geneva, 1981); Nutton, 'Continuity or rediscovery', and Italian bibliography therein; McVaugh and García-Ballester, note 12 above.

question the eagerness of such practitioners to monopolize the practice of healing, and their wish to subject it to norms decided by academic bodies composed exclusively of those who had been trained in similar circumstances.[24]

An interesting feature of this period is that it allows the historian to find out how this medical system reacted when the society was subjected to an abnormal event, one that was perceived as abnormal by that society itself, as was the plague of 1348. The system and those physicians and surgeons forming part of it were put to the test. Their opinions were sought, and the procedures they designed to confront this new illness (if they did indeed consider it to be such a radical novelty) were accepted. The intellectual resources (the explanations they offered of the mechanism of the illness) and the practical ones (the specific therapeutic steps) were adopted and considered to be fairly satisfactory. And, although it takes us beyond our chronological limits, we can state that the survivors of 1348 continued to ask for the technical services of the university physicians with the same conviction as before.[25]

ARISTOTELIZATION AND GALENISM

What do we understand by the 'university physician or surgeon'? Simply the individual trained in the *studia generalia* – the universities – after having followed the medical studies laid out in the *syllabi*, which, by the early fourteenth century were more or less uniform in faculties of medicine in the whole of this area of Europe.[26] This university form of medicine could count among its achievements the conversion of the empirical act of healing into a true *scientia* that was respectable in both intellectual and social terms. Intellectual respectability was achieved by establishing both the patient–physician relationship and the natural phenomenon of illness itself on Aristotle's *libri naturales* and the doctrines of Galen and Arab physicians, whose writings were fully assimilated in Latin Europe in the last third of the thirteenth century. Its social respectability was achieved because the professionals were able to provide a satisfactory response to the specific

[24] See, for example, the fights between the guild of physicians (*collegium*) of Barcelona (with a high percentage of non-university members) and the king (supporter of the university doctors): L. García-Ballester, 'Los orígenes de la profesión médica en Cataluña: el *collegium* de médicos de Barcelona (1342)', in *Estudios dedicados a Juan Peset Aleixandre*, 3 vols. (Valencia, Universidad de Valencia, 1982), vol. II, pp. 129–55. For the problem in the Kingdom of Valencia, see García-Ballester, McVaugh, and Rubio, *Medical licensing and learning*.

[25] For example, the municipal council of the town of Castelló d'Empúries sent a messenger to Avignon in January 1350 to look for a university physician and to contract him (Arxiu Històric de Girona, Castelló d'Empúries, reg. 2062, *s.f.*, 2 February 1351); see García-Ballester, 'Medical ethics in transition'.

[26] A good survey is Nancy Siraisi, *Medieval and early Renaissance medicine. An introduction to knowledge and practice* (Chicago and London, 1990).

daily challenges that illnesses presented through involvement in a complex system of medical care and attention, which, as has already been mentioned, seems to have been successful. At least the controlling social groups, from royalty down to the increasingly powerful bourgeoisie, supported this new *scientia medica* and those who based their professional activity on it.

Aristotle's works were received among circles interested in medicine, both directly and indirectly, over a long period (from the time of Boethius onwards but especially between the end of the eleventh century and the last third of the thirteenth century). This reception did not take place only within academic institutions. Nevertheless, the universities and their faculties of arts were the bodies that formulated a clear program for the 'Aristotelization' of the Latin intellectual world, and invented or reformulated intellectual analytical tools that turned out to be efficient.[27]

'Aristotelization' went beyond what is generally understood as the natural world: it extended to the rational analysis of the nature of man and of his relationship with his surroundings (usually his physical surroundings) and with the cosmos itself. This 'nature' of man was liable to fall ill, but was also capable of recovering good health and maintaining it; and this was achieved simply by means of human resources, which depended exclusively on the activities of man. Such activity was significant for the individual of the Middle Ages because it involved both the microcosm (man himself and the physical environment in which he moved) and the macrocosm (the universe in which man exists). 'Aristotelization' also included a way of understanding and organizing society and social life,[28] which was closely related to the organization of this same social body through Roman Law. Aristotle's books on ethics and politics were fervently debated in university circles in the second half of the thirteenth century, and we are sure that the intellectual innovation of *quaestiones* affected medical practice itself. For this reason, it is valid to point out in this context that Aristotle's *Politics* repeatedly emphasizes the responsibility on the part of those wielding power in society to supply technically qualified medical attendance. This point was discussed by such influential commentators as Albert the Great and Thomas Aquinas himself.[29] This program was derived from combining the Greek Aristotle with the commandments of Christian charity. The implementation of this program in a society which had made Christianity its basis and which was dominated by the poverty of the majority of its

[27] L. Minio-Paluello, 'Aristotle: tradition and influence', in C. C. Gillispie (ed.), *Dictionary of scientific biography* (*DSB* hereafter) (New York, 1980), vol. I, pp. 267–81; J. A. Weisheipl (ed.), *Albertus Magnus and the sciences*; Guy Beaujouan, 'Une lente préparation au "décollage" des sciences', in R. H. Bautier (ed.), *La France de Philippe Auguste* (Paris, 1983), p. 860, reprinted in Guy Beaujouan, *Par raison de nombres: collected studies* (Aldershot, 1991), item IV.

[28] See J. A. Weisheipl, 'The life and works of St Albert the Great', in Weisheipl (ed.), *Albertus Magnus*, pp. 13–51, on pp. 30–1, and pp. 575–6 (Appendix I).

[29] García-Ballester, 'Medical ethics in transition'.

population was one of the problems confronting both society and these new practitioners. It is, however, an issue that we do not cover in this volume.

A new stage in medical knowledge in the West was marked by the translations made by Constantine (d. *c.* 1087)[30] (especially that of the *Pantegni* of Haly Abbas (al-Majusi), but also that of Ibn al-Gazzar's *Viaticum* and of Johannitius' *Isagoge*), the later translations by Gerard of Cremona (d. 1187)[31] (chief of which was Avicenna's *Canon*), and the continued movement of translating from Arabic into Latin, including several works by Rhazes. For these produced a great torrent of terminology, methods, medical doctrine characterized by a logical and coherent structure, and evidence of the clinical success of a rational form of medicine. Galenism, which constituted the common doctrinal foundation of all of them, demanded a direct knowledge of the medical works of Galen himself, either translated from the Greek or approached by means of Arabic versions. The whole universe of Greek medicine, including the Hippocratic tradition, was covered by the shadow of Galen, and this state of affairs was something that the Latin West inherited from their Islamic teachers.[32] Paradoxically, although Galen was undoubtedly the most widely admired author and an obligatory point of reference in medical matters by the mid thirteenth century, he was still a completely unknown historical figure up until the last years of that century, as Arnau de Vilanova admitted.[33] Galen's works, basically those of a clinical and therapeutic nature, entered the learned medical world of the Middle Ages relatively slowly until the 1270s and 1280s when an intellectual movement, which we may call the 'new Galen', suddenly burst on the academic scene.[34] The availability of this considerable corpus of teachings allowed those physicians who had access to it to reconsider old questions, to formulate new readings of old texts and to make reflections and offer bold solutions which served to widen the intellectual horizons of the academic community and also of the

---

[30] M. McVaugh, 'Constantine the African', in *DSB*, vol. III, pp. 393–5; Heinrich Schipperges, *Die Assimilation der arabischen Medizin durch das lateinische Mittelater* (Wiesbaden, 1964), pp. 17–54; Jacquart and Micheau, *La médecine arabe*, pp. 96–118. See also H. Bloch, *Monte Cassino in the Middle Ages* (Rome, 1986), vol. I, pp. 93–110, 127–34.

[31] R. Lemay, 'Gerard of Cremona', in *DSB*, Supplement I, vol. XV, pp. 173–92; Schipperges, *Assimilation der arabischen Medizin* pp. 147–53; Marie-Thérèse d'Alverny, 'Translations and translators', in R. L. Benson, G. Constable, and G. D. Lanham (eds.), *Renaissance and renewal in the twelfth century* (Oxford, 1982), pp. 421–62, on pp. 452–4.

[32] Owsei Temkin, *Galenism, rise and decline of a medical philosophy* (Ithaca and London), 1973.

[33] 'Tercium est que sit causa efficiens huius libri, quia Galienus quis autem fuerit ignoramus; verum modo tamen certa penitus auctoritate antiquorum exoprimitur ipsum divitum parentum filium excesisse et eruditum fore erudicione mirabile', *Commentum super librum Galieni de morbo et accidenti*, attributed to Arnau de Vilanova, Cracow, Jagiellonian Library 781, lib. I, fol. 131r. We give particular thanks to Fernando Salmón, who called our attention to this passage.

[34] L. García-Ballester, 'Arnau de Vilanova (*c.* 1240–1311) y la reforma de los estudios médicos en Montpellier (1309): el Hipócrates latino y la introducción del nuevo Galeno', *Dynamis*, 2 (1982), 97–158.

medical community subject to its direct or indirect influence. This medical community included a new type of surgeon, who found in this movement a way of distinguishing himself from those who wanted to maintain surgery at a purely empirical level and keep the process of learning at the level of a mere oral tradition, and a simple list of artisan-style techniques.

Assimilation of the 'new Galen', whose nucleus was composed of the works of Galen himself, but which also included the entire corpus of Arab medical works, demanded a detailed knowledge of the Aristotelian natural philosophy corpus on the part of the university physician; this equipped him with the intellectual tools without which it was impossible to understand the complex and unsystematic world of Galen's writings. There can be no doubt that such well-structured works as the *Pantegni*, the *Canon* or the *Isagoge* stimulated the Aristotelization of medieval Galenism.[35] The well-known organization of medical knowledge made by the Arab author of the *Pantegni*, straddling both theory and practice, is simply a transferral to medicine of Aristotle's doctrine, according to which the speculative foundations of a particular branch of knowledge (in this case the 'natural' part of philosophy) permit the rational development of a particular field of activity (medicine), whose goal is to maintain man's nature or to restore its integrity when it has been lost.[36] This gave rise to an 'ideology according to which *physica* had a moral imperative to devote its explanatory powers first of all to the human body and its health-related needs'.[37] In the first book of the *Canon* a summary is given of the structural and dynamic components of human nature (that is, those related to the natural part of philosophy), and when this began to be widely known from the first third of the thirteenth century onwards, it simply served to reinforce this organization of medical knowledge.[38] Johannitius' *Isagoge* popularized the same conceptual scheme of the 'naturals' (*res naturales, res non naturales, res preter naturam*) from the moment when it came to be known in learned circles in the twelfth century, and around it learned Latin physicians evolved their various doctrinal elaborations. This conceptual scheme came to be fully appreciated when Aristotle's *libri naturales* and other philosophical books became known; in these, subjects such as cosmology, physics and the theory of matter, especially of 'organic' matter, but also of ethics and political science, are dealt with. The reception of Aristotle's books might similarly be said to have built on the stimulus provided by the so-called

---

[35] Danielle Jacquart, 'Aristotelian thought in Salerno', in Peter Dronke (ed.), *A history of twelfth-century western philosophy* (Cambridge, 1988), pp. 407–28.

[36] 'Medicina est scientia cognoscendi dispositiones humani corporis in quantum sanabile, et conservandi sanitatem inventam in eo, et restituendi deperditam quantum possibile fuerit', *Arnaldi de Villanova Opera. Speculum medicine*, cap. 1 (Leyden, 1504), fol. 1ra.

[37] Jerome J. Bylebyl, 'The medical meaning of *physica*', in McVaugh and Siraisi (eds.), *Renaissance medical learning*, pp. 16–41, on p. 17.

[38] For an accurate description of Avicenna's *Canon*, and its role in medical teaching, see Nancy Siraisi, *Avicenna in Renaissance Italy* (Princeton, NJ, 1987).

Salernitan questions, partly derived from the tradition of the pseudo-Aristotelian *Problemata*.[39]

It is important to remember that to a medieval scholar astronomy/astrology, which were concerned with the mobile heavenly bodies, also came within the field of natural philosophy. The macrocosm and the microcosm, which were closely related, were the object of the intellectual curiosity of learned physicians. Medicine was an activity concerned with a particular body (that of man, in himself a microcosm) affecting situations of great personal and also social importance: those associated with health and illness. In this respect, medicine had no necessary connection with the natural part of philosophy. However, one of the intellectual innovations of the time was the use of the corpus of texts on the natural part of philosophy to give a theoretical analysis to the wide field covered by medical activity.[40] It was soon seen that all this speculative *rapprochement* had immediate practical repercussions in the real world, in the field of human activity, and in the physician–patient relationship. The result was that medicine from the twelfth century onwards was not only considered as an empirical activity, but also as an *ars*; in other words, as an operative or practical activity of a *rational* nature, with the capacity to detect, and to interfere in and alter processes at the core of human nature and in man's relationships with his immediate surroundings (microcosm) and with the universe as a whole (macrocosm), of both of which he formed part. Medicine was even considered as a *scientia*, that is, that medicine *is* the knowledge of the human body, in so far as the body is capable of recovering good health when it had been lost. Such knowledge was put into practice by means of the Aristotelian 'causes' (material, formal, efficient and final).

From this point onwards, the whole formal world of scholasticism placed itself at the service of analysing illness.[41] This approach became possible only when, from the second third of the twelfth century onwards, an ample corpus of Aristotle's works translated from the Greek began to be diffused from the south of Italy and the north of France.[42] An important role in this diffusion was played by the personal contacts between physicians from other areas of southern Europe (for example, the Ebro valley),

[39] Brian Lawn, *The Salernitan questions: An introduction to the history of medieval and Renaissance problem literature* (Oxford, 1963), p. 25 (rev. Italian transl. Salerno, 1969); and Brian Lawn (ed.), *The prose Salernitan questions* (London and Oxford), 1979, p. xxiii.

[40] See Bylebyl, 'The medical meaning of *physica*'.

[41] On the status of medicine *c.* 1300 in the faculty of medicine of Montpellier and Padua, see Michael McVaugh, 'The nature and limits of medical certitude at early fourteenth-century Montpellier', in McVaugh and Siraisi (eds.), *Renaissance medical learning*, pp. 62–84, on pp. 80–2.

[42] On the development and propagation of Graeco-Latin versions of Aristotle in twelfth-century Latin Europe, see Lorenzo Minio-Paluello, 'Iacobus Veneticus Grecus, canonist and translator of Aristotle', *Traditio* 8 (1952), 265–304, repr. in L. Minio-Paluello, *Opuscula: the Latin Aristotle* (Amsterdam, 1972); for *Aristoteles Latinus* manuscripts, see Minio-Paluello, *Aristoteles Latinus*: Codices, pars prior (Rome, 1939), *Pars posterior* (Cambridge, 1955), *Supplementa altera* (Bruges and Paris, 1961), repr. in 3 vols. (Leyden, 1979).

who were familiar with Arab Galenism in its highly developed form and with the natural part of Greek philosophy.[43] This introduction of the corpus of Aristotle's work gave rise to a particular form of medical knowledge whose fundamental characteristic was that it could be transmitted and taught as a written and rational body of knowledge.[44] This had evident social and economic repercussions, to which both physicians and society itself were very sensitive.

TOWARDS A PHILOSOPHICAL NATURAL MEDICINE IN SALERNO:
AN OPEN HISTORICAL QUESTION

One of the European intellectual innovations developed in the field of medicine from the twelfth century onwards that we have emphasized so far was the deliberate search for support for professional activity from the 'natural' aspect of philosophy. It seems logical to enquire about its origins. This change could be seen to be personified in those individuals in the south of Italy who, around the mid 1060s, found Greek culture to be both the intellectual stimulus for this search and, from their own point of view, the source from which to endow medicine with the support it needed. From the Abbey of Montecassino, Abbot Desiderius, and, from the city of Salerno, the Montecassino monk, physician and archbishop, Alphanus, undertook this quest, jointly so it would seem. The person who made it feasible was Constantine, a monk at Montecassino, where almost all of his work was carried out and which resulted in the collection of medical works translated from Arabic known as the *corpus Constantinum*.[45] The nucleus of

---

[43] The clearest example of such contact is the physician Petrus Alfonsi (b. in Huesca, 1062 or 1063), an Aragonese Jew who lived in the learned court circle in the Muslim-ruled cities of Huesca and Zaragoza. He had a good scholarly education and was familiar with Aristotelian and Galenic sources. Christians conquered Huesca in 1097 and Zaragoza in 1118. Petrus Alfonsi, whose Jewish name was Moshe ha-Sephardi, converted to Christianity in 1106. From this moment onwards he had contacts with England and the north of France. The author of the most complete study of Alfonsi's work says, 'More striking still is the almost total dependence on work unknown in the west at that time and, in some cases, never transmitted, of mediaeval Jewish and Muslim scientists and philosophers. His range is very wide, covering astronomy, cosmology, cosmogony, elemental theory, meteorology, psychology, medicine, and the occult.' See Jacqueline H. L. Reuter, 'Petrus Alfonsi: an examination of his works, their scientific content, and their background', unpublished Ph.D. thesis (Oxford, 1975), p. iii.

[44] In his commentary to Aristotle's *Metaphysics* (written in 1267), Thomas Aquinas underlines this characteristic of the *artifex*'s knowledge – for instance that of the physician – as well as pointing out the proper intellectual tool to be used in scholastic teaching: 'Signum scientis est posse docere: quod idea est, quia unumquodque tunc est perfectum in actu suo, quando potest facere alterum sibi simile, et dicitur quarto *Meteorum* ... Artifices autem docere possunt, quia cum causas cognoscant, ex eis possunt demonstrare: demonstratio autem est syllogismus faciens scire, ut dicitur primo *Posteriorum*'; see R. M. S. Spiazzi and M.-R. Cathala (eds.), *In duodecim libros Metaphysicorum Aristotelis expositio* (Turin, 1971), Lectio I, 1, 29, p. 10.

[45] The literature on Constantine and the so-called 'School of Salerno' is very large. It was collected by Gerhard Baader, 'Die Schule von Salerno', *Medizinhistorisches Journal*, 13

this corpus was directly concerned with works whose Arab authors came from or were in some way connected with Kairouan, in present-day Tunisia, the North African centre of Islamic culture. Constantine's personal relationship with Kairouan and with the Abbot Desiderius and archbishop Alphanus made it possible for him to offer to medicine not only the doctrinal support of Greek (basically Aristotelian) philosophy, but also the intellectual means to advance further along the path of the natural part of philosophy as applied to medicine. The diffusion of Constantine's works in southern Italy – and more precisely around Salerno itself – marks the beginning of this development.[46]

However, in the search for Greek culture via the vehicle of Islamic transmission, unsuspected new visions of man and of medicine itself were encountered (for example, the relationship of men and women to their sexuality; the structure of medical knowledge; a new, theoretical pharmacology; a rational arrangement of medical pathology), all contained in these Islamic medical works, which were thus recognized to be fulfilling a more substantial role than simply relaying Greek culture.[47] One can see this in the complex intellectual world of the *Pantegni* or in the apparent simplicity of the *Isagoge*.

Nevertheless, as will be seen below, this was not enough. Certainly the availability of a doctrinal corpus translated into Latin was necessary (the works translated from the Greek and circulating throughout the south of Italy and Sicily),[48] but it is not enough to explain the extent of the phenomenon. In addition to the existence of this doctrinal corpus, there

(1978), 14–145, and there is an up-to-date bibliography in Baader and Keil, *Medizin im mittelalterlichen Abendland*, pp. 13–23. On Constantine the African, see Bloch, *Monte Cassino in the Middle Ages*. Paul O. Kristeller called attention to these questions and stressed the importance of developing more research on them. See his article, 'The school of Salerno. Its development and its contribution to the history of learning', *Bulletin of the History of Medicine*, 17 (1945), 138–94 (repr. and rev. in Italian translation, 'La scuola di Salerno. Il suo sviluppo e il suo contributo alla storia della scienza', in *Studi sulla schola medica salernitana* (Naples, 1986). We shall use the Italian version), p. 34. On Alphanus, see his preface to *Nemesii episcopi Premmon physicon . . . a N. Alfano . . . in latinum translatus*, ed. by C. J. Burkhard (Leipzig, 1917), pp. 1–4. See Constantine's preface to Desiderius in *Omnia opera Ysaac*. Pars II: *Liber Pantegni Isaac Israelite . . . quem Constantinus Aphricanus monachus Montis Cassinensis sibi vindicavit* (Leyden, 1515), fol. 1. As we shall see later, Kristeller's urgings have been followed in recent years.

46 D'Alverny, 'Translations and translators', pp. 422–6, and the literature and MSS therein.
47 Enrique Montero Cartelle, *Constantini liber de coitu. El tratado de andrología de Constantino el Africano* (Santiago de Compostela, 1983); Monica Green, 'The *de genecia* attributed to Constantine the African', *Speculum*, 62 (1987), 299–323; D. Jacquart and C. Thomasset, *Sexualité et savoir médical au moyen âge* (Paris, 1985); E. Montero Cartelle, 'Encuentro de culturas en Salerno: Constantino el Africano, traductor', in *Rancontres de cultures dans la philosophie médiévale. Traductions et traducteurs de l'antiquité tardive au XIVème siècle* (Louvain-La-Neuve and Cassino, 1990), pp. 65–88. On the Arabic influences on the doctrine of grades in medieval theoretical pharmacology, see M. McVaugh, Introduction to *Arnaldi de Villanova, Aphorismi de gradibus* (Granada and Barcelona, 1975).
48 G. Cavallo, 'La transmissione scritta della cultura greca antica in Calabria e in Sicilia tra i secoli X–XV. Consistenza, tipologia, fruizione', *Scrittura e Civiltà*, 4 (1980), 157–246.

was needed the circulation between the principal European intellectual centres of a sizeable proportion of Aristotle's writings (both on logic and the so-called *libri naturales*) translated from Greek, into which the Arabic-Latin translations were incorporated.[49] The existence of a school system was also essential, though its origins and nature in the case of Salerno continue to be obscure.[50] Furthermore, the application to this corpus of the pedagogical and investigative technique of commentary structured around *questiones* was also necessary.[51] This last procedure proved to be extremely fertile and was the decisive internal factor in a process for those who, probably in the first half of the twelfth century, began to apply this technique in a systematic fashion to some or all of the five works that later came to be known by the name of the *Articella*. In these commentaries, master physicians living in Salerno for the first time integrated the natural part of philosophy of the new Aristotle with Constantine's Aristotelian Galenism.[52] At this point it would seem logical for the historian to enquire into the nature of the social factors that made the initiation and subsequent development of such an important intellectual process possible in twelfth-century Salerno. But this is a question to which historians have not managed to provide an answer as detailed as they have for the intellectual side.[53]

Constantine's disciples, Afflacius and Azus,[54] continued translation activity at Montecassino for thirty or forty years after his death in about 1087, but apart from this we find no intellectual activity concerning medicine in the south of Italy which took into account any of the medical works translated by the Montecassino circle, or indeed by anyone in the wider area of the whole of southern Italy.[55] We have to wait until sometime in the first half of the twelfth century to find clear signs of contact between Latin medical literature translated from Greek or Arabic and the intellectual activity of Salernitan physicians. It was also at this date that, according to the view most widely held among historians, there appeared the first writings in the form of commentaries on works translated by Constantine, such as Johannitius' *Isagoge*,[56] or on works that were

[49] Jacquart, 'Aristotelian thought in Salerno', pp. 407–28.
[50] Kristeller, 'The school of Salerno', pp. 56–8.
[51] See Lawn, *The Salernitan questions*.
[52] We are referring to the commentaries written by the twelfth-century Salernitan masters; see pp. 19–28.
[53] Kristeller had already suggested the convenience of combining both approaches: see 'The school of Salerno', pp. 14–18.
[54] On Constantine's students, see Bloch, *Monte Cassino in the Middle Ages*, pp. 102ff.
[55] Kristeller, 'The school of Salerno', p. 36.
[56] P. O. Kristeller spoke of this version as a probability: 'Bartholomaeus, Musandinus and Maurus of Salerno and other early commentators of the Articella', *Italia Medioevale e Umanistica*, 19 (1976), 57–87. (Italian transl. and rev., in *Studi sulla scuola medica salernitana*, pp. 97–151. We shall follow the Italian version, p. 114.) D. Jacquart has confirmed it; see her article, 'A l'aube de la renaissance médicale des XI–XIIème. siècles: L'*Isagoge Johannitii* et son traducteur', *Bibliothèque de l'Ecole de Chartres*, 144 (1986), 209–40.

circulating in southern Italy (Philaretus' *De pulsibus*, Theophilus' *De urinis*, Hippocrates' *Aphorismi* and *Prognostica*, and Galen's *Tegni*.[57] Such commentaries were also produced by Salernitan physicians and they were given a scholastic technical framework and methodology; in addition to displaying clearly the educational aim of basing medicine on the natural part of philosophy, they were both fairly sophisticated and obviously inspired by Aristotle's works.[58]

If the Salernitan physicians did not demonstrate the slightest interest in the natural part of philosophy and rational methods of analysis before the second or third decade of the twelfth century, and if Constantine's contemporaries in Salerno remained (as the available evidence suggests they did) indifferent to or ignorant of the work of this Benedictine monk at Montecassino, what was the reason for the sudden and surprising change in both attitude and activity? What connection, if any, was there between the Salernitan physicians of the second half of the eleventh century (Gariopontus, Petrocellus, the author of the *Anatomia porci*, the author or authors of collections of receipts and prescriptions such as the *Antidotarium magnum*) and the intellectual authors of the Salernitan commentaries of the twelfth century? Where did the authors of these commentaries come from? How and when was an organized group formed in Salerno, a group which based preliminary medical training upon these five or six texts, the main one of which was the *Isagoge*? Were the twelfth-century Salernitan commentaries the result of an open model in medical education, where teaching activity reflected the interests of an individual teacher, not the requirements of a set curriculum? Why were commentaries always focused on these five or six medical texts headed by the *Isagoge*? These are difficult questions and a satisfactory answer to them would shed much light on this period, which is without doubt an important one in the intellectual history of Europe. However, in view of the present state of research, it is not possible for us to answer all these questions. One of the main difficulties is simply the establishment of a chronology, not just of the Latin translations, both from the Greek and the Arabic, that circulated in southern Italy between the last third of the eleventh century and the first half of the twelfth century, but more especially of the twelfth-century Salernitan commentaries themselves.

But the achievements of recent scholarship allow us to reduce to three

---

[57] On Galen's *Tegni*, see Richard J. Durling, 'Corrigenda and addenda to Diels' Galenica, 1: Codices Vaticani', *Traditio*, 23 (1967), 461–76, on p. 463; and his 'Lectiones galenicae: Téchne iatriké', *Classical Philology*, 63 (1968), 56–7. Theophilus is Theophilos Protospatharios, a Byzantine physician from the sixth/seventh century. Philaretus is an unknown medical author. His Latin text is derived from the pseudo-Galenic *De pulsibus ad Antonium*. See Kristeller, 'The school of Salerno', pp. 108–13, and John A. Pithis, *Die Schriften Peri Sphygmon des Philaretos. Text, Übersetzung, Kommentar* (Husum, 1983), pp. 187–94.

[58] Another problem is that related to the origins of the *Articella*: see Augusto Beccaria, 'Sulle tracce di un antico canone latino di Ippocrate e di Galeno', *Italia Medioevale e Umanistica*, 2 (1959), 1–56; 4 (1961), 1–73; 14 (1971), 1–23; Kristeller, 'The school of Salerno', pp. 107ff.

the number of hypotheses that might be put forward to explain the appearance of these medical commentaries, in which, for the first time in Europe, the natural part of Aristotelian philosophy was used to provide a basis for the physician's activity. The commentary model also exhibits a methodology with clear educational techniques being used for the same purpose as before, while at the same time it proved itself to be an efficient tool for intellectual research and questioning. Moreover, this methodology had its own originality, for it had as its principal analytical tool the *quaestio*, which was already demonstrating its value in the fields of theology, the liberal arts and law. Two of these hypotheses emphasize the local character of this twelfth-century phenomenon in Salerno, in the sense that all the factors, and especially the intellectual ones, that were drawn upon in order to undertake and continue the process, already existed in Italy. The third hypothesis points out that this Salernitan originality was the result of an encounter between the medical texts circulating in these lands in southern Italy and the newly arrived physicians trained in the scholastic method-ology (commentary, with heuristic techniques such as the gloss and the *quaestio*) recently created and developed in French and British centres, men who were also aware of the new Aristotle being spread in these same centres in northern France. Their arrival coincided with the existence in southern Italy of a series of social and political circumstances that favoured and made use of this intellectual development. The various explanations in turn emphasize different evaluations of the role of Islamic culture in the origins of the particular form of medicine that emerged in Latin Christendom from the twelfth century onwards. Let us examine these hypotheses in turn.

(i) The first hypothesis[59] emphasizes the intellectual dominance of Arab medicine evident in Constantine's Latin translations. On the one hand, there is the personal role of Constantine, a key individual in the cross-fertilization between two intellectual centres – the southern Italian one represented by Desiderius and Alphanus, and the Islamic one in Kairouan, a city known for its medical activity. (Indeed it is possible that Constantine himself may even have emerged from the small Christian community of Kairouan, and acquired his medical background there.) The second leading role was that of the new circle of physicians in Salerno, which was to dominate intellectual medical activity in the part of southern Italy that was in Norman hands from the end of the eleventh century onwards. The Arabic works of medicine, once translated into Latin, served as a Trojan horse which carried into the interior the stimulating and fertile strength of Islamic medicine. This would have been represented not only by the *Isagoge*, but more especially by al-Majusi (Haly Abbas)'s *Pantegni*, Ibn al-Gazzar's *Viaticum*, *De gradibus*, *De melancholia* and *De coitu*, and Isaac

---

[59] Jacquart and Micheau, *La médecine arabe*, pp. 87–129, and the literature cited there.

Israeli's *De febribus*. This would deliberately have been a Galenism, but one with hardly any contribution from Galen himself, an author whose works, even in the best of cases, Constantine did not find particularly manageable.[60]

In this interpretation, Islamic medicine must have been the true driving force of the changes that took place in Salernitan medicine from the twelfth century onwards. The doctrinal components derived from the natural part of philosophy – including the elements, qualities, complexions, vital force, the position of man in the cosmos, the polarity of theory–practice, even the very vocabulary itself contained in works such as the *Isagoge* or the *Pantegni* – supplied the Salernitan physicians with material and confronted them with questions whose solution could be found only in the works of Aristotle, whose philosophy of nature underlay the Arabic texts.[61] These works must have circulated in Salernitan circles in translations from the Greek that were probably made by anonymous translators in Italy, as well as others from northern France, to which were added, in the last decades of the century, translations from Arabic carried out in Spain.[62] Thus, the new Salernitan masters of this century were the first physicians in the Latin West to link medicine (with its inevitable practical dimension) to the natural part of philosophy (in this case the Aristotelian form).[63] In spite of various disagreements, Western medicine was never to abandon this approach. The *medicus* was definitively transformed into the *physicus*.[64] If Galen and his medical works had remained on the other side of the boundary established by Constantine, by contrast the new Galenism that was now being developed in twelfth-century Salerno demanded direct knowledge of Galen. It is in this intellectual context that we should place the translations from the Greek by Burgundio of Pisa, who was in contact with Bartholomaeus,[65] another individual whose knowledge of Greek seems to have been far from negligible.[66]

What could have been the origin of the special feature of Salerno according to this first hypothesis? This special feature was not only the use of the natural part of Aristotelian philosophy as a basis for medical practice, but also, and more especially, the circulation of a genre of medical literature

---

[60] Jacquart and Micheau, *La médecine arabe*, pp. 103–4.

[61] Jacquart, 'Aristotelian thought in Salerno', pp. 412–16.

[62] D'Alverny, 'Translations and translators', pp. 436 and 458.

[63] Jacquart, 'Aristotelian thought in Salerno', p. 413; Jacquart and Micheau, *La médecine arabe*, p. 127.

[64] See Kristeller, 'The school of Salerno', p. 45; Bylebyl, 'The medical meaning of *physica*'.

[65] 'Explicit Tegni Galieni secundum antiquam translationem sed postea M[agister] Borgundius rogatu M[agistri] Bartolomei transtulit quod sequitur', Vienna, Österreichische Nationalbibliothek, cod. 2504, c. 39, quoted by Durling, 'Corrigenda and addenda to Diels' Galenica', p. 463. See Kristeller, 'Bartholomaeus, Musandinus and Maurus of Salerno', p. 106, n. 23.

[66] Kristeller, 'Bartholomaeus, Musandinus and Maurus of Salerno', pp. 106 and 137–8 (Appendix III).

(the commentary, with the *quaestio* as a key tool) that exhibited such great intellectual vitality. The answer is fairly clear. The Aristotelian link was already expressed in the writings of Constantine himself. The conventionalism of the commentary (something more than mere rhetorical adornments), and the fact that five or six brief medical texts formed the core of the Salernitan commentaries, was nothing other than the renewal of a tradition created in Ravenna in the fifth and sixth centuries,[67] as expanded in twelfth-century Salerno with the diffusion of Constantine's works in the medical circles of that town and by its own tradition in the use of *questiones*. For this reason, this might be called the 'renewal theory'.

(ii) The second of the hypotheses[68] explicitly considers the origins of the medical commentary in Salerno and more directly the chronological relationship between the twelfth-century examples currently known. In order to provide an answer to the problem of origins, what we might call the 'reinvention theory' has been developed.[69] According to this, the learned scholar of Salerno must have reinvented, on the basis of Constantine's writings (the *Isagoge*, the *Pantegni*) and of the medical literature and works of the natural part of philosophy (fundamentally Aristotle's works) circulating in the south of Italy, a complete approach to medical pedagogy which led them to create the literary genre of the commentary in the medicine of the Latin West. The currently available evidence does not allow us to establish the chronology of the twelfth-century Salerno commentaries directly. This has to be established by means of a combination of conjecture and inference. After detailed internal comparative analysis of the contents of surviving commentaries, the author of this second hypothesis proposes the following chronological sequence: in the first place stand the so-called 'Digby commentaries', thus named because of the Oxford manuscript in which they are to be found.[70] These commentaries cover Hippocrates' *Aphorisms* and *Prognostics*, Johannitius' *Isagoge*, and the brief works by Theophilus on urines and of Philaretus on pulses. The author of these

---

[67] 'They were renewing a tradition established in Ravenna in the fifth and sixth centuries', Jacquart, 'Aristotelian thought in Salerno', p. 412.

[68] Mark D. Jordan, 'Medicine as science in the early commentaries on "Johannitius"', *Traditio*, 43 (1987), 121–45; Jordan, 'The construction of a philosophical medicine. Exegesis and argument in Salernitan teaching on the soul', in McVaugh and Siraisi (eds.), *Renaissance medical learning*, pp. 42–61.

[69] 'The differences between the development of *physica* at Salerno and at other centers – Chartres, Paris, Toledo, Hereford – are due in some way to the requirements placed on the reinvention of physical knowledge within the context of medical pedagogy': Jordan, 'The construction of a philosophical medicine', p. 61.

[70] Oxford, Bodleian Library, Digby 108, fols. 4–26 (*Johannitius*), fols. 26–76 (*Aforismi*), fols. 76–91 (*Theophilus*), fols. 91–106v (*Prognostici*), fols. 106v–112 (*Philaretus*): see Kristeller, 'Bartholomaeus, Musandinus and Maurus of Salerno', pp. 115–16; list of copies in other libraries, in Appendix Ib, p. 124, revised list on pp. 139ff. In these additions to the Italian edition, Kristeller reproduces a personal communication from Dr Brian Lawn about the Salernitan origin of the Digby commentary according with its medical doctrine (p. 142).

commentaries should be placed in the first decades of the twelfth century[71] and whose identity has still not been established, must have been the same person as the author of the so-called *Second anatomical demonstration* of Salerno.[72] These commentaries were soon to be known beyond the Alps. This would appear to be demonstrated by the painstaking reconstruction and internal comparative analysis of the 'Chartres commentaries' (named from the manuscript from that cathedral lost during the Second World War).[73] These commentaries include the same five texts mentioned above and must have been a teaching summary, in the form of a primer, of the other works.[74] The second group of Salerno commentaries must be dated to just after the middle of the century. Their author was an enigmatic Archimatthaeus, whose commentaries only covered the *Isagoge*.[75] The third set of twelfth-century Salerno commentaries had Bartholomaeus as their author, and they were most probably drawn up in the 1160s or 1170s. Their contents, in addition to extending the commentaries on Galen's *Tegni*, were more complex and more intellectually mature, especially as regards the use of the *quaestio* as an intellectual tool of analysis and the role played by the 'new Aristotle'. This set of commentaries has been preserved in two versions, one of them reported or redacted by Peter Musandinus, another contemporary Salernitan physician,[76] The fourth and last of the groups of Salernitan commentaries from this century is that belonging to Maurus (d. 1214).[77] His commentaries present a certain dependence as

---

[71] See Lawn, *The prose Salernitan questions*, pp. xx, 2–16.

[72] Jordan, 'The construction of a philosophical medicine', p. 48.

[73] Kristeller identified copies in other libraries except that on Johannitius: see 'Bartholomaeus, Musandinus and Maurus of Salerno', pp. 115 and 123 (Appendix 1a). A copy of the first part of that commentary was later found in a marginal note of a manuscript which is now in the private London collection of Mr Philip Robinson (formerly Helmingham Hall 58): see pp. 141, 151 (additions to Italian edition).

[74] Jordan, 'The construction of a philosophical medicine', p. 53.

[75] Trier, Bibliothek des Priester-Seminars, 76, fols. 1–53v. It was personally checked by Kristeller in 1976. His opinion was that this commentary attributed to Archimatthaeus was written before that of Bartholomaeus: see 'Bartholomaeus, Musandinus and Maurus of Salerno', p. 143. Jordan's analysis is in 'The construction of a philosophical medicine', pp. 53–6.

[76] Winchester College, The Warden and Fellows' Library 24, fols. 22v–166v, found by Kristeller in 1952: see P. O. Kristeller, 'Nuove fonti per la medicina salernitana del secolo XII', *Rassegna storica Salernitana*, 18 (1957), 61–75; Kristeller, 'Beitrag von Schule von Salerno zur Entwicklung der scholastischen Wissenschaft im 12. Jahrhundert', in J. Koch (ed.), *Artes Liberales von der antiken Bildung zur Wissenschaft des Mittelalters* (Leiden and Cologne, 1959), pp. 84–90; Kristeller, 'Bartholomaeus, Musandinus and Maurus of Salerno', where he gives the copies dispersed in libraries, pp. 124–6, 136, 150. See also Jacquart, 'Aristotelian thought in Salerno'; Jordan, 'The construction of a philosophical medicine', pp. 57–60.

[77] Paris, Bibliothèque Nationale, Lat. 18499, fols. 1–209. The first description was given by K. Sudhoff, 'Die vierter Salernitaner Anatomie', *Archiv für Geschichte der Medizin*, 20 (1928), 33–50, on p. 38. His commentary on *Prognostici* was edited by M. H. Saffron, 'Maurus of Salerno, twelfth-century "Optimus physicus", with his commentary on the Prognostics of Hippocrates', *Transactions of the American Philosophical Society*, 62: 1 (1972).

regards subject matter and form on those attributed to the mysterious Archimatthaeus and those of Bartholomaeus.[78]

In spite of the apparent similarities with the educational process that had taken place in Alexandrine medicine in earlier centuries (the establishment of a canon of writings on which teaching was based, the use of the commentary) and of the fact that the Salerno commentators (e.g. Maurus) saw the *Isagoge* as a product of the Alexandrine school,[79] there does not seem to have been any connection between them, even though Arab medicine could also have served as a vehicle for knowledge of this pedagogical method.[80] The Salernitan writings, in this respect, were 'renewers' and were endowed with a creative strength and originality not found in Alexandrine commentary.[81] Both characteristics appear in the 'Digby commentaries', the first of the Salerno texts of this type. The medical doctrinal nucleus that these commentaries aimed to communicate to their readers was that formed by the writings of Constantine (the *Isagoge* and the *Pantegni*) and Nemesius (*Premnon physicon*), together of course with what was contained in the short texts that were the object of commentaries. The characteristics of the Salernitan pedagogy that began with these commentaries can be reduced to the following:[82] in the first place, there was an exegetical aim, by means of which the master proposed to clarify the text commented upon by glossing specific terms, the conclusion of the arguments, the establishment of textual relationships and the use of rudimentary forms of *quaestio* destined to answer apparent textual inconsistencies. The aim of the commentator was to offer an introduction to medicine for beginners that was simpler and more rudimentary than the schematic and laconic, but conceptually complicated, introduction to be found in the *Isagoge*. Secondly, the explicit introduction of the *quaestio*, although it must be admitted to have been still in an inchoate form without the complexity that it was to exhibit in the following century, was an intellectual tool that would allow these scholars to identify problems (initially those raised by conflict between different authorities), to treat them in depth and to develop and defend new responses. Here a phenomenon similar to that which was occurring in the fields of theology, the liberal arts and law in northern Italy and other parts of Europe, especially in France, was taking place in Salerno in the field of medicine. In the third place, the simple nature of the explanation, characteristic of a form of medical literature aimed at a public consisting of beginners, was compatible with the need that the commentator felt to resort to rational explanations based on the

---

See the list of copies in the libraries, in Kristeller, 'Bartholomaeus, Musandinus and Maurus of Salerno', pp. 126–7, 149–50.

[78] Jordan, 'The construction of a philosophical medicine', p. 56.
[79] Jacquart, 'Aristotelian thought in Salerno', p. 412, n. 25.
[80] Jordan, 'The construction of a philosophical medicine', p. 50, n. 31.
[81] Jordan, 'The construction of a philosophical medicine', pp. 60–1.
[82] Jordan, 'The construction of a philosophical medicine', pp. 49ff.

world of *physica* or of the *res naturales* applied to the human body (e.g. the doctrine of the four elements or the qualities). This meant that the intellectual skills of the audience, even though they were taking only their first steps in the area of medical knowledge, had to include a range of references to the natural part of Aristotelian philosophy, and this enabled beginners to appreciate the need for theoretical foundations for medical practice. This demand was also imposed by the need to understand the Aristotelian terminology used in the *Isagoge*, which was the subject of the commentary.[83] In fact, analysis of the Aristotelian references used by Bartholomaeus in his commentary on the *Isagoge* reveals that a substantial number of Aristotle's works were circulating in Salerno at the beginning of the second half of the twelfth century in their Graeco-Latin version (the *Physics, Categories, On generation and corruption, Metaphysics, Nichomachean ethics, On the soul*, among others).[84] It is obvious that these works must also have been accessible to those who made up the readership of the commentaries in the educational context. As the last years of the twelfth century are reached, it is possible that the range of Aristotelian references might also have started to include Arabic-Latin versions of Aristotle coming from Spain.[85] Whatever the case, Bartholomaeus' commentaries 'provide indubitable evidence that Latin versions of an Aristotelian corpus were consulted'.[86] The result was the elaboration in Salerno of a philosophical medicine characterized by shortening the distance between the world of Aristotelian causality and that of the particular phenomena of the human body. The concern with making the human body – the object of medical care – the final point of reference for their writings is something that can be noticed even in the case of Urso, the most speculative and latest of the Salernitan commentators, working in the late twelfth and early thirteenth centuries.[87] Some at least of the Salernitan physicians, on coming into contact with the natural part of philosophy basically contained in the medical texts of Constantine and Nemesius, must have brought about the 'reinvention of physical knowledge within the context of medical pedagogy'.[88] This approach was not shared by all the intellectuals from beyond the Alps. Hugh of Saint Victor (*c.* 1096–1141), probably a contemporary of the author of the 'Digby commentaries', in a controversy about the initial words of the *Isagoge*, in which a medical *physica* is presumed to exist ('*Medicina* is divided into two parts, namely *theory* and *practice*'), denied

[83] Jacquart, 'Aristotelian thought in Salerno', p. 413.

[84] Piero Morpurgo, 'Le traduzioni di Michele Scoto e la circolazione di manoscritti scientifici in Italia meridionale: la dipendenza della scuola medica salernitana da quella parigina di Petit Pont', in *La diffusione delle scienze islamiche nel medio-evo europeo* (Rome, 1987), pp. 167–91, on pp. 179–82; Jacquart, 'Aristotelian thought in Salerno', pp. 416–20, 423.

[85] D'Alverny, 'Translations and translators', pp. 457–9; Morpurgo, 'Le traduzioni di Michele Scoto', pp. 184–7.

[86] Jacquart, 'Aristotelian thought in Salerno', p. 426.

[87] Jordan, 'The construction of a philosophical medicine', p. 61.

[88] Jordan, 'The construction of a philosophical medicine', p. 61.

that medicine possessed its own theory and relegated it to the rank of mechanical art.[89] This controversy was left behind in the thirteenth century as a consequence of the new textual basis of Aristotle (in Graeco-Latin and Arabic-Latin versions), of Galen (likewise in both versions) and of the wave of works by Arab physicians (Alkindi, Ali ibn Ridwan, Serapion, Albucasis, Rhazes and Avicenna's *Canon*), to mention only those put into circulation through the translations by Gerard of Cremona (1157–87) and his colleagues (*socii*). The new-style university teaching was built on these texts, even though their entry into university circles on a regular basis was slow and rather late, being datable to towards the last third of the thirteenth century. It was during this period that the intellectual horizons of university physicians, and of those within their circle of influence, were noticeably widened.[90] Although we are not claiming to go beyond the novelty that twelfth-century Salerno represented for the intellectual and social definition of medicine, yet it is worth mentioning that hardly anything is known about the beginnings of the integration of medical studies in the new communities of masters and students that were formed in the Latin West from the early thirteenth century. The only centres for which we have any evidence that regular medical teaching was given are Paris, Montpellier and Bologna.[91] By the middle of that century the argument that had occupied the previous century about the overall position of medicine within knowledge as a whole no longer made much sense. Words such as the following, uttered by someone from outside the medical world (Albert the Great, in 1246), are a clear indication that the fields of natural philosophy and medicine were by then perfectly demarcated, once medicine had adopted Aristotelian assumptions:

I must point out that should problems arise concerning faith and custom, I am more inclined towards Augustine than towards the [natural] philosophers. If the problems are expounded in the field of medicine [*medicina*], I shall be inclined towards Galen and Hippocrates; and should we be dealing with things concerning nature [*de naturis rerum*], I shall follow Aristotle more than any other.[92]

(iii) The third hypothesis on the origins of the intellectual innovation that the twelfth-century Salernitan medical commentaries effected takes a

---

[89] *Hugonis de Sancto Victore Didascalion. De studio legendi: A critical text*, ed. by C. H. Buttimer (Washington, DC, 1939); V. Liccaro, 'Ugo di San Vittore di fronte alla novità delle traduzioni scientifiche greche e arabe', *Actas del V Congreso Internacional de Filosofía Medieval* (Madrid, 1979), vol. II, pp. 919–26.

[90] Nancy Siraisi, *Taddeo Alderotti and his pupils: two generations of Italian medical learning* (Princeton, NJ, 1981); García-Ballester, 'Arnau de Vilanova'; Jacquart, and Micheau, *La médecine arabe*, p. 176.

[91] See Vern L. Bullough, *The development of medicine as a profession* (Basle and New York, 1966); Siraisi, *Medieval and early Renaissance medicine*.

[92] *Super II Sententiarum*, d. 13, C, a.2, *Opera Omnia* (Paris, 1890–9), vol. XXVII, p. 247. The date 1246 is given in one of the arguments in book II of the *Sentences*: see Weisheipl, 'The life and works of Albert the Great', p. 22.

totally different approach from the previous two.[93] In addition to transferring the initial stage to eleventh- and twelfth-century French intellectual
circles and their relations with southern Italy,[94] it also sets out a new
chronology which is markedly different from that laid out by the previous
two hypotheses.[95] We could call it the 'breakthrough theory', because it
states that the appearance of the commentaries to the *Articella* in twelfth-
century Salerno was a real breakthrough in the earlier medical Salernitan
writings, as well as a novelty.[96] The line of argument of this new proposal
endeavours to integrate a series of conjectures resulting from the analysis
and rereading of an extremely complicated set of elements of a social and
intellectual nature over a longer period of time between the early Middle
Ages and the twelfth century, including the formal examination of this
literary genre as well as analysis of the palaeographic characteristics of the
codices containing the Salernitan commentaries and comparison with those
appearing in Paris based on the Bible. Among these elements we might
draw attention to the following: the works of French and British Latin
intellectuals living in the first half of the twelfth century, who enjoyed a
high degree of mobility (William of Conches, Thierry of Chartres, Hugh
of Saint Victor, Bernard Silvestris, Adelard of Bath and John of Salisbury,
among others); the possible role of the Alexandrine commentaries through
their Graeco-Latin translations deriving from fifth- and sixth-century
Ravenna; the renaissance of the gloss as a literary genre in French centres
(Paris, Tours), which also acted as centres of diffusion for this genre; the
diffusion of Graeco-Latin versions of Aristotle outwards from centres in
Normandy; the connections between Salerno and British and French
intellectual circles in the eleventh and twelfth centuries; the presence in
Salerno in the mid twelfth century of medical texts and others concerning
the natural part of philosophy translated from the Greek; and finally the
changing fortunes of the political and religious struggles of southern Italy
in the twelfth century.

The conclusions that this third hypothesis reaches are thus noticeably

93   Morpugo, 'Le traduzioni di Michele Scoto', pp. 180. 187–90; and *Filosofia della natura nella
schola salernitana*.
94   'Quanto abbiamo esposto offre elementi sufficienti perchè all'idea de Minio-Paluello
[*Opuscula: the Latin Aristotle*], che retineva che il centro di diffusione delle traduzioni
dell'Aristotele latino fosse la Normandia o l'Inghilterra, si possa affiancare la tesi di Hunt
[R. W. Hunt, *The schools and the cloister. The life and writings of Alexander Nequam*, ed. and
rev. by M. Gibson, Oxford, 1984] su un'origine francese della diffusione degli *accessus ad
auctores*, per poi verificare se da questo *milieux* siano partiti Bartolomeo, Mauro e Ursone alla
ricerca di nuovi testi', Morpurgo, *Filosofia della natura nella schola salernitana*, pp. 133, 150.
95   The Digby commentary could be related to and dependent on the Chartres commentary,
William of Conches and Dominicus Gundissalinus. See Morpurgo, *Filosofia della natura
nella schola salernitana*, pp. 163–5, 185–6.
96   'una rottura con la tradizione degli erbari e quindi con la medicina *practica* ... tra una
prima fase che vide l'attività di Constantino e di Alfano I di Salerno, e una seconda fase con
Bartolomeo, Mauro, Ursone e Pietro Musandino': Morpurgo, *Filosofia della natura nella
schola salernitana*, p. 179.

different from those put forward by the other two, which are to a certain extent complementary. The appearance in Salerno of commentaries on the writings in the *Articella* around the mid twelfth century meant a complete innovation, both as regards methods and doctrinal contents, compared to the medical literature previously produced in Salerno (Gariopontus, Petrocellus, anatomical works, and receipt literature).[97] The author of the 'Digby commentaries' would, in this case, not belong to the first decades of the century, and *a fortiori* he would not have had anything to do with the author of the second Salernitan anatomical text. Such an innovation could only be explained as a result of an encounter between the medical sources circulating in southern Italy – and more precisely in and around Salerno – and physicians trained at French centres.[98] It is at these centres – in particular at the school of the Petit Pont in Paris – that Bartholomaeus of Salerno and the other commentators would have received their medical knowledge, their training in the scholastic techniques of text access (the *accessus ad auctores*) and of commentary on the texts (from the system of glosses through to the commentary proper), and their familiarity with them.[99] Salernitan *glossule* would thus be the adaptation of developments in Biblical scholarship to medicine.[100] Intellectual curiosity would have been the personal motive that led them to settle in Salerno, capital of a Norman Duchy from 1075 onwards, in search of new manuscripts containing works of medicine and the natural part of philosophy.[101] It was there that they entered into contact with the whole rich tradition of medical texts in southern Italy, where Graeco–Latin versions of Alexandrine and Byzantine medical texts, some Hippocratic and Galenic works, Aristotle's natural writings and Constantine's Latin translations from the Arabic were all in circulation. These last would already have been diffused in the first decades of the twelfth century by centres in northern France such as Chartres, where commentary on five of the texts of the *Articella* (the 'Chartres commentary') had already even been tried out, totally unconnected with the subsequent commentaries which followed that by Bartholomaeus. With the intellectual armoury of the new Aristotle and scholastic techniques, Bartholomaeus of Salerno undertook a way of teaching in this city centred upon commentaries of six of the works that made up the *Articella*, and in this way laid the foundations of a school, 'the Salernitans' (*medici*

[97] Morpurgo, *Filosofia della natura nella schola salernitana*, pp. 179ff.

[98] Morpurgo, *Filosofia della natura nella schola salernitana*, p. 41, *et passim*.

[99] Morpurgo, *Filosofia della natura nella schola salernitana*, pp. 110, 125–6, 179ff, 225.

[100] C. F. R. De Hamel, *Glossed books of the Bible and the origins of the Paris booktrade* (Woodbridge, 1984). 'Il confronto tra quanto sostiene De Hamel e quel che emerge dalle *glossule* salernitane sembra confermare che Parigi fu proprio il centro di diffusione di questo genere letterario volto al commento dei testi letti nelle scuole': Morpurgo, *Filosofia della natura nella schola salernitana*, p. 98.

[101] 'il motivo che spinse questo gruppo di maestri a formare una 'schola' a Salerno sia stato proprio la ricerca di nuovi testi di medicina e di filosofia da tradurre o appena tradotti': Morpurgo, *Filosofia della natura nella schola salernitana*, p. 150.

salernitani), to which belonged Peter Musandinus, the author of the 'Digby commentaries', Maurus and Urso. What is more, in the Paris school from which Bartholomaeus came – that of the Petit Pont[102] – the canon of medical texts with which students of medicine had to take their first steps had already been tried out. This canon coincided with that of the *Articella*.[103] This is how Bartholomaeus and his disciples would have accomplished in Salerno the feat of establishing a philosophical medicine on the basis of the nature books of the new Aristotelian philosophy. The members of this school would have been called 'Salernitans' because of their link with the master (Bartholomaeus of Salerno, or the Salernitan) and not because they lived in the city.[104] The school must have been established in the mid twelfth century and would have had no connection at all with the physicians of Salerno nor with the earlier authors resident in Salerno, who have sometimes been brought together under the heading of a supposed 'Salerno school'. The literature generated by this supposed 'school' would have been contemporary with Constantine's and Alphanus' translation work, although no connection at all existed between them.[105] In the late twelfth century, the new influence of Aristotelian natural philosophy derived from the Arabic-Latin translations coming from Spain would have increased the wealth of texts circulating in southern Italy. The Normans' policies in Salerno, and in southern Italy as a whole, favoured the settlement of Bartholomaeus and his disciples, as well as the development of the new school in the twelfth century.

As for the role played by the medical corpus translated by Constantine and by the translations of Alphanus himself (the *Premnon physicon*), this hypothesis rejects any direct relationship between the Abbey of Monte-cassino and the physicians of the city of Salerno before Bartholomaeus' arrival there. Similarly, it rejects the idea of his role as an intellectual catalyst among the Salernitan commentators. As in the case of the Aristotelian texts and scholastic techniques (including the manner of approaching a text, the arrangement of the glosses, and the content of the commentary), the works of Constantine and Alphanus that are directly or indirectly referred to by the twelfth-century Salernitan medical commentators also came from the French contexts where these same commentators had been trained. In short, the Galenism transmitted in the translations of Constantine was known in the sphere of Salerno from the mid twelfth century onwards, but subsequent to its earlier diffusion by the intellectual centres of northern France and Britain in the first half of the century. The potential contained in Constantine's texts was thus made apparent only when it came into contact with the already sophisticated Christian scholastic world of beyond

---

[102] Morpurgo, *Filosofia della natura nella schola salernitana*, p. 120.
[103] Morpurgo, *Filosofia della natura nella schola salernitana*, pp. 166, 185.
[104] Morpurgo, *Filosofia della natura nella schola salernitana*, p. 46.
[105] Morpurgo, *Filosofia della natura nella schola salernitana*, p. 167.

the Alps, where the new Aristotle was playing a decisive role in the field of theology and the liberal arts.

(iv) According to the first two hypotheses, diffusion of Constantine's works took place simultaneously, during the first half of the twelfth century, at two points at least: one situated in northern Europe (Chartres, Tours, Paris); the other in southern Italy, basically in Salerno. In the case of the centres in northern France, it contributed to the establishment of the new intellectual boundary established by the contents of these medical texts based on the natural part of philosophy – which was Aristotelian cosmology.[106] The most widely known expression of this movement was the work of William of Conches (written between 1125 and 1145).[107] In Salerno, on the other hand, Constantine's works were integrated as part of a medical corpus elaborated on the principles of Aristotle's philosophy of nature; this had the clear educational aim of training physicians, a goal that did not exist in the French centres.[108]

However, we still do not know the institutional form that housed organized teaching in Salerno, the first evidence for which, according to the first two hypotheses, was the anonymous scholar of the 'Digby commentaries'. Identifying him as the same person as the author of the 'Second anatomical demonstration' is an important link in the connection between the Salernitan written tradition of the last third of the eleventh century – which was contemporary with Constantine, but still ignorant of his work – and the new world of the commentators. The pedagogical methods used for the first time in medicine in a systematic way (questions, glosses, the confirmation of contradictory opinions, the commentary) could trace their origins to the model of the pseudo-Aristotelian *Problemata*, as well as to the tradition of questions provoked by the *Isagoge*.[109] The commentaries that have come down to us must have been the result of the readings and of comments made by Salernitan masters on five basic texts around which teaching began to be based in Salerno at the beginning of the twelfth century. Were these commentaries given according to an open model of medical teaching, or with a fragile institutional framework, whose real nature is still unknown? According to the open model, the person who possessed medical learning transmitted it or imparted it, following his own personal criteria and without enjoying the protection of

---

[106] See D'Alverny, 'Translations and translators'; Jean Jolivet, 'The Arabic inheritance', in Dronke (ed.), *History of twelfth-century western philosophy* (Cambridge, 1988), pp. 113–48.

[107] William of Conches in his *Philosophia* (ed. by G. Maurach (Pretoria, 1980), pp. 26, 30) added the theory of the elements of the *phisicus* Constantine to those of *philosophi*: 'Constantinus ergo ut physicus de naturis corporum tractans, simplices illorum et minimas particulas, elementa, quasi prima principia vocavit'. See Heinrich Schipperges, 'Die Schulen von Chartres unter dem Einfluss des Arabismus', *Sudhoffs Archiv*, 40 (1956), 193–210, on pp. 202–4.

[108] Jacquart and Micheau, *La médecine arabe*, p. 128.

[109] See Lawn, *The Salernitan questions*; Jordan, 'The construction of a philosophical medicine', p. 56.

any institution. On the other hand, we cannot forget that towards the end of the eleventh century and throughout the twelfth century there accumulated in Salerno a rich stock of medical receipts (or recipes), which gave rise to a receipt literature that gradually put them into order (Gariopontus' *Passionarius*; *Antidotarium magnum*, c. 1100). This process culminated in the *Antidotarium Nicolai*, without doubt one of the most influential medical texts in medieval literature, and essential for both physicians and apothecaries,[110] and whose purpose was to provide a reliable guide to the ingredients required for popular remedies. It was drawn up in Salerno between 1160 and 1200 by a (still unidentified) medical teacher at the request of his students, who desired a plain guide to the constitution of remedies, although it also introduced identifiable measures of weight that were usable by physicians and apothecaries, as well as techniques for the storage of stocks.[111] We are thus moving in a medical world whose main aim was to heal. The receipt literature need not have been incompatible with, nor diametrically opposed to, elaborations of an intellectual nature; on the contrary, it was a type of literature which was able to incorporate lexical and technical innovations, new products, even new concepts (for example, the theory of the four degrees of Arabic theoretical pharmacology collected by Constantine), as is shown in Platearius' herbarium known by the name of the *Circa instans* (c. 1200).[112] This is the approach that is most widely accepted at present among specialists. Nevertheless, the problem of twelfth-century Salerno continues to trouble us; and a definitive solution requires further research on different fronts. The discovery of new documents, the systematic searching of the local archives, critical editions of medical texts (translations and commentaries) and comparative analysis of them, the in-depth study of specific intellectual processes and, in the case of translations, comparison of the new version or translation with the original text, whenever this is possible, are the only routes that can be taken in order to make further progress in our knowledge.[113] In fact, so far as we know, there is no study which combines in a satisfactory way evidence from local archives and other similar underexploited sources with the results of intellectual history built on a critical edition of the Salernitan commentaries.

The exposition of the three hypotheses dealing with the origins in Salerno of a new development that meant the appearance of a philosophical

---

[110] Willy Braekman and Gundolf Keil, 'Fünf mittelniederländische Übersetzungen des "Antidotarium Nicolai". Untersuchungen zum pharmazeutischen Fachschrifttum der mittelalterlichen Niederlande', *Sudhoffs Archiv*, 55 (1971), 257–320.

[111] Gundolf Keil, 'Zur Datierung des "Antidotarium Nicolai"', *Sudhoffs Archiv*, 62 (1978), 190–6; Dietlinde Goltz, *Mittelalterliche Pharmazie und Medizin, dargestellt an Geschichte und Inhalt des Antidotarium Nicolai* (Stuttgart, 1976); Hunt, *Popular medicine in thirteenth century England*, pp. 14–15.

[112] See Jacquart and Micheau, *La médecine arabe*, p. 124.

[113] Some of the ways of progressing in this specific topic were pointed out by D'Alverny, 'Translations and translators', p. 426.

form of medicine is a very illuminating example of the standard of discussion existing today on one of the decisive moments in the intellectual history of medicine in the Latin West. But it is also an example of how difficult it is to make headway in a period of medieval medicine in which the pre- and post-Constantinian manuscripts must be examined with much caution. Continuing research is constantly supplying new material, and, above all, it encourages scholars not to be satisfied with a simple, already established panorama of medieval medicine. This does not mean that medieval medicine is at present like a kaleidoscope, but it does indicate that further research (especially that dedicated to producing critical editions) requires us to follow the path of rigour and detailed analysis.

Finally, we should not forget that historically speaking there were other intellectual medical alternatives available during this same period, quite distinct from academic Aristotelianism and establishment-accepted Galenism. Movements such as empirical nihilism, the so-called Lullian school of medicine, the medical aspect of the alchemical movement,[114] and others, were suffocated or obliged to maintain a semi-clandestine existence in the extra-academic world, thus perhaps limiting the available intellectual possibilities and perhaps also restricting areas of social concern and public well-being at the time. None of these are covered in this volume. We have decided to focus our efforts on one area to which research has hitherto paid little or no attention: the subject of the relationship between the natural part of philosophy of an Aristotelian stamp and those medical practitioners who adopted it, and how the latter made it socially functional during the thirteenth and the first half of the fourteenth centuries.

[114] See, for example, the new perspectives offered by Michela Pereira, *The alchemical corpus attributed to Raymond Lull* (London, 1989).

1

Astrology in medical practice

ROGER FRENCH

INTRODUCTION: A PARABLE

Daniel of Morley's journey to Toledo is something of a parable for the topic of this chapter and perhaps for the book as a whole. It has lessons for us. Let us first hear the story and then draw the moral from it.[1]

As Daniel told the Bishop of Norwich (probably in the early 1170s) there was little about the state of learning in the West that he found exciting. Paris was full of lawyers, arrogant and with closed minds, marking minute changes in their texts with asterisks and obeli. He was more interested in the *doctrina Arabum* being taught by the wiser philosophers of the world (as he called them) and so he took himself off to Toledo, where Gerard of Cremona was expounding the *Almagest* to a class of pupils, apparently during the course of its translation.[2]

What was exciting about the Arabic doctrine of the heavens was the belief that events on earth, day-to-day or momentous, were caused by the motions of the celestial bodies. This causal relation was *necessary*, which meant that, if the motions of the superior bodies were known, events on earth could be *predicted*. Daniel was partly horrified and partly fascinated. Did not prediction deny free will, he asked of Gerard, quoting some homilies of St Gregory. Moreover, how could a man born under Aquarius in a Spanish town miles from the sea or a river *necessarily* become a fisherman? Gerard, smiling at the young man's presumption, answered that

---

[1] The moral of a story was its higher meaning. See B. Smalley, *The study of the Bible in the Middle Ages* (3rd edn, Oxford, 1983).

[2] Daniel's text is given in K. Sudhoff, 'Daniels von Morley Liber de Naturis Inferiorum et Superiorum', *Archiv für die Geschichte der Naturwissenschaften und der Technik*, 8 (1918), 1–40. See also R. W. Hunt, 'English learning in the late twelfth century', in R. W. Southern (ed.), *Essays in medieval history* (London and New York, 1968), pp. 106–28, who identifies Daniel's sources as twelfth-century Paris masters and the pseudo-Avicennan *De celo et mundo*. See also the classic paper by A. Birkenmajer, 'Le rôle joué par les médecins et les naturistes dans la réception d'Aristote au xiie et xiiie siècles', in his *Etudes d'histoire des sciences et de la philosophie du moyen âge* (Warsaw, 1970). This edition includes an assessment of Birkenmajer's work by D'Alverny. B. Stock, *Myth and science in the twelfth century. A study of Bernard Sylvester* (Princeton, 1972), dates Daniel's book at about 1175.

the man would necessarily be disposed to be a better fisherman, which would appear should he ever have the opportunity to fish. Very well then, said Daniel, what about the son of a king and the son of a peasant, both born under a royal sign. It would surely be the case that only the son of a king would grow up to be a king. Ah, said Gerard, but the young peasant would be a king among the peasants. Indeed, he added, I was born under a royal sign myself, and I am a king. Oh, said Daniel, somewhat nettled, and where do you reign? In my mind, said Gerard coldly.[3]

The lessons for us are firstly that the exciting thing about such translations was that they seemed to supply powerful and useful knowledge about the world. It was almost a question of forbidden fruit tasting sweeter, for predictive knowledge of this kind hovered on the denial of free will and even of God's providence. Moreover, it was clearly pagan knowledge. Daniel had to explain to the bishop in his book how it was that pagan knowledge could be used by a Christian. It was, he said, like the gold the Jews borrowed from the Egyptians before the exodus: it was not holy, but it was useful. The same image of Egyptian gold was used by many in the twelfth and thirteenth centuries to excuse the use of pagan philosophy. The most significant use of the image is that of Gregory IX, who in 1231 set up a commission to remove what was offensive to faith from Aristotle's physical works in order to render them useful – to find their gold – in education. This event is essentially the formal acceptance of Aristotle's physical works in the *studium* of Paris and shortly predates the masters' construction of natural philosophy[4] – and as we saw in the introduction to this book, the importance of the reception of Aristotle's works for medicine was immense.

The second lesson from the story of Daniel is that this knowledge was fetched and did not come of its own accord. The twelfth-century Western Latin translator was a man who left home, spent a great deal of time and money on difficult journeys to uncomfortably hot places on the very fringes of Christendom, and learned a difficult language in order to read a highly technical book with the help of a Jew.[5] For all that, he surely had a

---

[3] Sudhoff, 'Daniels von Morley Liber de Naturis Inferiorum et Superiorum', pp. 40ff.

[4] This topic will be dealt with at length in Roger French and Andrew Cunningham, *Before science. The invention of the friars' natural philosophy*, forthcoming. For Gregory IX's bowdlerizing committee, see *Chartularium Universitatis Parisiensis*, ed. Henri S. Denifle and Aemilio Chatelain, 4 vols. (Paris, 1889–97), vol. I, p. 143.

[5] Adelard of Bath, a generation before Daniel, was another Englishman who travelled into countries where Arabic was spoken, and he translated some tables and some Euclid, as well as Albumasar's short *Isagoge minor* (an introduction to the *Introductorium*: see R. Lemay, *Abu Mashar and Latin Aristotelianism in the twelfth century* (Beirut, 1962), p. xxx). He was tutor to the future Henry II. See D. Lindberg, 'The transmission of Greek and Arabic learning to the West', in D. Lindberg (ed.), *Science in the Middle Ages* (Chicago, 1978), pp. 52–90; see p. 62. The material brought back by Adelard, Daniel and others was used by men like Roger of Hereford, on whom see N. Whyte, 'Roger of Hereford's *Liber de astronomia iudicandi*: a twelfth-century astrologer's manual', M.Phil. diss. (University of Cambridge, 1991).

motivation greater than the intellectual curiosity that we are sometimes left with as a motive in the diffusion of an '-ism'. Indeed, the motives of the twelfth-century translators are rarely touched on in the extensive scholarship that has gone into this question. This gap leaves unanswered the question of the *kind* of enterprise the translators were engaged on.[6] It is clear that much of the ecclesiastical patronage of translation was concerned with getting to grips with Koranic materials for the purposes of refutation. It was also necessary to work out how the newly discovered philosophical Christianity of the Greek Fathers could be reconciled with Latin theology. Some Arabic star-lore was desirable for the construction of calendars. It is very likely too that the astronomical, mathematical and medical works had a direct utility that explains the eagerness which had made Adelard of Bath travel to Arabic-speaking countries and translate Albumasar's *Isagoge minor*, which drove Gerard to pursue the *Almagest*, and which lay behind the travel-and-translate activities of Alfred of Shareshill.[7] To the early part of this list of Northerners we can add Walcher of Malvern and to the end, Michael Scot. With the exception of Gerard, they happen to be all Britons, for whom any knowledge of Arabic was an exotic quality; Walcher, Alfred and Michael all needed the assistance of Jews to help them translate from the Arabic. The existence of Hebrew versions of Arabic works is not so much evidence of a stage in some process of 'diffusion' as of the practical utility of the translated works to the Jews as much as to the Christians.

The third lesson is that little distinction was made between what we call astrology and what we call astronomy. We shall return to this below.

The fourth is that the person most likely to put predictive knowledge to some use was the medical man. He had a commercial use for prognosis, and had already developed uroscopy as a highly visible prognostic device in the business of securing a reputation. What sold learned medicine to the patient was the display of knowledge, on the part of the doctor, that impressed and comforted the patient. The doctor whose prognostications came true *proved* his learning. Here in knowledge of the causal relationship between upper and lower worlds was a field of learning that took medical prognostication back to the very fundamentals of the world picture.

This was very important. Medicine, as a service that could be bought and sold, existed in the market place. A medical teacher not only had to satisfy his patients but needed to attract pupils. He could attempt both by

---

[6] Much material which could be used to answer this question has been provided by historians of translation. See the work of M.-T. d'Alverny, for example 'Translations and translators', in R. L. Benson, G. Constable and G. D. Lanham (eds.), *Renaissance and renewal in the twelfth century* (Oxford, 1982), pp. 421–62. See also Lindberg, 'Transmission of Greek and Arabic learning to the West', pp. 52–90.

[7] On Alfred, see J. K. Otte, 'The life and writings of Alfredus Anglicus', *Viator*, 3 (1972), 275–91.

his authority,[8] by his learning and by his rationality: he could, as indeed Galen himself had done,[9] not only persuade the patient and pupil that he knew by experience and reading about this or that disease, but that he could *explain* it on the basis of a chain of argument that reached from the patient's symptoms back to the very fundamentals of the world picture. An important part of what follows in this chapter is the claim that the medical man's need for a rationalist prediction provided an important motive for the study of the upper world. It was a medical student who first attempted a translation of the *Almagest*. The medical men found that Ptolemy's *Centiloquium* was addressed to them as much as to anyone.[10] Daniel treats *medicina* as one of the eight parts, indeed, of astronomy. The others are equally predictive. For him *medicina* and astrology are indissolubly linked; he who attacks astrology destroys medicine. For Daniel, by contrast, *physica* was a study of the physical world, upper and lower. The process whose beginning we are looking at here is the taking over of *physica* by the medical man, who thus became the *physician*.[11] At the end of the process will be the physician who has been formed by adopting the new Aristotle and the 'new Galen'.

In the relations of theory and practice of medicine in the Middle Ages there was more than one role for medical learning. We shall see in later chapters to what extent it reached the surgeon and the other categories of practitioner and how it was put to use. Here we are concerned with how medical knowledge could also be used to organize the academic profession of medicine and to attract patients and students.

'ASTRONODIA' IN THE WEST

In the 'high' Middle Ages authors did not have our distinction between astrology and astronomy. (It is a distinction made by post-Renaissance astronomers and post-Enlightenment historians.) Sometimes these terms were used in approximately our sense, sometimes in the reverse.[12] Some-

---

[8] The authority of the doctor, gained from his learning and rationality, was guarded by the ethics of the professional group for the often overt purpose of gaining advantage in the doctor–patient relationship.

[9] An interesting introduction to Galen's use of rational chains of argument to secure a reputation for himself is found in P. Brain, *Galen on bloodletting* (Cambridge, 1986). V. Nutton, *Galen on prognosis* (Berlin, 1979, *Corpus medicorum graecorum*) is also very useful.

[10] See C. Burnett, 'Adelard, Ergaphalau and the science of the stars', in C. Burnett (ed.), *Adelard of Bath. An English scientist and arabist of the early twelfth century* (London, 1987). Likewise the unpublished tract, *The reduction of the knowledge of astronomy to the faculties of medicine* (see pp. 53–5 below) freely quotes the *Centiloquium* for its medical content.

[11] For Adelard, *physica* consisted of two equal partners, *medicina* and *naturalis scientia*. See Saffron, note 33 below. See also J. J. Bylebyl, 'The medical meaning of *physica*', in McVaugh and Siraisi (eds.), *Renaissance medical learning*, pp. 16–41.

[12] Thus for Bartholomew of Bruges, discussing medical prognostication, it is the *astrologi* who agree with Galen on the influence of the moon, and *astronomi* who prognosticate on

times other terms were used for those who made predictive calculations, such as *mathematici*.[13] Sometimes the only distinction made was that the whole subject had practical and theoretical parts, like medicine.[14] Where judicial astrology was marked out for criticism it was *on moral or religious grounds*, not because it did not work, or was superstitious or fanciful. Indeed, almost everyone believed in 'astrology', and it can even be argued that our 'astronomy' was simply the necessary theoretical background to being able to practise 'astrology'.[15] The contemporary term 'astronodia' will be used here to cover all parts of the topic.[16]

These different terms were being used throughout the period we are concerned with. But the subject itself changed rapidly, from being qualitative and cosmological to mathematical and predictive. Before people like Daniel of Morley were seeking out Arabic works on the natural world, the West of the early twelfth century had some astronodial knowledge from authors like Macrobius, Chalcidius and especially Martianus Capella. It was largely Platonic, for the *Timaeus* was being used as a sort of secular and natural *Genesis*. In addition there were exerpts from Pliny's *Natural History* accompanied by characteristic diagrams expressing the order and periods of the planets, the harmonic intervals between their circular orbits and their ascent and descent across the latitude of the ecliptic.[17] Interest in astronodia in the West stirred before the first translations were made from the Arabic. Julius Firmicus' *Mathesis*, dating from the fourth century, is found in manuscripts in the West in the eleventh century. It was a work that made clear the possibilities of predictions, but on its own, without tables, it could

this basis. I am very grateful to Dr C. O'Boyle for providing me with a transcript of Bartholomew's as then unpublished commentary: see note 55 below.

[13] Hugh of St Victor said it was the mathematicians who regarded the superlunar world as 'nature' and the sublunar as 'the works of nature' – a common twelfth-century view and one which would accommodate well the later predictive *astronomia*. Taken together these two halves of a single philosophy of nature are *physica* or *physiologia*. Quoted by L. Thorndike, *A history of magic and experimental science*, vol. II (London, 1923), p. 10. See also J. Tester, *A history of western astrology* (Woodbridge, Suffolk, 1987), esp. chapter 5.

[14] The *Ergaphalau* text says that 'astronomy' is practical, being based on the use of instruments, and 'astrology' is theoretical (intellectual and mathematical). Raymond of Marseilles has an *astronomia contemplativa* and *activa*, the latter the making of talismans and images. See Burnett, 'Adelard, Ergaphalau and the science of the stars', pp. 133–45.

[15] Thus the Italian commentators on Sacrobosco were primarily interested in astronomy as an introduction to judicial astrology. In general 'astrology' seems to have been a greater reason for studying 'astronomy' than was the need to construct a calendar and determine the date of Easter. See C. A. McMenomy, *The discipline of astronomy in the Middle Ages*, Ph.D. thesis (University of California, Los Angeles, 1984) (University Microfilms International), pp. 182, 522. On the widespread belief in astrology, Thorndike's famous survey, *A history of magic and experimental science*, is still very valuable.

[16] The term is used in the text beginning 'Ut testatur Ergaphalau'. See Burnett, 'Adelard, Ergaphalau and the science of the stars'.

[17] See B. Eastwood, 'Plinian astronomical diagrams in the early Middle Ages', in Edward Grant and John E. Murdoch (eds.), *Mathematics and its applications to science and natural philosophy in the middle ages* (Cambridge, 1987), pp. 141–72; and the same author's chapter on this topic in R. French and F. Greenaway (eds.), *Science in the early Roman Empire: Pliny the Elder, his sources and his influence* (Beckenham, 1986), pp. 207–12.

not be used to make them. But the very possibility of prediction was scandalous enough. Both Daniel and Gerard had read it and had perhaps been enthused by it to look further; John of Salisbury thought that 'mathesis' with a short 'e' was the equivalent of 'doctrine', and with a long 'e' was vanity and superstition; most scandalous of all was the Archbishop of York who died with the book under his pillow.[18]

The well-known 'nature poets' of twelfth-century Chartres also provided a picture of the celestial world. Their prosimetrons incorporated the device of allegory, which enabled nature and figures from the pagan pantheon to exist and act within a Christian world. The device was necessary, for the planets were called by the names of and often identified with the gods of the ancient world: Jove was not only the planet Jupiter, but the principal god of the Romans. Of the Chartrians we need only mention Bernard Sylvestris, for whom astronodia and medicine were the chief parts of philosophy, dealing with the macrocosm and the microcosm.[19]

Twelfth-century discussions of the kinds of knowledge, such as that of Bernard, are very much to the point here. They are not classifications of types of knowledge, but rather divisions of a single philosophy. The purpose of this philosophy was the religious one of repairing the damage done to the soul of man by the Fall. Gundissalinus, Hugh of St Victor, Robert Kilwardby in the next century are clear that 'perfection of the soul' and preparation for eternal life are the purposes of philosophy.[20] Astronodia and medicine – whether *medicina* or *physica* – are part of this philosophy. So were the quadrivial arts. Part of the quadrivium was *astronomia*, a knowledge of the heavens and their parts (just as geometry, at least in part, was a knowledge of the sphere of the earth and its parts). But *astronomia* – qualitative and cosmological – was neither physical, in the Aristotelian sense, nor mathematical and predictive in the sense that was to become clear from Arabic sources. Indeed, the nature of the quadrivium in general in the twelfth century is not entirely clear. There is a presumed prehistory in classical culture, particularly in late antique Roman civilization with

---

[18] For Bernard see Stock, *Myth and science*, esp. p. 26. The pre-Aristotelian nature of these views appears particularly in the belief that the heavenly bodies are animated and that they are composed of the four elements (views shared to a greater or lesser degree by Adelard, William of Conches and Raymond of Marseilles). See Lemay, *Abu Mashar*, and Thorndike, *A history of magic and experimental science*, vol. II, pp. 40, 56. Also useful, particularly on the relationship between the idea of nature and of law, is B. Stock, 'Science, technology and economic progress in the early Middle Ages', in D. Lindberg (ed.), *Science in the Middle Ages*, pp. 1–51.

[19] For Bernard Sylvester (more correctly Sylvestris) see P. Dronke (ed.), *Bernardus Sylvestris Cosmographia* (Leiden, 1978).

[20] D. Gundissalinus, *De divisione philosophiae*, in C. Baeumker and G. F. von Hertling (eds.), *Beiträge der Philosophie des Mittelalters* (Münster, 1906), vol. IV; C. H. Buttimer (ed.), *Hugonis de Sancto Victore Didascalicon. De studio legendi*, Studies in Medieval and Renaissance Latin, 10 (Washington DC, 1939); R. Kilwardby, *De ortu scientiarum*, ed. A. G. Judy (Toronto, 1976).

Boethius and Cassiodorus. There seems to be continuation with Isidore. But all this may be a construction of the newly vigorous schools of the twelfth century. The twelfth-century division-of-the-sciences literature, associated with and sometimes emanating from the schools, has an air of unreality. Gundissalinus gives an idealized system. Hugh of St Victor may well have been promoting the school at St Victor. All may have been involved with finding a formula with a Church that needed to control teaching, for which a history of the subject could have functioned as a partial justification. There is evidence[21] that some form of the quadrivium was taught in the early University of Paris and examined by the chancellor, but it is unlikely to have been in any thoroughgoing sense, either physical in the Aristotelian sense or mathematical and predictive in the Arabic sense.[22] No doubt some Capellan-Platonic or Chartrian alternative would have been acceptable, and so would a Sacroboscan one before mid century.

So prediction was not part of earlier twelfth-century astronodia. Arabic prediction relied on tables carrying the positions of the planets. These ultimately relied on observation, and had to be changed by calculation to adapt to places distant from where the observations were made. The astronodia sought by Daniel of Morley in the 1170s was being changed in this way by his countryman Roger of Hereford, who observed an eclipse and calculated tables for the meridian of Hereford in 1178.[23] Roger was among the first generation of Englishmen to be able to cast nativities and answer elective questions.[24] He certainly taught some form of astronodia in the cathedral school of Hereford; but, as the English schools came to be overshadowed by the two *studia generalia*, Oxford and Cambridge, astronodia seems to have been temporarily pushed to one side by the early thirteenth-century introduction of Aristotle's natural works, including his physical, non-mathematical treatment of the heavenly spheres.[25]

---

[21] C. Lafleur, *Quatre introductions à la philosophie au xiie siècle* (Montreal and Paris, 1988). The introductions discussed by Lafleur are partly examination guides.

[22] It is unlikely that the Church would have encouraged predictive astronodia, and the physical works of Aristotle were banned in Paris in 1210 and 1215.

[23] See for instance the MSS in Cambridge University Library 1.11.1 and Gg.6.3; Oxford, Bodley, Selden supra 76. For a preliminary interpretation of Roger see Whyte, 'Roger of Hereford's *Liber de astronomia iudicandi*'. It is hoped that a further treatment of Roger will appear in a joint publication by Nicholas Whyte and Roger French.

[24] A nativity was the act of describing the astronodial circumstances at the moment of birth with a view to prediction; elections were answers to questions posed to the astrologer by his client.

[25] Some of the material discussed by Lafleur, *Quatre introductions*, was composed of guides to the examination held by the chancellor. The chancellor was the bishop's representative and granted the licence to teach. He did not need to issue statutes and favoured an education that included the old liberal arts. The university statutes, in contrast, were drawn up by the masters, and concern the procedures necessary for inception into the masters' *consortium* and rely almost entirely on Aristotle. The masters also taught what was necessary for the chancellor's examination, but did so less formally, often in their own houses or colleges and on feast days and vacations. This included astronomy. See G. Beaujouan, 'Motives and

The physician at the time of the schools and the early *studia* thus had available to him two ways of developing his subject, and in so doing no doubt made it more attractive. By the 1160s or 1170s commentators on the *Articella* in Salerno were using the physical works of Aristotle to expand the theory of their subject:[26] finding value in the physical works, the medical men made the effort to go and find and use them. At the same time they had the possibilities of prediction, being used in the same period by the astrologers. What seems to have happened is that those physicians who guided their subject into the universities chose Aristotle as their vehicle. But the close ties between astronodia and medicine did not dissolve and university medicine was to become increasingly astronodial in the fourteenth century. Further evidence of this is provided by manuscript illustrations of the zodiac man, rarely found before the twelfth century and only incidentally concerned with medicine. However, after the translations from the Arabic, the figure took on its familiar form of showing relationships between the parts of the body and of the heavens. It is then clearly a medical illustration and served no doubt not only to prompt the memory of the doctor but to impress the patient. The coloured diagrams, the astrological volvelles carried by the visiting physician and the zodiac men that were used as posters in bath houses were all good advertising for the newly astrological medical man.[27]

The two ways open to the medical man to enrich and lend authority to his subject interacted to a certain degree. It was Aristotle's physical doctrines that persuaded the doctor that the planets, once thought animated and elementary, were quintessential and so not subject to decay. Their effect on earth was now not so much the sympathy exerted by their elements or souls but was derived from their 'aspects' to each other and to the earthly 'houses', a highly mathematical argument that could be deployed in an impressive way.

DANIEL ON THE UPPER AND LOWER THINGS

Having given the bishop a brief answer to his question on the relationship between upper causes and lower effects, Daniel extended it into a small book. This is essentially the translation of Arabic astronodia for a Christian context.[28] The Muslim emphasis on the unreachability of God enabled Arabic astronodia to be very deterministic. Avicenna, for example, had

opportunities for science in the medieval university', in A. Crombie (ed.), *Scientific change* (London, 1963), pp. 219–36.

[26] Birkenmajer, 'Le rôle joué par les médecins'.

[27] For details see C. W. Clark, *The zodiac man in medieval medical astrology*, Ph.D. diss. (University of Colorado, 1979).

[28] Raymond of Marseilles similarly used Albumasar's texts and adapted them to Christian purposes, claiming, for example, that the sun stopped at the birth of Christ. Lemay, *Abu Mashar*, p. 141; Clark, *The zodiac man*, p. 239.

taught that God created only the outermost sphere or intelligence, which then created all below it, in a necessary fashion: God was not concerned with the particulars of creation.[29] Such a view could not be sustained in the Christian West, and Daniel, whose hesitations over determinism we have already met, found it necessary to establish the proper creational framework for his account. First defending his use of pagan philosophy with the story of the Egyptian gold, he sets out the Christian view of the world as created directly by God as the habitation of man. God's wisdom and bounty to man, says Daniel, are evident everywhere. The world, the *aula mundi*, is the image of God's will. That is, God uses the mechanisms of upper to lower causality to achieve what he wishes: nothing could be more directly opposed to deterministic Arabic astronodia.[30]

It is in this way that Daniel's astronodia is a complete account of the heavens and earth. It is introduced as a complete philosophy of God and his works, like the philosophy of other twelfth-century writers mentioned above, and like theirs has the overall purpose of remedying the natural defect of man's condition (in this case that he is partly corporeal). It also becomes a point of doctrine for Daniel that the world is not eternal (which would have been the Aristotelian position of some of his Arabic sources) and that God created it not by rearranging pre-existing matter (the Platonic position within surviving Western astronodial sources) but by creation *ex nihilo*. Daniel's knowledge of Aristotle's physical works is mostly second-hand,[31] and we would not agree with his analysis of Aristotelian causality; but it is important for his account that God created upper and lower realms together, so that the flowing down of causes from the higher has been the mode of God expressing his will from the start. The law that God gave for the continuation of the process is Nature.

Daniel frequently refers to the *physici*, whose concern with the physical world dealt with this point where the attractions of the old Western Platonic explanation of the world were being rivalled by the attractions of Arabic astronodia and its still largely hidden Aristotelian component.[32] As observed above, it seems that it was the business of the *physici* that the medical men took up when turning themselves into physicians. The important connection between the concerns of the *physici* and the *medici* that Daniel makes, following Albumasar, is to establish that the moon is not only an important celestial body for the *physici*, but the signifier of the

---

[29] See, for example, J. Weisheipl, 'Aristotle's concept of nature: Avicenna and Aquinas', in L. D. Roberts (ed.), *Approaches to nature in the Middle Ages* (New York, 1972).

[30] Islamic astronodia also had to be recalculated in terms of the Christian calendar; and the starting point for the Great Conjunctions was calculated back to the moment of Creation.

[31] Birkenmajer, 'Le rôle joué par les médecins', p. 3.

[32] Daniel quotes Albumasar freely, and it is likely that his knowledge of Aristotelian doctrines comes from the almost wholly unacknowledged use of them by Albumasar and others. Despite Lemay's emphasis on Albumasar as a vehicle of Aristotelianism into the West, very few western readers would have identified the Greek source of the doctrines. See Lemay, *Abu Mashar*.

querent (the client) in judicial astrology, and in addition the signifier of the
acutely ill patient. This enabled the medical man to bring into the equation
the Galenic rationale and calculation of the Hippocratic critical days. As
Daniel sees, it is in the calculation of critical days that astronodia and
medicine were indissolubly linked. It is here that he says that to attack the
one is to destroy the other.

Daniel's astronodia moves without distinction from the physical description of the heavens (in which the ultimately Aristotelian spheres are
combined with mathematical epicycles) and the great terrestrial circles to
the medically important correlation between the signs of the zodiac and the
parts of the body and between the planets and bodily functions. He does
not enlarge upon the list of correlations he supplies, but it is clear the
interest is in the *necessary* connection, giving the possessor of such knowledge the practical power of prediction.

THE 'ASTRONOMY OF HIPPOCRATES'

In treating the moon in this way Daniel was partly depending on an earlier
and non-predictive medical planet-lore. Twelfth-century medical men like
Maurus, in Salerno,[33] believed that Hippocrates had not only recommended that medical men should know astronodia, but that he had himself
written a text on the subject. That Hippocrates himself should be seen to
endorse astronodia was no doubt an additional reason for the medical man
to be interested in acquiring further astronodial knowledge. This *Astronomia Ypocratis*,[34] apparently well known before Maurus, is not, therefore,
predictive in the way that later medical astrology is. It is not concerned
with the planets, their aspects and positions, but with the position of the
moon in cases of illness. The reasoning here is that the moon clearly causes
the sea to swell up – an effect taken to be greater at the full moon – and that
there is a monthly periodicity in the growth of blood, leading to superfluity. As a cardinal humour the blood has a direct effect on the other three.
Since the moon is held to be the cause of these things, then the celestial
circumstances in which the moon finds itself reflect also upon the effect of
which it is the cause, that is, the behaviour of the humours in illness.

Thus, should a disease begin when the moon is in Aries, together with
the sun or Mars, then the patient's condition reflects the fact. His disease will
be in his head, since – as the medieval zodiac figures demonstrate – Aries has
control of the head (see Figures 1 and 2). It will be a hot disease because of

---

[33] M. H. Saffron, 'Maurus of Salerno. Twelfth-century "Optimus physicus", with his
Commentary on the *Prognostics* of Hippocrates', *Transactions of the American Philosophical
Society*, new series, 62: 1 (1972), 5–104, at 55.

[34] Included in the *Regimen sanitatis* of Magninus Mediolanensis (Lyons, ?1505), unpaginated.
Maurus refers to other commentators who said that Hippocrates encouraged the use of
astrology. The text has an editorial beginning which suggests that it was written round a
remark by Hippocrates that the physician should look at the moon when it is full because
the blood and the medulla increase and all things grow on earth and the sea increases.

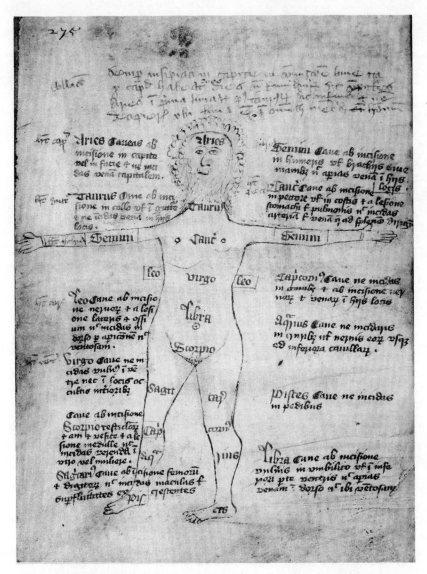

Figure 1 Zodiac man from a French *Miscellanea Medica* of the early fourteenth century.

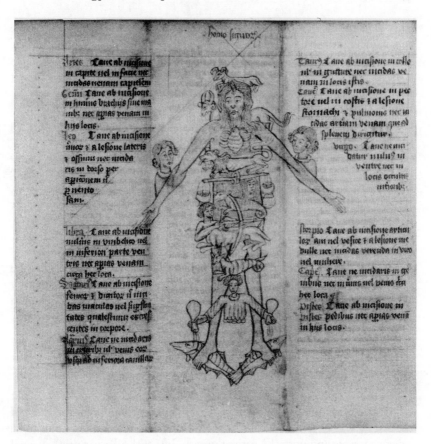

Figure 2 Zodiac man from a fifteenth-century calendar.

As in the case of the 'blood-letting men' (see figs. 4, 5 and 6 of Chapter 4 below) there was a standard 'zodiac man' illustration with a traditional text. The names (or pictures) of the signs of the zodiac are written on the human figure and the figure is surrounded by twelve sentences each headed by the name of a sign. These sentences offer surgical advice, that is, not to incise a part of the body when its corresponding sign was astrologically significant.

These figures are closely related to the phlebotomy figures, not only in the characteristics of the human figure, but because the astrological impediments to surgery applied also to blood-letting. These captions routinely advise when not to let blood. Like the phlebotomy figures, these do not represent the learned medicine of the early universities but an older and alternative tradition.

the warmth of the sun or of Mars. The treatment is to reduce the sun-induced heat by reducing the more readily available hot humour, the blood, and by the use of a 'cold' diet.

Mars and Saturn were regarded as evil planets – the Infortunes. Their position in regard to the moon was therefore critical. Should the waxing moon, drawing the disbalance of humours with her, be in Aries with Saturn and Mars, then the patient would die in seven days. That is, seven days is a quarter of a month and the moon is at 45 degrees or 'square' to the sun. This is a bad aspect and the full power of the Infortunes is exerted via the moon to the patient. If the moon in Aries is at square to Saturn, then the patient survives, but is driven mad: again the moon represents the patient, Aries specifies the part of the body, the planet in aspect determines the nature of the disease and the nature of the aspect determines its strength. Likewise the terrestrial, secondary cause, the excess of a particular humour, is determined by the elementary qualities of the planets and the signs.

In other words, the 'astrology of Hippocrates' is medical astronodia at a fairly simple and early level: the planets have their effect by elementary sympathies and by virtue of only the simplest relational positions: being in the same sign or at square. Such calculations as it uses are concerned only with critical days.

MAURUS ON THE *PROGNOSTICS*

Much use is made in the *Astronomia Ypocratis* of the future tense. It is not only a case of telling what will happen to the patient, but what the cause of the disease will be and what the disease will look like. That is, it seems to be a device for dealing with the patient unseen. Just as the doctor was expected to be able to say everything about a distant patient from a sample of his urine, so here what is on display and on trial is the doctor's use of technical knowledge. What we are seeing here is the sale of *rational* medicine: the doctor impresses his patient with a display of erudition that links the patient to the very workings of the world; the doctor proves his knowledge by the outcome of his prediction. Maurus, discussing prognostication, expressly says that one of its benefits is that the doctor collects 'praise and glory'.[35]

Maurus' commentary on the Hippocratic *Prognostics* is related in some ways to the *Astronomia Ypocratis*. Both texts are based on the motion of the moon; but Maurus does not describe the qualities of the planets, their aspects or relationship to parts of the body. He is in fact writing a tract on critical days. The Hippocratic authors had written that crisis in a fever happens most often at fixed times, such as the seventh, fourteenth or twentieth days, but had studiously avoided giving any reason for it. Any *rationalist* doctor, explaining and impressing his patient with natural

---

[35] Saffron, 'Maurus of Salerno', p. 22: *laus* and *gloria*.

reasoning, had to have an explanation for this fixed periodicity. The great rationalist himself, Galen, was clearly exercised to find a rationale, and so were our twelfth-century doctors.

Maurus' problem is to explain how in fever the twentieth day is critical, since a periodicity of a week would suggest the twenty-first. (He also wants to include an explanation of why sanguineous and phlegmatic apostemes erupt on the twentieth day, bilious on the fortieth and melancholic on the sixtieth.) His explanation consists of a brief introduction to astronomical calculation. He distinguishes between a solar week (one fifty-second of 365¼) and a lunar week (one quarter of the 29½ days it takes the moon to move across the zodiac). The first calculation gives him a week of six days and sixteen hours, three of which weeks are short enough to approximate to three weeks of normal speech each consisting of seven whole days. (It also comes close enough to explain the periodicity of the rupture of apostemes, allowing for some Hippocratic inconsistency.)

Maurus also had a doctrine of daily dominance of the humours which was his own invention.[36] Maurus divided the day into four six-hourly parts, during each of which a different humour became dominant in the body in accordance with the dominating elementary qualities of the ambient air. The doctrine was significant for his practice of bleeding, purging and so on, but it is not directly astronodial.

JUDICIAL ASTROLOGY

A man who was ill at the time of Maurus and later might well not have had the opportunity to seek Salernitan help. If there was no medical help available he might go instead to a practising astrologer. Such a man had a number of ways of predicting what would happen, even if he did not, in his own trade, have remedies to suggest. His predictions, later adopted by medicine, were now more mathematical and planetary than the early medical astrology based on the moon and the calculations for critical days.

The astrologer depended on a system of Houses of the heavens. This was essentially a grid that divided the sky up into twelve parts. The grid was fixed in relation to the earth by the points at which the ecliptic joined the horizon – broadly speaking where the sun rose and set, the east and west – and the top and bottom of the sky – that is, above and below the observer.[37] So the visible sky occupied half the Houses, and all the heavenly bodies passed in twenty-four hours through the twelve Houses. Each House, being terrestrial, related to aspects of life on earth. Family, fortune, friends all belonged to their proper Houses. This grid of Houses was the

---

[36] At least according to Gentile da Foligno, whom we shall meet below.

[37] The seasonal variation in the length of the day and the midday height of the sun led to many attempts to specify the extent of the earthly Houses more precisely. No single account became predominant.

astrological fine-tuning device that could locate celestial and terrestrial events down to a second or even trice of time. What the astrologer did when consulted was to see where the moon was at that time. He also made a note of what sign of the zodiac was rising in the east. This told him which was the important planet in the sky, because each sign had a special relationship to a planet. That planet was then the Lord of the Ascendant, which had a role similar to that of the moon in the *Astronomia Ypocratis*, that is, it signified the patient. The astrologer might find that the moon or Lord of the Ascendant was in the House of Life, or of Death. The outcome also depended on how far through the House the Lord of the Ascendant had proceeded; on what sign of the zodiac he was in; on aspects he had with Fortunes or Infortunes and so on. The astrologer depended utterly on ephemeris tables calculated for his degree of latitude, and the energetic ones, like Roger of Hereford, modified extant tables of Toledo or Marseilles for their home town.[38]

Astrological doctrine, used by such non-medical authors as Roger of Hereford, contained much material that related to health and disease. Each planet exerted its influence over a part of the body, so that, for example, Mars controlled the head, Saturn the chest, Jupiter the abdomen and so on to Venus, who had charge of the feet. The correlations between the planets and the parts of the body shifted as the planets moved through the different Houses, so that, for example, in Taurus Venus' connection was with the head, while in Cancer it was with the arms. These connections are the subject of many medieval figures in which the signs of the zodiac are imposed on parts of the body (see Figure 1) which indicated when surgery or blood-letting should be avoided.[39]

WILLIAM OF ENGLAND IN MARSEILLES

Marseilles in fact seems to have been a not unimportant centre of astronodial activity.[40] Here we have to locate the story a little more closely in time and space. We are in the Latin Mediterranean. We shall find in fact that the relationships between astronodia and medicine are different here from those further north. We are also at that time when the *studia* are emerging as formal and legal structures, in Italy and Montpellier as well as in the

---

[38] Roger of Hereford was a contemporary of Daniel of Morley and seems have been gripped by the same excitement about the predictive power of the new Arabic learning. Nothing he wrote has been published, but a number of MSS survive. I have not included a discussion of them here because Roger remained to the north of the Mediterranean, perhaps at the school in Hereford. Nor did he use his judicial astronodia in a medical context. I hope to publish something on Roger in the future.

[39] Roger of Hereford, 'De astronomia iudicandi', Cambridge University Library, MS I.I.I, fols. 42v, 43r.

[40] Thorndike describes a MS from Marseilles that claims to make the first use of Arabic astronodia (in either 1111 or 1139): *A history of magic and experimental science*, vol. II, p. 92.

north, and this also had its effect on the relationship between astronodia and medicine.

Marseilles was not only the place from which Roger of Hereford took his tables, but was home too, a few years later perhaps, to his countryman, known to us as William of England.[41] 'English by nation, medical by profession and astrologer in opinion', William wrote in 1219 a little book called *De urina non visa*, 'On unseen urine'. It is a predictive text, clearly designed to exploit the reputation-building potential of rationalized prognostication of both astrology and uroscopy. As William says, the medical man who can foresee the nature of the disease, devise a remedy and stipulate a suitable future moment for its consumption will deserve the praise he will receive. Glory (*gloria*) follows both astronodial and medical predictions.[42] His text became so useful in this respect that it came to be prescribed by statute to be read in the *studium* of Bologna.[43]

William emphasizes the links between medicine and astronodia. Did not Ptolemy record that the Egyptians practised the two arts in conjunction, to be more certain of their predictions? William of course is particularly interested in the links between the medical man's prognostication from urine and astronodial prediction. Both activities are parts of a range of natural operations: William stresses that the upper 'root' or ultimate cause is the motion of the heavenly bodies. Because they are perfect, their causation is perfect; but their effects, the lower root or secondary cause, operate in the realm of imperfect, corruptible matter. It follows that prediction can never be perfect since lower, terrestrial, corruptible things are subject to accident. Like Gerard of Cremona, and other writers, William has here a mechanism that will explain how prediction cannot in practice be perfect. It is also a mechanism that saves free will and providence: the planets provide invariant *dispositions* towards action in matter, but both accidents and determination in our material circumstances can overcome this disposition.

The corruptibility of matter was not only a reason for a lack of total precision in astronodial prediction, but it was also of course central to medical theory. Corruption of the air and of water, of which William writes, was a recognized cause of disease, leading to a corruption of the humours of the body. William has adopted the doctrine of the Great Conjunctions from Albumasar, a doctrine that lays down that the rare conjunctions of the Infortunes cause major political and natural disasters,

[41] There was a school at Marseilles, where William and a close relative were educated. Perhaps it was here too that Raymond of Marseilles wrote his astronodial text in about 1139–40. It is based on Albumasar's *Introductorium* and the *De magnis conjunctionibus* in an emphasized Christian framework. See Lemay, *Abu Mashar*, p. 141.

[42] Manuscripts of the work exist in astronodial collections from Rome to Cracow. I have used Vienna, National-Bibliothek, 5207; Cambridge, Trinity College, 0.8.31.

[43] McMenomy, *The discipline of astronomy*, pp. 452ff.

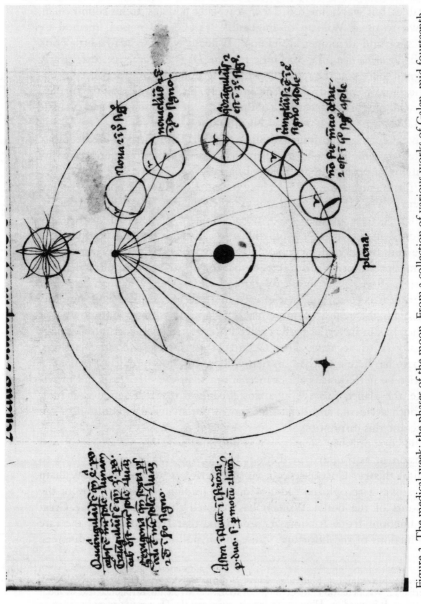

Figure 3　The medical week: the phases of the moon. From a collection of various works of Galen, mid fourteenth century. For explanation see foot of next page.

and particularly, by corruption of the air, plagues.[44] A related doctrine used by William is that lunar eclipses have similiar effects. The moon was, after all, the signifier of the patient and the cause of terrestrial growth. Its sudden and unusual loss of virtue was seen as a cause of evil.

A large part of William's text is taken up, as are many such texts, with a systematic exposition of the linkages between macrocosm and microcosm. Each planet (chapter 3) has particular influence on a part of the body, its function and its characteristic diseases. This link allows the macrocosmic system of aspects and the circumstances of the Lord of the Ascendant to relate to the anatomy of man. In a similar way each part of the body and its illnesses are distributed among the Houses (chapter 4), which provides an hourly guide for prediction. A third link is the special relationships each of the planets have with the parts of the body while the planets are passing through the signs of the zodiac in turn. After discussing the Lord of the Ascendant, William finishes indeed with an account of how to predict, astronodially, the nature of urine. It is 'unseen' urine because it is not yet in the jordan for inspection. But William knows what it will be like, because he can tell the qualitative nature of the heavens at some future time. He is bringing his astronodia to bear in particular upon the liver, of which he is concerned to find the macrocosmic place. It was in the liver that the production of urine was held to take place, as a superfluity from the fundamental process of the generation of blood. In normal uroscopy the colour, substance and contents of the urine told the doctor what was going on in the liver, where the natural faculty was making blood; William has reversed the process and is predicting both the state of the liver and the nature of the urine.[45]

In short, then, William's book represents the adoption of mathematical

---

[44] The doctrine of the Great Conjunctions became an important medical topic after the Black Death of 1348, right at the end of our period. Thereafter it became a common explanation of *epidemics*, that is, where normal horary, judicial and individual-centred astronodia could supply no explanation. It was concerned with cycles of very long duration (for example 960 years) between the conjunctions of the Infortunes and Jupiter at various positions in the zodiac.

[45] The text by Theophilus on urines was a standard part of the medieval textbook of medicine, the *Articella*. Occasionally it was replaced by a text by Gilles de Corbeil.

> The earth is in the centre of the diagram and the sun at the top and its increasing light on the moon is shown in the descending positions of the moon as it moves from new to full. The new moon is the first of the five intermediate positions. The moon between its two extremes is 'quadrangular' because a square can be drawn (and has been) with its corners on the dark moon, the full moon and the two positions of the half moon; in other words, the half moon is a 'square' to the earth. In a similar way the other aspects of the moon are represented by triangles. The full and dark moons may be omitted in calculating the medical week.

prediction into medical astronodia. William would have needed ephemeris tables to know when planets were in conjunction. He would also have needed tables to tell what sign was rising at what particular moment and thereby to identify the Lord of the Ascendant. Marseilles was one of the few places with local tables.

MEDICINE AND ASTRONODIA IN THE *STUDIA*

When medicine became a university subject in northern universities like that of Paris, it does not seem to have been very astronodial. The picture we have of medicine in the early northern universities is one of a common curriculum, the *Articella*, expounded by commentary and disputed questions. Nothing in the *Articella* is astronodial. Since astrology could arouse as much criticism as medicine itself, perhaps the medical men took care not to encounter a double criticism by making their medicine astrological.[46] The picture we have of northern medicine being largely innocent of astronodia has perhaps also been rather cultivated by historians anxious to see medicine shaking off so unscientific a business. But we should remember that right at the end of our period the Paris medical faculty proclaimed that the plague was due to Great Conjunctions. How much and what kind of astronodia was taught in the liberal arts in the northern universities before the mid thirteenth century is not clear.

In contrast, some of the southern *studia* had started life as separate academic incorporations of law and of medicine combined with arts, and it was not a question of medicine *entering* them. Such medicine may have been more closely associated with astronodia than that of the north, perhaps because it found a natural place in the associated arts course. Evidence for what was taught in the early Italian *studia* is very scanty[47] but by the mid 1260s predictive astrology in Italy was of concern to the Dominicans. The order was spread throughout Europe and so in a position to make comparisons: it is significant that it is Italy and not the towns of the north that attracted their censure. The new master of the order in 1264 instigated a new Dominican astronodia, designed to replace the mathematical, predictive, deterministic and noxious *scientia* of the 'enemies of Christianity' with something more suitable.[48] Bologna had a full astrological course by 1405 – including the text of William of England – and the evidence points to growth of medical astronodia only in the later thirteenth and the fourteenth centuries. McMenomy found few manuscripts of

---

[46] For the attacks on medicine and astronodial/physical branches of knowledge, see S. C. Ferruolo, *The origins of the university: the schools of Paris and their critics, 1100–1215* (Stanford, 1985).

[47] See N. Siraisi, *Arts and sciences at Padua. The studium of Padua before 1350* (Toronto, 1973).

[48] M. Grabmann, 'Die "Summa de Astris" des Gerardo da Feltra OP', *Archivum Fratrum Praedicatorum*, 11 (1941), 58–82; see also R. Creytens, 'Hugues de Castello astronome Dominicain du xive siècle', *Archivum Fratrum Praedicatorum*, 11 (1941), 95–108.

'medical astrology' in the thirteenth century. Perhaps, then, medicine became astronodial only after the faculties had become well established; and this was in the later thirteenth century, later than hitherto thought.[49] The standard teaching texts of *studia* astronodia are also comparatively late; at least they postdate the origin of the Paris and Italian *studia*. Sacrobosco's *Sphere* was written sometime between 1215 and 1235, and the other main source of medieval astronodia within the *studia*, the anonymous *Theorica planetarum*, dates from between 1260 and 1280.[50]

This mathematical astronodia was matched within the *studia* by the more physical accounts of the heavens, based on Aristotle's *De caelo*. This text was part of the natural philosophy of the later part of the arts course in Paris, specified in the mid 1250s and soon copied in many European universities. Natural philosophy came to Padua in Taddeo's time[51] when, perhaps, *De caelo* was added to the astronodial works of the medicine-and-arts course. All in all then, it looks as if the southern pattern may have been that the twelfth-century interest of the medical man in the single *philosophia* of the world and in Arabic prediction persisted in the *studia* and was supplemented by the addition of Aristotelian physical works in the later thirteenth century. In contrast, the natural philosophy of the later arts course in the north was astronodial only in so far as commentaries on *De caelo* became predictive rather than physical. Even this preceded and was not part of the medical course. It seems general that the development of astronodia in medicine was the product of the fourteenth and fifteenth centuries.

To dwell for a moment on commentaries on *De caelo*, there are several manuscript examples of a regent master's commentary being written down, to say nothing of the exceptional and famous commentaries by people like Aquinas. These commentaries are 'physical' in the Aristotelian sense, rather than mathematical and predictive. The manuscripts are examples of the physical *corpus* of Aristotelian nature books that formed the textbook of natural philosophy of the Middle Ages. In the generous margins of these volumes, and sometimes on the flyleaves, is found material that is distinctly unAristotelian but which represents the efforts of thirteenth-century teachers to place Aristotle in a context that is both Christian and astronodial. Sometimes the *Sphere* of Sacrobosco appears. The front leaves of such a volume annotated in Oxford fill out Aristotle's creatorless world with a discussion, based on Plato, of the divinity of natural things.[52] It proceeds to an astronodial description of the upper and perfect causes and

---

[49] See C. O'Boyle, 'The founding of the French university faculties of medicine. The life and work of Bartholomew of Bruges', Ph.D. diss. (University of Cambridge, 1987).

[50] McMenomy, *The discipline of astronomy*, pp. 16, 127.

[51] N. Siraisi, 'Pietro d'Abano and Taddeo Alderotti: two models of medical culture', *Medioevo*, 11 (1986), 139–62: 147.

[52] London, British Library MS Royal 12 G v; 12 G II and III contain postils and glosses also derived from lectures.

of their effects among lower corruptible matter, dealing in particular with the nature of the planets and of the people who are influenced by them. As time went on this process of adding different material to the simple list of Aristotle's nature books specified in the mid thirteenth century was institutionalized. The Oxford statutes of 1350 add Sacrobosco's *Sphere*, a compotus and Euclid's geometry to the traditional thirteenth-century list of the nature books (reflected in the *statuta antiqua* of 1340). The statutes of Paris of 1366 have something similar.[53]

Montpellier in some respects followed the northern pattern, and the statutory medical course in 1340[54] contained no astronodia. Masters are said to have used the subject in discussing critical days and bleeding and we would expect extensive use of it when the new Galenism arrived and the masters had to comment on Galen's *Critical days*. Bartholomew of Bruges provides a detailed mathematical analysis of the Hippocratic-Galenic problem of calculating critical days, but this is in a commentary on the *Prognostics*, and he is not concerned with planetary aspects and qualities. In the south, Gentile da Foligno has a similar treatment of critical days.

THE CALCULATION OF CRITICAL DAYS

Bartholomew of Bruges[55] provides a worthwhile example of the medical use of astronodia.[56] He was an exponent of high scholastic medicine at the end of our period, having taught arts in Paris and medicine in Montpellier. He taught the new Galenism, which transformed the old curriculum based on the *Articella*. He was heir, then, to rational medicine in the sense used in this chapter, that is, medicine whose intellectual connections to other branches of knowledge made it attractive to patient and students, justified it institutionally and laid the basis of common professional belief and practice. We can emphasize again the importance of prognosis in a medicine of this kind, and that no kind of prognosis in medicine was much more important than the prediction of critical days, the days that dramatically sealed the fate of the patient.

It will be useful to compare what Bartholomew has to say on critical days with Gentile da Foligno's *quaestio extravagans* on the same topic.[57]

53 McMenomy, *The discipline of astronomy*, appendix.
54 L. Demaitre, 'Theory and practice in medical education at the university of Montpellier in the thirteenth and fourteenth centuries', *Journal of the History of Medicine*, 30: 2 (1975), 103–23, at 110.
55 See C. O'Boyle, *Medieval prognosis and astrology: a working edition of the* Aggregationes de crisi et creticis diebus: *with introduction and English summary* (Cambridge, 1991) (Cambridge Wellcome Texts and Documents, no. 2).
56 Bartholomew of Bruges, *Dicta super* Prognostica, Österreichische Nationalbibliothek, Vienna, MS Vind. Pal. 2520, 50v–68r.
57 Gentile da Foligno, *Quaestiones et tractatus extravaganates* (Venice, 1520). In this collection, Gentile's tract on critical days follows his commentary on chapter one, tract four of the 14th fen of the *Canon*.

Both were teachers at the end of our period, when medicine was firmly Galenic and its theory was firmly based on the natural part of Aristotle's philosophy. This made Gentile's handling of critical days different from that of Maurus, whose arguments about critical days Gentile dismisses as rhetorical and vulgar in not proceeding from propositions in a demonstrative way with proper use of logic. In fact he links Maurus with many other earlier writers whose explanations lay in the power and perfection of numbers, such as the superiority of odd numbers like 7 which consists of 4 and 3. Such numerology for Gentile is not only insufficiently based on Aristotelian demonstration, but has no connection with the physical world. This brings him, in the company of Bartholomew, to Galen. In Bartholomew's Montpellier, the bachelor of medicine becoming a master[58] had to have read Galen's *Critical days*, and we would therefore expect that it was the job of regent masters to comment on it. In fact Bartholomew's treatment of the Galenic text is part of a larger commentary on the Hippocratic *Prognostics*. Since much of Galen's own writing on crises is a Hippocratic commentary, Gentile and Bartholomew have a strongly Galenic style of rationalizing commentary.

It is with Galen that they base the calculation of critical days not on a numerology that Gentile attributes to most earlier writers, but on physical arguments. The centre of their attention is the moon. This is partly because of the normal astronodial use of the moon as the signifier of the patient and the controller of his humours, and partly because the periodicity of the moon can be mathematically related to the Hippocratic critical days. Bartholomew sets up the physical situation in astronodial language: the *radix superior* consists of the heavenly bodies, the *radix inferior* the generable and corruptible material things of earth; *all* motions, if controlled at all, are controlled from above.[59] As Gentile says, the relationship between the upper cause and the crisis is necessary, *ordinatus*. What happens on the non-critical, or intercadent days, says Bartholomew, has its (secondary) causes in the lower *radix* and so is variable and uncertain.

Of the celestial bodies, our authors say, the sun controls chronic diseases with its yearly cycle, while acute diseases follow the shorter lunar cycle. Since the phases of the moon depend on the sun, the sun is not without influence in critical days, both in this physical sense and in the mathematical techniques of calculating. Bartholomew and Gentile, like Maurus and Galen himself, are engaged in the exercise of rationalizing the Hippocratic critical days. What, they ask, is the physical reason that explains the crises of the seventh, fourteenth and twentieth day? If the number seven is important why is not the twenty-first day critical? (or why does Hippocrates say that three weeks are completed in twenty days?).

The physical answer they were seeking is the one we have already met, that the moon has a special relationship to the patient and his humours. The mathematical problems are solved by an elaborate analysis of the moon's periodicity. Apart from the calendar month, which Bartholomew calls 'artificial' because of its different lengths, and the 'month' of common speech that was thirty-two days, our authors have at least four different kinds of months. The first is what Gentile calls the month of conjunction, which is, as we can read in Bartholomew, the month in which the moon goes through all the astronodial aspects to the sun: conjunction, sextile, square, at triplicity and opposition. These are the phases of the moon as it goes through the angles of 45, 90, 135 and 180 degrees on the fourth, seventh, eleventh and fourteenth day. From this position, full moon, it returns in reverse order to conjunction.[60] The second kind was the 'month of peragration' in which the moon completed a circuit of the signs of the zodiac. (This was also called the month 'of proper impression'.) This, say our authors, is twenty-seven days and eight hours. The third kind was the 'month of common impression' or the 'manifest vision'; that is, while the moon's means of influencing us, its light, was apparent. This month did not include the period when the side of the moon facing us was not illuminated by the sun. This month was reckoned to be twenty-six days twelve hours.

In fourth place was the medical month. This was calculated by the medical man, says Bartholomew, from the second and third kind of natural month as follows: compare the length of both; divide the difference – twenty hours – into two and add ten hours to the month of common impression, making a month of twenty-six days twenty-two hours. So the medical month was ten hours longer than the month of common impression and ten hours shorter than the month of peragration. Since it was also shorter than a month of four weeks each of seven whole days, there were 'medical weeks' and 'medical days' each proportionally shorter than natural weeks and days. Thus medical days did not coincide with natural days, and so provided an alternative way of counting when calculating critical days. It was also possible to count 'continuously' or 'discretely', the second of which is what we would now call an 'inclusive' week ('from the first to the seventh inclusive') which meant in practice taking day seven as the last day of the first week and the first day of the second week. All in all these procedures enabled the rationalizing doctor of the first half of the fourteenth century to explain Hippocratic critical days, and particularly why three weeks added up to twenty days, on the basis of what we might want to call physical astronomy. The reason for doing so was, it can be argued, to enhance medicine by means of an attractive story about its macrocosmic 'fit'.

It is for this reason that Bartholomew and others do not make a distinction between astronomy and astrology in which historians of science

---

[60] Bartholomew of Bruges, *Dicta super* Prognostica, fol. 61r.

could look for signs of emancipation of science from superstition. Bartholomew's purpose is rather to strengthen medicine with knowledge about the natural world. The very sun and moon are vitally important in medical matters, as in the world at large. The sun makes the seasons and causes animals to generate, as Bartholomew read in Aristotle. The moon causes the tides, menstruation and swelling of the brain. The primary mechanism of this causation is the light of the moon, which varies as the moon passes through different aspects to the sun. In describing the moon's motion round the zodiac, Bartholomew passes without hesitation into what we would call astrology. He does not have this distinction, and indeed for him it is the *astronomi*[61] who predict and the *astrologi* who study the active influence of the moon. According to Bartholomew, it is not only the relative amount of light sent to us by the moon that determines the course of a disease, but whether the moon, when the disease began, was in a sign together with a Fortune – Jupiter, Mercury or Venus – or an Infortune, Mars or Saturn.[62] Bartholomew proceeds to nativities with the same confidence. If a man is born, he says, when there is a Fortune in Aries and an Infortune in Taurus, then his disposition will be good when the moon – as always, his signifier – moves into Aries or into one of the two signs having the good aspect of square to Aries. For similar reasons his disposition will be bad when the moon enters Taurus, and these reasons govern the course of a disease that starts at an identifiable moment.

Bartholomew claims that most of this can be found in Galen, and it is at this point, he says, that Galen becomes oblique in his language. Having given here, he says, what the good medical man needs, Bartholomew recommends that anyone who wishes to understand what Galen is being obscure about should study *astrologia*. But Bartholomew is not separating medical knowledge from superstition, but recognizing there are practitioners of prediction – he calls them again *astronomi* – who are not medical men. The medical man should be prepared, he says, to accept from the *astronomi* what is established in their field. The difference between the two kinds of prediction is that 'astronomical' prognostication concerns only the future influence of the planets – what Gerard of Cremona would have called the necessary forming of a disposition – while the medical man has to balance the strength of the disease against that of the influence of the planets.

THE *REDUCTION OF THE KNOWLEDGE OF ASTRONOMY TO THE MEDICAL FACULTIES*

This unpublished text represents a further degree of integration of the theory of medicine with that of astronodia.[63] It was written probably in the

---

[61] Bartholomew of Bruges, *Dicta super* Prognostica, fol. 61v.

[62] Bartholomew of Bruges, *Dicta super* Prognostica, fol. 62r.

[63] I have used Cambridge, Trinity College, MS 0.8.31, fols. 132v–133v. L. Thorndike and P. Kibre, *A catalogue of incipits of mediaeval scientific writings in Latin*, 2nd edn (London,

early fourteenth century, and certainly after the time of Bernard of Gordon, whose book on prognostics it cites. It comes, that is, from the time when the 'new Galenism' of the fourteenth century had been developed, and its doctrines bind up the Galenic system of faculties with astronodial systems.

The author justifies his work by Hippocrates' recommendations of prognostication and on Bernard de Gordon's observation that the medical man is expected, whether he likes it or not, to know the nature and complexions of the signs and planets. As in the *Astronomia Ypocratis* and our other sources, the moon is the most important of the planets, not because of its size but because it is closer to us. 'Nature and complexions' of the signs and planets are the key to this marriage of medicine and astronodia, because the four Galenic faculties are also said to have qualitative causes. The faculty of attraction is in this way said to achieve its works by the hot and the dry, that of retention by cold and dry. The digestive is correspondingly warm and wet and the expulsive cold and wet. In this way the four faculties correspond to the four sets of 'trigons' or 'triplicities', each of which is a group of three signs having two elementary qualities in common. The hot and dry attractive virtue thus corresponds to Aries, Leo and Sagittarius, the hot and dry signs. In a similar fashion Taurus, Virgo and Capricorn control the retentive faculty, Gemini, Libra and Aquarius the digestive, while the expulsive is governed by Cancer, Scorpio and Pisces.

Naturally enough the hot and dry planet Mars relates to attraction, Saturn to retention, the sun, Jupiter and Venus to digestion and the moon to expulsion. These simple correspondences give shape to the practice of medicine recommended by the author. Despite the relation of the moon to expulsion it remains, as in other schemes, the signifier of the patient. So, when the doctor wants to strengthen the attractive virtue, he does so when the moon is in one of the three signs that favour attraction. If the Lord of the Ascendant is with the moon, so much the better, and better still if the sign ascending is one of the triplicity of the faculty in question. This formula is repeated for each of the three remaining faculties.

In addition the author's practice is shaped by the relationship between, on the one hand, the humours that are to be evacuated by his therapeutic techniques and, on the other, the planets. Blood, being hot and wet, is favoured by the sun (hot) and Venus (wet). When blood is in excess and has to be removed, then it should be done when the planets that favour it are weakened by reason of their celestial aspects. Jupiter is said to strengthen all natural things, including the faculties and humours, so any attempt to

1963), give the alternative title *Virtues and signs of the planets*. The work is found also in an Oxford MS: Bodley, Digby, B Ld 29, fifteenth century, fols. 179r–181. See also the short but learned article by C. Burnett, 'Astrology and medicine in the Middle Ages', *Bulletin of the Society for the Social History of Medicine*, 37 (Dec. 1985), 16–18.

remove a humour and restore a balance while the influence of Saturn is strong will not be successful. Not dissimilar arguments are used for the proper times of taking medicines: the watery triplicity will aid the dispersal of an ingested medicine, and the Lord of the Ascendant, if below the earth, will draw the medicine down. Should it be above the earth, vomiting will ensue. Lastly, astronodially suitable times should be selected for the preparation of medicines (which of course operate by reason of the elementary qualities).

PIETRO D'ABANO

The period covered by this book begins when the first translations from the Arabic were being added to the descriptive astronodia of the pre-*studia* West. It ends when the Black Death all but disrupted the universities, in which mathematical and predictive astronodia was an established and statutory study. We can gain some insight into this change by looking at Pietro d'Abano, because he defended the increasing use of astronodia within medicine.

We have seen that astrology may have been more a feature of the south than the north. Pietro taught astrology (and medicine and philosophy)[64] in Padua, in a country, that is, where astrology was already in demand in court circles.[65] He had also been to Paris, where we may suppose he became familiar with the northern style of university.[66] His *Conciliator* was finished in 1303, but he claimed to have been working on the material for ten years.[67]

Pietro announces his enterprise in terms that had been used by those who wrote in the twelfth century about the 'divisions of the sciences'. That is, he saw philosophy as single, knowledge-as-a-whole that had the purpose of perfecting man's nature or at least remedying the faults caused by the Fall. Its ultimate purpose was religious, both for the twelfth-century authors and for Pietro: 'All branches of knowledge agree in one purpose', he said, 'which is the acquisition of perfection of the human soul that prepares it for future happiness'.[68] But, unlike his twelfth-century predecessors, Pietro's apparatus for explaining and achieving this is Aristotelian. It is to the *Ethics* and *Politics* of the arts course that Pietro refers when explaining man's desire to 'live well and be happy'. 'To live' is the form of the living, says Pietro from *De Anima*, and 'to live' for the living means to strive for a more perfect and divine state: the ultimately religious nature of philosophy

---

[64] See Siraisi, 'Pietro d'Abano and Taddeo Alderotti', p. 142.
[65] Siraisi, *Arts and sciences*, p. 72.
[66] Siraisi, *Arts and sciences*, p. 282.
[67] *Conciliator*, prologue.
[68] 'Omnes scientiae communicant in una utilitate, quae est acquisitio perfectionis animae humanae praeparantis in effectu eam ad futuram foelicitatem', *Conciliator*, p. 4r.

is not far below the Aristotelian surface in Pietro. Indeed, while he thinks of happiness as an operation of the soul in terms of Aristotle's *De Anima*, and of man's desire to know in terms of the *Metaphysics*, yet the 'happy life' acquired through philosophy can culminate in beatitude of a religious kind, a perfect state of the aggregation of all that is good.

But, continues Pietro, man's basic desire for life and happiness is not enough. Things can go wrong. In a word, *differences* appear. It was his purpose in putting together his *Conciliator* to remove some of these differences, particularly those that arise in medicine between philosophers and physicians. The *Conciliator* consists of 210 'differences', each treated in a formal disputational way. For Pietro it is Aristotelian methods of argument and Aristotelian philosophy that provide the power – *potestas* – to bring the basic desire for life and happiness to actuality. Part of this discipline of living is the need to know the good and evil influences of the stars.[69] It is Pietro's view of the oneness of philosophy that directs his arguments for regarding astronodia as useful to, essential to, and indeed part of medicine. He represents medicine as that which, of all the *scientiae*, is the most devoted to particulars. It relies, then, upon more general *scientiae* that deal with universals, that is, upon natural philosophy and the seven liberal arts. Even the trivial arts, like logic, are for Pietro part of the philosophical enterprise: 'Logic is an organic part of the whole of philosophy, defending us from evil in practice and from the false in theory.'[70] The quadrivial arts, especially astronodia, are equally necessary, but it is plain from Pietro's treatment that his interest lay primarily in astronodia. Arithmetic is said to be useful simply for calculating critical days, and geometry for assessing the size and shape of wounds. As for music, Pietro simply refers to a separate *differentia*, and says nothing about its relation to medicine.

The formal principles on which Pietro constructed the *Conciliator* obliged him to lay out the most fundamental differences first. The first ten *differentiae* form a complete section of the book and are concerned with the nature and relationships of medicine; the doctor should be familiar with the other theoretical *scientiae*, including logic; his medicine is indeed such a *scientia*, theoretical as well as practical; at the same time it is the most excellent of the arts. Its subject is the human body, which is best committed to the care of a single doctor, who should be aware that, for philosophical and religious reasons, it is now more fragile than in ancient times. The final 'difference' of this first section is whether the doctor's astronodia can help cure his patients.[71]

---

[69] Ibid., prologue.

[70] 'Logica est pars organica totius philosophiae defendens nos a malis in practicis et a falsis in speculativis', ibid., p. 3v. (*Differentia* 1: does the medical man need to know the other *scientiae*?).

[71] Not included in the list of *differentiae* given here is Pietro's long discussion of that widely debated question on what Galen intended by the three 'orders' or 'doctrines' by which he began the *Tegni*: it is number eight.

Pietro's formal principles also oblige him to begin the discussion of each disputed question with an account of the arguments against the position he is defending. This is a device of the schools, but it is probable that some of these arguments in favour of a negative resolution of the question were those used by the opponents of Pietro's position. Thus the arguments *against* the doctor knowing other subjects are arguments against medicine being learned, that is, a university subject. They may well have been used by those who did not wish to see medicine taught in institutions that they felt served religious purposes.[72] According to Pietro, they centre on the empirical nature of medicine and its status as a manual craft. Had not the great Hippocrates avoided theory?

In answering such questions in the first section of the book, Pietro is leading up to the final treatment of astronodia. The other *scientiae* are the necessary preliminary steps for the medical man. He should be familiar with them but not study them for their own sake. 'Don't grow old in arts', was the cry of the ambitious teaching master in Paris, who wanted to proceed to higher studies. Pietro says the same – 'neque antiquandum est in aliis scientiis'[73] – for excessive concern with the subtleties of language or of universals discourages the attention to sensory observation and particulars that is so fundamental to medicine. While the other disciplines are preliminary for medicine, Pietro argues that astronodia is part of medicine. He was encouraged in this assertion by his belief that Hippocrates himself had written on astronomia: it is the text we have looked at above.

Having thus arrived at the medical uses of astronodia, what does Pietro say? How is this most particular of disciplines, this most excellent of arts informed in its practice by the *scientia* of the heavens and earth? The answer is: not very much. In general, says Pietro,[74] the astrologizing doctor can foretell the qualitative changes of the air and so adjust the regimen of his patients. Astrology also provides suitable times for providing medicines.[75] It shows when the moon is tempered by the Fortunes. It explains why the effect of purges (as we have seen) is diminished when the moon is with Jupiter. It supplies some rules for surgery (including phlebotomy),[76] for 'it is horrible to take the knife to any part when the moon is in the sign of that part'.[77] But this is not very much when compared, for example, with his enormous digression on the 'three doctrines' of Galen. It is clear that Pietro is concerned with the *principle* that astrology is part of medicine, and not with details of astrological practice of medicine.

Some of the reasons for adopting this principle were external to the

---

[72] For the opposition to medicine as a learned, university subject, see Ferruolo, *The origins of the university.*
[73] *Conciliator*, p. 4r.
[74] Ibid., p. 17v (*Differentia* 10).
[75] Ibid., p. 3v.
[76] Ibid., p. 17v.
[77] Ibid., p. 3v.

perceived technical superiority of astrological medicine. Some had to do with the expectations of the patient, for, as Pietro says,[78] the doctor must be able to deal with a patient who has already seen an astrologer. It was expected that the doctor knew his astrology, and many would have agreed with Pietro's advice that no one should put themselves in the hands of a doctor who was ignorant of astrology.[79] Indeed, Pietro makes it plain that part of the doctor's authority derived from his impressive knowledge of the stars.[80] His authority with the patient was an important part of the doctor's armoury: Pietro goes into some detail in giving what was probably a standard account of medical ethics, a great deal of which was concerned with the building and defence of the doctor's reputation. The doctor with authority was in control of the relationship between himself and the patient, particularly if he was in sole charge of the patient (as Pietro argues in the seventh *differentia*). He could influence the patient in the matter of fees. The very authority of the doctor generated a confidence in the patient which itself helped him to recover. For Pietro this authority – the doctor's reputation – could be increased in a number of ways. Treatment of the poor without a fee 'generates fame'.[81] His modest behaviour in civil life demonstrates that he is worthy of faith and confidence. And Pietro's preferred route to a reputation is through prognostication. Joy for the doctor and glory for his reputation are the results of successful prognosis.[82] Use of astrological signs not only reinforces the doctor's own confidence but enables him to convince the patient and the assistants, and to build his reputation, says Pietro explicitly.[83] But the hazards are considerable, and rules must be obeyed in order to avoid disaster. The doctor and the astrologer should never be absolute but always tie their predictions to conditional circumstances, says Pietro; the patient must be obedient, and the assistants skilful. Nothing is certain, especially in acute cases; but, if death looks certain, advises Pietro, then change your expression and say with an assumed grief to the assistants, 'Only a divine miracle can restore health'. The result is a prognostication that does not detract from God's freedom of action and which is good for the reputation of the doctor.

CONCLUSION

So what, ultimately, is the moral of the story of Daniel's journey to Toledo – what different message does this way of looking at the story give us? At

---

[78] Ibid., p. 4r.
[79] Ibid., p. 4r: 'Cuiusmodi est medicus, qui astrologiam ignorat, nullus debet se in eius manus ponere.'
[80] Ibid., p. 4r: Doctors, says Pietro, ought to know the *scientia* of the stars 'ut per eam sciant sui magisterii radices certissime'.
[81] Ibid., p. 5r.
[82] Ibid., p. 5r.
[83] Ibid., p. 17v.

his time, the *moral* reading of a story, perhaps a parable, was held to give a higher meaning than the *literal* reading.[84] To transfer this distinction to modern scholarship: a *literal* reading of the history of translations and translators gives us an event which is often called 'the reception of Greek and Arabic science'. Perhaps the *moral* reading shows us that there was a different kind of historical dynamics at work than some mysterious 'reception'. For, to be able to predict the future gives one power. This is the moral reading, this gives us the cause and reason why people translated Greek and Arabic works in the Middle Ages. If we are looking for causes of the medieval reception of someone else's 'science' then, in terms of excitement and practicality, the practical need to foretell the future comfortably beats as an explanation the desire just to curl up by the fire with Aristotle's *Physics*.

Finally, and to repeat an earlier point, this chapter has not sought to give a systematic account of medical astrology in the period. It points indeed to a gap at that particular spot in the literature and suggests that it might be plugged by a more detailed look at the manuscript sources, some of which are briefly examined here, and by a re-evaluation of the historical dynamics of translation, 'transmission' and 'assimilation'. In relation to the connections between learned and practical medicine from Salerno to the Black Death, it suggests an alternative view of the uses of medical learning in the medical market place.

[84] See Smalley, *Study of the Bible*, esp. pp. 26ff.

2

The science and practice of medicine in the thirteenth century according to Guglielmo da Saliceto, Italian surgeon

JOLE AGRIMI and CHIARA CRISCIANI

I

In this chapter we want to examine some aspects of the image that a professional physician and author of practical medical texts – Guglielmo da Saliceto (1210–1276/80) – presents of his knowledge, and also to investigate the forms of the transmission of this knowledge, and the position it holds in the wider doctrinal medical tradition of the time. Therefore, our research is directed to answering questions such as these: What image of knowledge does Guglielmo uphold? How does he perceive the relationship between the doctrinal aspects of medicine and its practical aims? How does he represent his role as operator and what are the characteristics of the model of physician that he introduces? In what cultural context does he place his successes and his limitations? What are the rules that embody and transmit this knowledge? What are the difficulties that undermine it? The analysis of Guglielmo's position, dealt with from this point of view, is part of a more general evaluation we are offering both of the characteristics of scholastic medicine between the thirteenth and the fifteenth centuries and of the relationship between medicine and natural philosophy in the late medieval Latin culture of Italy. There are two obvious features of the medicine of the thirteenth century which make it homogeneous with scholastic culture. On the one hand there is the strong link between *scientia* and teaching, thanks to which what counts as authentic knowledge is (and this becomes increasingly the case) what can be transmitted according to well-defined institutional procedures and structures of teaching. On the other hand there is the organization (which is progressively more articulated) of medical knowledge into epistemological levels – *scientia*, *ars scientifica*, *operatio*. This permits the ascription of relative values of truth, efficiency and cultural value as deemed appropriate to different fields and texts, and it also permits the ascription of relative value to different social roles and figures which have to do with medicine. It seems useful to dwell upon the initial stages of this process of integration between medical knowledge and scholastic culture, at the time when this organization still appears very flexible in both its doctrinal and institutional respects, in order to throw light on its development and later results.

The course we follow here unfolds along these two specific lines: (a) The identification of the characteristics of practical medicine in Guglielmo da Saliceto's writings, in particular its place with respect to the relationship between the theoretical and practical parts of medicine, the *pars theorica* and *pars practica*. (b) A comparison between the *Cirurgia* of Guglielmo and his *Summa* on the one hand; and between the *Cirurgia* of Guglielmo and that of Lanfranco on the other. In this way we intend to find out how the shift of epistemological level in the first case, and the presence of stronger teaching institutions in the second, bring about changes in the epistemological definition of practical medical knowledge among the hierarchy of professionals, and in the criticism and exclusion of those operators who are now defined as inexpert and therefore ignorant and illegitimate.

II

It is difficult to define Guglielmo's institutional position precisely. It is no accident that Sarti – an erudite eighteenth-century historian of Bologna University – includes Guglielmo da Saliceto among the renowned *medicinae professores* of Bologna University, even though he can find no evidence of his medical degree ('licet doctoris titulo insignitum non reperiam'). Sarti has stronger evidence with respect to the lasting value of Guglielmo's writings. His *Cirurgia*, printed several times between the fifteenth and sixteenth centuries, was translated into several languages for wider use ('ut exteris hominibus usui esse posset'). His *Institutiones medicae* were widely studied and appreciated, according to Sarti, until the ancient medical theories were superseded by new theoretical and practical knowledge ('quoad antiqua medendi ratio novis inventis exclusa non est'). Sarti refers also to a document which mentions the presence of 'magister Guilielmus medicus de Placentia' in Bologna in 1269.[1] Probably 'magister' here is not an academic title, but refers to someone who works as a practitioner (and is therefore *medicus*) and simultaneously teaches the medical art (and is thus *magister*). Rather, the term 'magister' refers here to forms of private teaching which are rooted in the tradition of the schools, or *scholae*, of independent teachers. Courses were held, often in the houses of the most renowned physicians and surgeons, for groups of students – *socii* – under private contracts or arrangements.[2] These *socii* had to possess a basic level of

[1] M. Sarti, *De claris Archigymnasii Bononiensis professoribus* (Bologna, 1769), p. 466.
[2] See G. Zaccagnini, 'L'insegnamento privato a Bologna e altrove nei secoli XIII e XIV', *Atti e memorie della R. Deputazione di storia patria per le provincie di Romagna*, 4th series, 14 (1923–4), 261–2; Zaccagnini, *La vita dei maestri e degli scolari nello Studio di Bologna nei secoli*

education and know Latin; they had to follow the teacher's lessons and assist him in his professional activities.

One of the strongest traditions of this kind of teaching in the field of surgery, after Parma and Salerno, is to be found precisely in Bologna. Indeed, the school of surgery praised by Guy de Chauliac in the prologue of his *Inventarium sive collectorium cirurgie*[3] was founded in Bologna during the thirteenth century. It grew around very reputable teachers: firstly Rolando and Ugo Borgognoni, then Teodorico (Ugo's son) and Guglielmo da Saliceto. It had the form of a *societas*, that is, a didactic and professional community identified mainly by the operating methods, the *modi operandi*, and the ways of teaching of its 'master-physician', its *medicus magister*.

Nevertheless, the establishment of a doctrinal tradition in the fields of surgery and practical medicine, together with the creation of a learned didactical literature, indicated that there was a growing need for a more regular and methodical mode of teaching. In fact, the surgery texts we are referring to here are written in Latin. Guglielmo's works share the same specialized vocabulary as the contemporary university practical medical texts and make increasingly precise references to the authorities, the *auctores*. The importance of teaching – *docere* – that is, the insistence on a more organic and structured relationship between teacher and student, is clearly being emphasized: one writes on request and for the benefit of one's pupils, one's *socii*.[4] But one writes above all to transmit practical knowledge to future practitioners, that is, a competence, a skill (even manual skill), acquired during the many years of one's professional practice. Here lies the distinctiveness and the flexibility of these texts and of this school. We have chosen to concentrate on Guglielmo da Saliceto precisely because this author epitomizes and symbolizes the characteristics of this process of institutionalizing the profession of the physician and of restructuring and regulating the teaching of surgery.[5] This restructuring and this regulation were brought about by stressing surgery's continuity and unity with the doctrinal tradition of practical medicine; therefore it was inevitable that it would be influenced in some way or other by the evolution of the teaching of practical medicine in the new university curriculum.[6]

According to his biographers, Guglielmo came to Bologna for the first time around 1230. Here he must have followed (we say 'must have' because we have no clear evidence about his training) the lessons of Ugo Borgog-

XIII e XIV (Geneva, 1926), pp. 111–12; N. Siraisi, *Taddeo Alderotti and his pupils. Two generations of Italian medical learning* (Princeton, NJ, 1981), pp. 14–15; Nancy Siraisi, this volume.

[3] *Cyrugia Guidonis de Cauliaco* (Venice, 1498).

[4] See J. Agrimi and C. Crisciani, *Edocere medicos. Medicina scolastica nei secoli XIII–XV* (Milan and Naples, 1988), pp. 163–7.

[5] See Siraisi, *Taddeo*, pp. 18–20; Siraisi, this volume.

[6] Siraisi, this volume, pp. 88–109.

noni and perhaps, though this is less likely, those of Bono del Garbo.[7] Along with Rolando, Ugo has traditionally been considered the founder of surgery in Bologna; he was paid by the Italian *Comune*, and was the prototype of the *medicus-magister* before the establishment of the universities, since he performed the two activities – not yet separated – of practising and teaching at the same time. The same is true of Guglielmo, who, in many autobiographical passages, insists on placing his own writings in the framework of both knowledge and practice: *doctrina* and *usus*. His texts, with their illustrative case histories, give a vivid account of the various places where he practised and of his travels as a practitioner. In some cases, he was paid as a physician by the *Comune*; in other cases he worked also as a teacher. He practised in Piacenza, Milan, Cremona, Pavia, Bologna and Verona, where we can find him active in prisons and hospitals, 'in palatio communis'[8] and 'in domo canonicorum' – in the communal palace and in the house of the canons. He was called to treat friars and abbots, criminals and soldiers, women and children. He had professional relations with important political figures, such as Oberto Pelavicino, the imperial representative and *podestà* in many of the towns mentioned above, and Martino della Torre, the *Signore del popolo* of Milan.[9] He was appreciated as a physician in the houses of rich and powerful families, such as the Scotti of Piacenza, the Guidoboni of Parma and the de Advocatis of Cremona. He mentions the successful operations he has performed, and also claims that teachers and students of the University of Bologna can bear testimony to some of them. Sometimes Guglielmo was called in for a consultation by other physicians, for instance by 'magister Octobonus de Papia', and also collaborated with them in the treatment which ensued. Very often Guglielmo was helped in his professional activity by assistants or disciples, who are sometimes referred to as *medici manuales* or *ministri*.[10] But we want to draw attention to a significant difference between Guglielmo and his (presumed) teacher Ugo Borgognoni: Ugo did

---

[7] A. Boreri, *Guglielmo da Saliceto. Studio storico-critico* (Piacenza, 1938), p. 12; M. Tabanelli, *La chirurgia italiana nell'alto medioevo*, (Florence, 1965), vol. II, p. 501; T. Zucconi, 'Guglielmo da Saliceto e il progresso della medicina', in *Storia di Piacenza* (Piacenza, 1984), vol. II, pp. 404, 408.

[8] In the MS. Bergamo Gamma VI.6 we read 'in platea communis, in qua eram cum quodam domino' (fol. 41va).

[9] On Oberto Pelavicino and Martino della Torre see *Storia di Milano* (Milan, Fondazione Treccani degli Alfieri, 1954), vol. IV, pp. 274–300.

[10] We have used the text of the *Cirurgia* and the *Summa conservationis et curationis* as printed in the Venice edition of 1490, checking passages of the *Cirurgia* quoted or discussed against MS. Bergamo Gamma VI.6, fols. 1–78. Medical cases can be found in the *Cirurgia*, I.1, fol. t2vb; I.3, fol. t3rb; I.20, fols. t5b–t6ra; I.27, fol. v1ra; II.5, fol. x5ra–b; II.7, fol. x5va; II.15, fol. y2rb–ca; III.26, fol. z4ra; these can all, except one, be found in the first version of the *Cirurgia*; the missing one (Book I, chapter 20), which was added in the later version, is dated 1279 in some manuscripts and printed editions (see also Siraisi, this volume, pp. 88–109). *Summa*, I.10, fol. b4rb; I.120, fol. g2rb; I.176, fol. 15rb; III.22, fol. 06ra; IV.3, fol. p3ra.

not leave any writings. Indeed, Ugo actually made his disciples swear to keep secret and not to reveal his techniques and remedies. But his surgical and medical procedures were indeed revealed later by his son Teodorico and by Bruno and Guglielmo – by writing them in texts. This was the first radical transformation of the educational model typical of the familial and shop-apprenticeship kinds of teaching (from father to son, from *mastro* – trainer – to apprentice), based on oral transmission and practical training, into more regulated forms of instruction and professional training. The composing of texts can be seen as a fundamental turning point towards more ordered systems of studies which are able to establish a new kind of *societas*, one no longer based on private familial relationships.[11]

Guglielmo wrote the first version of the *Cirurgia* in Bologna in 1268 for the sake of students, 'ad utilitatem studentium'.[12] He finished the second version in Verona in 1275, where he retired, exiled from Bologna for political reasons, and where he was paid by the *Comune*.[13] In the *explicit* of the text he reminds us that he had compiled it ('ordinavimus cursorie')[14] in Bologna over four years. He probably wrote the long *Summa curationis et conservationis* between the two versions of the *Cirurgia* (there are frequent references to the *Cirurgia* in the major work),[15] in order to respond to the demands both of Ruffino (the prior of St Ambrogio's in Piacenza, where there was a hospital where Guglielmo probably worked) and of his *socii*. He dedicated this *Summa* to his son Leonardino, whom he wanted to steer

---

[11] See Agrimi and Crisciani, *Edocere medicos*, pp. 185–8.

[12] 'Explicit Cyrurgia magistri Guillelmi Placentini de Saliceto, quam ipse compilavit in civitate Bononiensi ad utilitatem studentium Millesimo ducentesimo sexagesimo octavo.' See MSS. Erfurt, Amplon. F 270; Modena, Bibl. Estense, 251 (2.1.12); Milan, Bibl. Trivulziana, 836; Città del Vaticano, Bibl. Apostolica Vaticana, Lat. 4468; Ross. Lat. 974.

[13] 'Sigillavimus et complevimus emendative librum cirugie nostre die sabbati VIII die junii in civitate Verone in qua faciebamus moram eo quod salarium recipiebamus a communi anno currente MCCLXXV. Verum est quod ipsum ordinaveramus cursorie ante hoc tempus in Bononia per annos quatuor.' See Venice edition, 1490; MSS. Cesena, Bibl. Malatestiana, Plut. XXIV (dextr.), 4; Bergamo, Bibl. A. Mai, Gamma VI.6; Verona, Bibl. Civica, 610 (733). A new version, which can be placed between the two previously mentioned ones (1273 is the date written in the manuscript), has been identified by T. Pesenti (*Le origini dell'insegnamento medico a Pavia*, in *Storia di Pavia*, vol. III, part 2 (Milan, 1990), p. 457) in MS. Vat. Palat. Lat. 1309. In this version, the request to write the *Cirurgia* is reported to have been made to Guglielmo by the Emperor (Frederick II, whom Guglielmo may have met in Pavia). However, it should be mentioned that this manuscript is the only one that gives evidence of this dedication. This manuscript is very late (1407) and it is a copy made by a German student, who corrupted or omitted a great number of proper nouns to be found in the text. Perhaps this student transcribed the date wrongly and also added Frederick's name. This version of the *Cirurgia* is dedicated, like the *Summa*, to Ruffino and not to 'Bone' (Bono del Garbo, that is), as has been maintained hitherto on the basis of printed editions and some manuscripts (in the MSS. Bergamo Gamma VI.6 and Milan Trivulz. 836 we find 'bene').

[14] In the MS. Bergamo Gamma VI.6 we can read 'ordinavimus consumare' (fol. 78rb), perhaps for 'consummare'.

[15] *Summa*, Prologue fol. a2ra: 'Feci enim alium librum in quo de his que pertinent ad manualem operationem seu cyrurgiam secundum meam possibilitatem complete determinavi'; see also 1.10, fol. b4rb; 1.189, fol. k1rb.

toward the profession of medicine, 'ad professionem artis medicinalis'.[16] The institutional fluidity of Guglielmo's writings now becomes clear: on the one hand, the readers of the *Cirurgia* – physicians, *medici manuales*, *restauratores* – are deliberately described in scholastic terms (as *studentes*). On the other hand, in the case of the *Summa* – that is, in the case of a genre, the *practica*, traditionally more structured (and, as we will see, more similar to university texts in the order of its contents, in treatment and in method) and written for the rational physicians, the *medici rationabiles* – Guglielmo immediately took care to put the text into the professional framework of practice in hospitals and of the professional transmission of knowledge and skills from father to son. Again, in the *Summa*, to the term *magister* Guglielmo sometimes preferred the term *prior*, derived from other associated forms (ecclesiastical and professional), and which was then adopted by later *Collegia medicorum* to indicate the oldest and most venerable *magister*.[17]

The rising institution of the university influenced Guglielmo more and more, by inserting the disciplinary tradition of surgery into a wider context with new texts and new philosophical perspectives.[18] Apart from references to the specialized medical authors in the *Cirurgia* (Hippocrates, Galen, Rhazes and above all Avicenna and Albucasis), whom Guglielmo mentions with a reverence which does not prevent him making his personal judgement of them, there are in the *Cirurgia* and in the *Summa* specific allusions to the new cultural context of the university. Indeed, he uses the new Galen (he mentions the *De crisi*).[19] But above all he refers to Aristotle, the 'new Aristotle', including the versions that Frederick II could have sent to Bologna through Michael Scot, according to a well-known tradition in political hagiography. The Aristotelian biological and psychological works (*De anima, De sensu, De somno et vigilia, De animalibus* – 'secundum diversas translationes') are frequently quoted, and so are the *Physica*, the *Metaphysica*, and the fourth book of *Meteors*.[20] And this is not all: Guglielmo confronts many problems, for instance that of the role of the woman in generation, which were then usual topics of scholastic discussion in the university faculties of arts and medicine. And he solves them by using the equally usual conciliative exegesis typical of university teaching.[21]

Guglielmo's texts were as much appreciated as he was famous. Amongst others, Michele Savonarola is loud in his praises of Guglielmo, 'that fellow

---

[16] Ibid. fol. a2ra. On the hospital attached to the Monastery of St Savino, and which stood beside the Church of St Ambrogio, see Zucconi, *Guglielmo da Saliceto*, p. 430. On Leonardino, see Boreri, *Guglielmo da Saliceto*, p. 19.

[17] See O. Weijers, *Terminologie des universités au XIIIe siècle* (Rome, 1987), pp. 71, 277–8.

[18] See also Siraisi, this volume, pp. 88–109.

[19] *Summa*, II. 7, fol. 14vb.

[20] See *Cirurgia*, II.24, fol. y4ra; *Summa*, Prologue, fol. a2ra; I.1, fol. a6va; I.7, fol. b3ra; I.59, fol. d4vb; I.176, fol. i4ra.

[21] See below pp. 79–80, 82–3. Another example of this conciliative exegesis can be found in the *Cirurgia*, II.24 (fol. y4ra), where the disagreement to be reconciled is between Avicenna (*Canon*, 'Cap. de solutione continuitatis nervorum') and Aristotle (*De anima* and *De sensu*).

from Piacenza, gifted with good judgement and real knowledge' ('Placentinus noster vir certe optimi iudicii et verae scientiae').[22] However, despite
– or perhaps just because of – its affinity with other *Practicae* written in the
university context (above all with that of Guglielmo Corvi), and despite
the fact that it was mentioned in the statute of 1405 among the good copies
(the *peciae* 'de bona littera et bene correctas') which the *bedelli* had to keep
available for the students of medicine at Bologna University,[23] the *Summa
conservationis et curationis* (or more simply the *Gulielmina*) experienced a
handwritten and printed tradition less rich than the more adaptable *Cirurgia*; and so it was to have fewer readers. The *Cirurgia* in the versions of 1268
and 1275, both in the Latin of the originals and in the later translations into
the vernacular, has been transmitted in twenty-two manuscripts (according
to the recent but not completely satisfactory survey by Tabanelli).[24] To this
list we must add the manuscripts already described by Thorndike and
Kibre.[25] Moreover, we must take into account other Latin manuscripts,
which have never been mentioned up to now and which are to be found in
the A. Mai Library in Bergamo and in the Biblioteca Apostolica Vaticana.[26] Another vernacular manuscript can be found in the Passerini Landi
Library in Piacenza.[27] This latter manuscript is very interesting because,
like the Putti 9 manuscript from Bologna, which was studied by Altieri
Biagi,[28] it presents some features which aid us in recognizing the different
levels of use of this work by a very diverse public, and the nature of its
audience among practitioners. It is a simplified text, in which the more
specifically epistemological and theoretical parts are left out, as are also the
sections devoted to the illustrative case histories, while over forty folios are
added in which some 'Experimenta Guillelmi' are reported. The *Cirurgia*,
in both the Latin and the vernacular versions, was printed several times
between the fifteenth and sixteenth centuries. There was also a contemporary French version (Lyons, 1492), to which Sarti was perhaps making
reference when he wrote about translations of this work into various
languages. Finally, better to understand the public and the audience for this
Cirurgia, we must note that the first printed edition was the *Guglielmo
volgare* (Venice, 1474), followed two years later by the *princeps* of the Latin

---

[22] Michele Savonarola, *Practica Major* (Venice, 1559), fol. 267rb.
[23] C. Malagola, *Statuti delle università e dei collegi dello Studio Bolognese* (Bologna, 1888),
p. 284.
[24] *La chirurgia italiana*, vol. II, p. 513–17.
[25] L. Thorndike and P. Kibre, *A catalogue of incipits of mediaeval scientific writings in Latin*
(London, 1963), col. 1141; we refer to MSS. Vienna 5154; Oxford, Bodleian, and St John's
College 76.
[26] For Bergamo MSS. Gamma VI.6 and Sigma VII.5 see J. Agrimi, *Tecnica e scienza nella
cultura medievale. Inventario dei manoscritti relativi alla scienza e alla tecnica medievale (secc.
XI–XV). Biblioteche di Lombardia* (Florence, 1976), pp. 29, 37. The Biblioteca Apostolica
Vaticana MSS. are Lat. 4488; Ross. Lat. 974; Pal. Lat. 1299, 1306, 1307, 1308, 1309, 1322.
[27] MS. Pallastrelli 75
[28] M. L. Altieri Biagi, *Gugliemo volgare. Studio sul lessico della medicina medievale* (Bologna,
1970).

text (Piacenza, 1476). The relative influence of the *Summa*, on the other hand, appears to be attested to by just five manuscripts and four printed editions of the fifteenth and sixteenth centuries.[29]

The *fortuna* of Guglielmo's *Cirurgia* is surely due to the comparatively poor textual tradition in surgery and also to the increasing demand for manuals by a growing specialized professional readership which had not always been trained at universities. This *fortuna* is also related to Guglielmo's fame, which had spread not only in Italy but also abroad (above all in France) through the evaluations of Lanfranco of Milan, Henri de Mondeville, and Guy de Chauliac, who considered him a founder of the Italian surgical tradition. These later authors referred to this Italian tradition in order to link to it the rising learned French surgical tradition, and thus give credentials to the latter.[30] In his 'history' of the surgical discipline, in his description (modelled after the Galenic description of the medical sects of his own time) of the three major Italian schools – the *sectae* – Guy points out the central role played by Guglielmo and Lanfranco in relation to the preceding school of Salerno, on the one hand, and to Ugo and Teodorico Borgognoni on the other. He describes Guglielmo and Lanfranco as wishing to mediate between these, 'volentes mediare inter istos.' This means that they knew how to co-ordinate doctrinal traditions, reason and experience, and thus elevated surgery to the level of an operative science. And it is exactly for this reason that we have focused our attention on Guglielmo da Saliceto. Let us now define more closely the features of this practical science, as viewed by Guglielmo.

III

If it is obvious that the characteristics of Guglielmo's surgery and practical medicine need to be analysed in the whole of his two texts, it is however in the prologues of these two works that he deals more explicitly with the epistemological definition of what the subjects of his treatises are: surgery and *ars medicinalis*.[31] In his view, surgery and practical medicine have the characteristics of *scientia operativa* (as Guglielmo himself defines it.)[32] This is the level of medical knowledge which has a relatively restricted but

---

[29] See Tabanelli, *La chirurgia italiana*, vol. II, pp. 520–2.

[30] See J. L. Pagel (ed.), *Die Chirurgie des Heinrich von Mondeville (Hermondaville) nach Berliner, Erfurter und Pariser Codices zum ersten Male herausgegeben* (Berlin, 1892), p. 138: 'Secunda secta fuit Magistri Guilielmi de Saliceto et Magistri Lanfranci et suorum sequacium. Et isti fuerunt minus defectuosi quam primi et primam sectam aliquantulum correxerunt.' See also Guy de Chauliac, *Cyrugia*, fol. 3ra; Guy affirms also that 'Guielmus de Saliceto valens homo fuit, et in physica et in cyrugia duas summas composuit, et iudicio meo quantum ad illa que tractavit satis bene dixit.'

[31] Guglielmo uses this term as well as *medicinalis operatio* in the *Summa*, Prologue fol. a2ra, a2rb. See also Siraisi, this volume, pp. 88–109.

[32] *Cirurgia*, Capitulum primum de diffinitione cyrugie et admonitionibus necessariis et utilibus operatoribus, astantibus et infirmis, fol. t2ra.

well-defined scope, different both from the more general notions of theory, the *pars theorica* (that is, the level of medicine linked to natural philosophy) and from the precise individual acts of surgical intervention (that is, the level of pure manual work, or *opus*).

We must point out right away that in Guglielmo's two prologues we do not find that elaborate and stereotyped kind of reflection on medicine as a *scientia* or an *ars*, on its theoretical and practical parts, and on the hierarchy of the parts, which would allow us to link natural philosophy to *operatio*. That kind of reflection is to be found, from the end of the thirteenth century, both in commentaries for teaching theoretical medicine and in texts dedicated more to practical medicine (we have in mind certain works of Arnau de Vilanova, the *Sermones* of Falcucci, the *Collectorium* of Bertrucci or even the later *Cirurgie*).[33] This fact is a first hint that Guglielmo's writings belong to an epistemological and institutional context which is not yet well defined and certainly not yet bound within a rigid framework.

However, this does not mean that Guglielmo shows any lack of reflection or lack of awareness of the structure of the knowledge that he was going to write about. Firstly, surgery is knowledge (*scientia*), and moreover it is knowledge of how to operate ('scientia docens modum operandi'). Indeed, it has its being in the mind ('esse in anima'), and therefore like all true knowledge it is not concerned with the particular ('non constet de particulari'). This is therefore a theoretical knowledge to be learned and transmitted through the use of reason ('per rationem'). It is based on principles and interweaves concepts and causes: that is, it offers universal directions which are theoretical, but related to *operatio*. These directions are related to the manual intervention, better still they may be said to regulate it, but they are separate from it. The *scientia operativa*, the operative knowledge – as Guglielmo often reaffirms – is not the same as 'operatio particularis que fit cum manu particulari', the particular operation which is made with the individual hand; it does not deal only with 'rem sensibilem corruptibilem', corruptibles and sensibles, nor is it identified with the irrational chance happening of a particular act of surgical intervention. On the contrary, the *scientia operativa* aims to give the particular interventions meaning, to orientate and to direct them, by relating them to the universals of true knowledge: 'sed bene dependet operatio particularis ex cirurgia que est scientia sicut particulare ab universali'.[34]

The *scientia medicinalis*, which is the subject of Guglielmo's *Summa*, is defined along the same lines. Here too the chance character of mere action is contrasted with the intervention performed according to considered rules which is effective because it is based on science (*scientia*), that is on the knowledge of definite causes.[35] In this text, however, the features of

[33] For these reflections see, among others, Agrimi and Crisciani, *Edocere medicos*, chapter 1.
[34] For these definitions see *Cirurgia*, Capitulum primum de diffinitione cyrugie, fol. t2ra.
[35] See *Summa*, Prologue, fol. a2ra.

practical medicine which make it a learned discipline are stressed much more. Guglielmo insists on the doctrinal teaching by which one can master the arts that have to do with operation or reflection, the 'artes operativas seu considerativas', among which is practical medicine. The group of disciples is here portrayed around the teacher, who is 'prior et melior', superior to and better than them; from him they learn the causes, the principles, the universal rules and the specialized terminology of the art ('vocabula arti propria'). These they learn *doctrinaliter*, that is, according to already tested didactic techniques and from already written texts which contain the results of an *usus rationalis* acquired over the long years of the teacher's healing activity.[36] These are the features that make practical medicine a *doctrina*, a structured discipline which is part of a more institutional *docere* or teaching.

The structure and the epistemological place of surgery and of operative medicine are now clear. Surgery (and we will dwell upon this because, as we said before, the scheme of *Summa* is already part of a better-established tradition) is a particular science which is included in and depends on more general medical knowledge (it is 'sub medicina'). The individual surgical interventions, in turn, depend on and are regulated by surgery. Thus, surgery has an indispensable intermediate function between too general notions and too particular acts, since it works from the former to the latter: it is able to 'adaptare vel contrahere quod docetur in universali ad particulare quod medicatur'[37] and it follows rules of reason which are directed towards intervention. Thus, the rules can direct the intervention but they are also subject to correction and confirmation ('rectificatio' and 'confirmatio'), which are imposed not by the *opus*, the particular act in itself with all its uniqueness, but by the *usus*, the continued practice, because a continuous *usus* promotes generalizations and allows for comparisons and corrections.[38]

What is the co-ordination of sensory, intellectual and manual functions (senses and reason, *usus* and *auctores*, *cogitatio* and *manus*) and what are their mutual adjustments and reinforcements that allow this interlacement between *ratio* and *operatio*? To answer this question, it is necessary to go beyond the two prologues and peruse the two texts more deeply.

IV

In Guglielmo's surgical treatise we can notice a persistent and recurrent orientation which we would like to define as a type of 'concrete epistemology'. By this we mean the process through which Guglielmo very often links rational criteria and procedures belonging to the experience of the

---

[36] Ibid., fol. a2vb.
[37] *Cirurgia*, Capitulum primum de diffinitione cyrugie, fol. t2ra.
[38] Ibid.; see also Siraisi, this volume, pp. 88–109.

senses and unites them strongly so as to create very meaningful lexical connections between terms from the domain of reason and terms of experience. Therefore, procedures of investigation and confirmation, such as *investigare, inquirere, determinare, perpendere* (which can usually be found in a purely theoretical and rational framework in not much later texts) are here connected, immediately and for the most part, to a concrete sensory apparatus. In the same way, some terms which are peculiar to the technical domain (like *ingeniare, machinare, temptare*) are used here to define intellectual procedures.[39] Thus the processes through which knowledge is acquired, through which what is hidden and latent becomes clear and evident to the physician, are seen not as merely logical argumentations but as explorations of the intelligent senses and of a sensory reason. The *inquisitio* is brought into act through the senses – sight, touch and hearing[40] – of the physician, who however knows what to look for and how; or through those artificial senses which are the instruments,[41] the artificially constructed intelligent extensions of the senses. As an example of this, we mention here the exploratory instruments *tentae* and *tenaculae*,[42] which are primarily means of knowledge, and means of intervention only after that. Therefore Guglielmo can speak about 'rational instruments', *instrumenta rationabilia*,[43] used by the surgeon, and about a surgical instrument used 'wisely' (*sapienter*).[44] Again, from the same point of view Guglielmo writes about *operatio manualis*, manual action (it must be borne in mind that such an operation depends on *operatio universalis in mente*);[45] it can be divided into *operatio docta*, that is learned, competent and therefore legitimate *operatio*, and *operatio indocta*,[46] that is unlearned, without order, and therefore dangerous.

Expressions like *operatio indocta* (unlearned operating), *usus rationalis* (rational practice) and *doctrina per visum et usum* (knowledge by seeing and doing) can be defined as oxymorons;[47] they could certainly have been defined in this way in texts of authors writing a little later (where such concepts and expressions are definitely not common), where the separation between the theoretical and the practical aspects of medicine is made more

---

[39] For occurrences of these terms see *Cirurgia*, 1.47, fol. v4rb; II.1, fol. x2ra; II.3, fol. x4ra; II.4, fol. x4rb; II.6, fol. x5rb; II.12, fol. y1ra; III.14, fol. z1vb.

[40] For some examples of the essential role of the senses in the surgeon's activity, see *Cirurgia*, 1.3, fol. t3ra; 1.4, fol. t3va; 1.9, fol. t4ra; 1.10, fol. t4rb; 1.16, fol. t4vb; 1.22, fol. t6ra; 1.28, fol. v1rb; 1.57, fol. v5vb; III.2, fol. y5rb; III.11, fol. z1rb; III.16, fol. z2rb.

[41] About the instruments, see *Cirurgia*, 1.9, fols. t3vb, t4ra; II.4, fol. x4rb; II.5, fol. x5rb; II.24, fol. y4ra; II.14, fol. z2ra.

[42] See, for instance, *Cirurgia*, 1.57, fol. v6ra; II.3, fol. x4ra; II.4, fol. x4rb.

[43] Ibid., II.5, fol. x5ra.

[44] Ibid., 1.26, fol. v1ra.

[45] Ibid., Capitulum primum de diffinitione cyrugie, fol. t2ra; II.1, fol. x2rb.

[46] Ibid., 1.44, fol. v3vb.

[47] For these expressions see *Cirurgia*, 1.9, fol. t4ra; 1.44, fol. v3vb; *Summa*, Prologue, fol. a2ra. An oxymoron is a rhetorical figure by which contradictory terms are joined together in one statement.

neatly and more definitely. This distinction certainly does not exclude appropriate mediations and articulated relationships between the two parts of medicine, which is in any case aimed at practical goals. What appears peculiar to Guglielmo's view is the immediate connection, almost a fusion, of those two aspects. In our opinion it indicates that medical knowledge is conceived by him as being all placed on a single level which is intrinsically and organically made up from knowing and acting, or, to put it better, from knowing how to act. Here, what is shown by the senses is already a *doctrina*, and a *doctrina* is not something merely rational or only based on *traditio* from authorities; here an *operatio* is not a chance or repetitive acting but a learned and wise action which produces knowledge.

To understand better this orientation of Guglielmo's knowledge, an orientation which is neither rationalistic nor based on authorities, it suffices to mention the recurrence in his text of a kind of concrete *questio*. In such cases the forms canonically used to introduce the question and pose the problem (*utrum . . . an, videtur quod*: whether, whether or not, it seems that) and the various positions which are discussed, do not refer to sentences taken from texts, but to instances of behaviour and to procedures actually adopted by various practitioners (*quidam, alii*) or to actual stages of a process of surgical intervention, of which Guglielmo points out the route and the chosen or rejected solutions.[48] Guglielmo acknowledges that the physician's intervention is in some cases (for example, in the reduction of fractures) based mainly on the sensory data, on *visus* and *tactus*, sight and touch, while in other cases (for example, in the choice of remedies and diets) on the intellectual indication of *cogitatio* and *imaginatio*.[49] At all events, he is firmly convinced that an intermediate route is to be followed, which excludes any strict adherence either to the directions of mere theory and of the *auctores*, the authorities, or to an irrational and therefore chance-based practice. Thus, in a particularly difficult case of an arrow wound he states that 'ex parte cognitionis contracte ex scientia' (that is, according to prognosis derived from rational knowledge, from *scientia*) the situation should be defined as a fatal one and therefore the physician should not intervene. But, despite this *iudicium scientiale*, this scientific judgement, he advises the physician to carry out the intervention. However, he does not suggest just proceeding without using scientific judgement, which would mean emphasizing the self-confidence and the primacy of *praxis* in itself, but rather he advises relying on a *cogitativa scientia*.[50] Indeed, this course of action is halfway between a possibly surer but more abstract knowledge on the one side, and a casual and unsure practice on the other, and hence it is

[48] For an example of this kind of 'concrete question', see *Cirurgia*, II.1, fol. x2rb; for an example of a customary *questio* (in the standard meaning of the term), in which the opinions and sentences of authors are examined according to rules of argument, see ibid., II.24, fol. y4ra.

[49] See, for these examples, ibid., III.2, fol. y5rb.

[50] This medical case can be found in *Cirurgia*, II.4, fol. x5ra.

the only one which can suggest a *medicamen rationabile*, a rational medical remedy.

In this intermediate zone we can find all the main concepts of Guglielmo's epistemology, both those dealing with criteria and with ways of producing knowledge, and those organizing and defining the results of this production, that is, with the contents of this knowledge. As to the production of knowledge, we can notice that Guglielmo seldom (at least in the *Cirurgia*) refers to *ratio* or *intellectus* as the agents most responsible for surgical knowledge. *Cogitatio, imaginatio, inquisitio* (thought, imagination and enquiry) are rather ascribed to *ingenium*,[51] whose main attribute is *subtilitas*, subtlety.[52] On the one hand, *ingenium* is an *intermediate* intellectual function; it produces notions, perhaps not necessary but effective ones, which are linked to the data of the senses, by which they are corrected (they undergo *rectificatio*) without however merely mirroring them; on the contrary, these notions are able to steer decisions and to organize operative sequences in surgical intervention, when the physician is faced with different possibilities, not all foreseeable at the beginning or predictable at the moment of defining the clinical case. One the other hand, *ingenium* is a *connecting* function which essentially mediates between experience and reason, knowledge and intervention, natural processes and the practitioner's initiatives, and finally between him and the patient. Above all, *ingenium* helps the physician to choose and connect the different criteria at his disposal – author's accounts, rational considerations, experiential proofs, artificial instruments – and to balance the two attitudes of the practitioner – boldness and prudence[53] – so that he can proceed firmly – *secure*;[54] for, while he is not supported by absolute certainties, yet he is not exposed to excessive risks either.

The way – or, better, the ways – which the *ingenium* fashions and which

---

[51] *Ingenium* is a manifold and meaningful concept in the text of the *Cirurgia*. Along with its derivatives, it occurs very frequently. It refers either to the instruments and the technical procedures used in diagnosis and therapy, or to the varied and concealed ways through which nature herself can promote health in the patient, or – finally, and mainly – to the skill of the operator, which is intellectual and manual at the same time. On this theme see D. Jacquart, 'La notion d'"ingenium" dans la médecine médiévale', in S. Knuttila, R. Työrinoja, S. Ebbesen (eds.), *Knowledge and the sciences in medieval philosophy. Proceedings of the Eighth International Congress of Medieval Philosophy* (SIEPM), vol. II (Helsinki, 1990), pp. 62–70. On *ingenium* and *subtilitas* see also J. Agrimi and C. Crisciani, 'Doctus et expertus': la formazione del medico tra Due e Trecento', *Quaderni Fondazione G. G. Feltrinelli* (Milan), 23 (1983), esp. pp. 162–3; see also Peter Murray Jones, this volume.

[52] On *subtilitas, ingenium* and the astute behaviour of the surgeon, see for instance *Cirurgia*, II.16 and 17, fol. y2vb; II.24, fol. y4ra; II.5, fol. x5ra; II.6, fol. x5rb; III.17, fol. z2va; I.1, fol. t3ra; I.43, fol. v3vb.

[53] On these two attitudes, so frequently alluded to in the *Cirurgia*, see for instance, I.1, fol. t3ra; I.g, fol. t3vb; I.34, fol. v2rb; I.44, fol. v3vb; II.4, fol. x4rb; II.6, fol. x5rb; II.13, fol. y1rb. See also Jones, this volume.

[54] Along with his own honour and success in the interventions, 'security' is the value to which the surgeon must pay the utmost attention. See for instance *Cirurgia*, I.1, fol. t2vb; I.44, fol. v3vb; II.1, fol. x2rb; II.13, fol. y1va; II.24, fol. y4ra; III.3, fol. y6va.

allow the practitioner to proceed and choose (*eligere*) securely, are the *regulae*,[55] that is, rational directions or rules. In this case too what is strictly interlinked and intertwined on the same level by Guglielmo, will be articulated more distinctly and above all more rigidly by later epistemological reflections. Thus, the rules are at one and the same time the results of a cognitive process which collects the constant features from among the disorder of the single facts and data (and they are therefore called general or common, *generalia*, *communia*), and they are also the proven and written contents of knowledge, which can be transmitted in the process of teaching (and therefore Guglielmo calls them *documenta*). Moreover, the rules are general criteria by which the individual surgical interventions are directed, and at the same time they derive from therapeutical practice because they emerge reliable from a long *usus*, which they in turn consolidate.

The final result, obtained by the *ingenium* of the physician through such rules, is the truth; a special truth, inasmuch as Guglielmo calls it *veritas operationis*, the truth of operation.[56] Once more, we are faced with a terminological juxtaposition which the later tradition will manage to resolve when it interprets the truth as the result of theoretical research and ascribes the successful result of the *operatio* to the carrying out of this truth. For Guglielmo, by contrast, the truth is immediately equivalent to efficacy; an effective result is clear and acceptable to knowledge because of its very effectiveness, and also a valid notion is immediately embodied into successful therapy.

v

These epistemological factors – *ingenium*, *regulae*, *veritas* – therefore have linking functions and are not structured in rigid schemes. If we now consider the structure of the text in which they are embedded, and the image of the practitioner who puts them into action, we will be able to recognize similar aspects of fluidity both in the style of writing and in the way the medical profession is depicted. The text of *Cirurgia* is, in fact, composed of treatises dealing with different subjects.[57] But in each treatise the different chapters do not always follow a set sequence of definitions, signs, causes and therapeutical prescriptions. Rather, they are characterized by various procedures of writing, which are not assumed at the outset, but are chosen each time in relation to the level of knowledge pertinent to the subject under consideration. Statements of general rules and *documenta* can be found along with discussions of genuine *quaestiones* and descriptions of

---

[55] On the *regulae* (also called *generalia*, *communia*, *documenta*) see for instance *Cirurgia*, 1.41, fol. v3va; 1.57, fol. v6ra; 11.1 fol. x2ra; 11.2, fol. x2va; 11.2, fol. x3rb; 11.3, fol. x3vb; 11.5, fol. x5ra; 11.6, fol. x5rb; 11.7, fol. x5vb; 11.8, fol. x6va; 11.16, fol. y2va; 11.27, fol. y4vb; 111.9, fol. y6vb.

[56] Ibid., v.1, fol. z2ra. On the 'concreteness of the truth' see also *Summa*, 1.176, fol. 15rb: 'Illud vero quod nostro fecimus tempore et in quo in multis fecimus veritatem est quod...'

[57] See Siraisi, this volume, pp. 88–109.

illustrative *exempla*.[58] The lists of opinions and sentences of authoritative writers, *auctores* – when available – seem to have a cognitive value which is equivalent, or at least comparable, to that of the narration of symptoms delivered by a patient, when interpreted by a physician. The opinions expressed by rationally acting operators, the *rationabiliter operantes*,[59] that is, the different therapeutical and doctrinal trends in the scientific communi-ty,[60] are compared not only with the perspectives offered by the *traditio* of the written authorities, but also and above all with the frequent and detailed presentation of medical cases treated with success by Guglielmo himself[61] and therefore used as *exempla*. More generally, the text of the *Cirurgia* seems to be in a borderline position with respect to the doctrinal dignity which is given to a disciplinary field by the very fact of its being written down.[62] On the one hand Guglielmo is aware of his role as a writer: notions and results up to now shaky because they have been entrusted only to speech, *sermo*, are made stable and authentic by him, through his writing them down. In this way he can refer to his own text (in later passages of the same work and in the *Summa*) as to an authoritative one; and, by writing them down, he can transform the general directions into *documenta*, that is, into stable rules which can be taught and transmitted. On the other hand, this process is just at its beginning and is a relatively new one. What Guglielmo transforms into writing, *scriptum*, is not yet – but is just becoming – a doctrinal tradition, and is still linked with the peculiarity and concreteness of *talking* and *doing*. This is why Guglielmo warns against the erroneous *sermo* (and not against the texts) of some of his adversaries, and often refers to a remedy or an intervention as 'said or done in chapter x' ('dictum vel factum in capitulo de . . .').[63]

Intermediate as he is between oral and written tradition through his

---

[58] For a list of these medical cases see note 10 above; on their didactic role see Siraisi, this volume, pp. 88–109; for more on the use of *exempla* in practical medicine, see Agrimi and Crisciani, *Edocere medicos*, esp. chapters VI and VII.

[59] *Cirurgia*, 1.44, fol. v3vb.

[60] On the role of the scientific community, mainly in the development of practical medicine, see M. R. McVaugh, 'The *Experimenta* of Arnald of Villanova', *Journal of Medieval and Renaissance Studies*, 1 (1971), 107–18; McVaugh, 'Two Montpellier recipe collections', *Manuscripta* (1976), 20: 175–81; Agrimi and Crisciani, *Edocere medicos*, esp. pp. 117, 229–38. In order to stress the comforting approval of the scientific community, Guglielmo refers to the agreement among the operators, that is, to the therapeutical line shared and agreed upon by many of them (*multi conveniunt*). This agreement makes the cure an approved, and hence a surer, one (see, for instance, 1.1, fol. t2vb; v.1, fol. z2ra).

[61] Guglielmo is very careful to stress the success obtained in medical cases, and the honour, fame and praise (and money) which the physician can gain as a consequence. See, for instance, *Cirurgia*, 1.20, fol. t5vb; 1.57, fol. v6ra; II.5, fol. x5ra; II.6, fol. x5rb; III.26, fol. z4va.

[62] On the role and importance of the written form for the institutionalization of medical studies see, among others, Agrimi and Crisciani, *Edocere medicos*, esp. chapter IV, part 4, and pp. 153–5, 185–7, 232–4.

[63] For these occurrences see, for instance, *Cirurgia*, 1.14, fol. t4vb; 1.33, fol. v2ra; II.13, fol. y1vb; III.14, fol. z1vb.

texts, between rules and intervention through his *ingenium*, the ideal practitioner whom Guglielmo describes, while describing himself and his own activities, is a complex figure, not very rigidly defined and the pivot of various relations. First, the image of the physician in the *Cirurgia* is not defined by a title, or by a single univocal term; he is sometimes called *medicus* (physician), *operator*, *magister* (master), *sapiens restaurator* (wise restorer), only sometimes *cirurgicus* (surgeon).[64] These are titles and terms referring to the multiplicity of functions (not yet separated) which he performs at the same time. Moreover, his identity and above all his authority are based on many factors, which are not hierarchically arranged but which reinforce each other and seem to have the same value as each other. Indeed, the knowledge and the doctrine of the physician are of the utmost importance, provided they are not separated from either the skill of his hands and senses or, and above all, from the long *usus* (the structured and continual practical performances, where his knowledge is put into action and corrected). Thus, a good physician is rightly called 'wise and expert' 'sapiens et usualis'.[65] What is more, doctrine and skill, besides not being values hierarchically arranged, are not even consistent if taken on their own. They must be validated, that is, they must produce concrete and evident effects, in the professional and social contexts themselves. Therefore worthy of trust as an authority – *auctorizabilis* – is the physician who, as *sapiens* and *usualis*, is successful and thus earns fame and honour, as well as large fees, 'bonam remunerationem et optimum stipendium'.[66]

As we have seen, in the practitioner as described by Guglielmo we can find, in a complex unity, many aspects which would in the near future be submitted to an analytic and often drastic separation. The figure of the practitioner is, on the other hand, the centre of a variety of manifold and flexible relationships. Since he has many functions – from teaching to operating – we are not surprised to find him in many places. It was to be suggested later that an indispensable aspect of the training and the activity of the physician-surgeon is his mobility. For instance, Henri de Mondeville was to claim that satisfactory surgeons, *cyrurgici sufficientes*, are only those who have passed 'through the schools of medicine as well as through tournaments and through the other most dangerous actions of war' ('discurrunt per studia medicinae, et per torneamenta et per cetera gesta armorum periculosissima'). Many surgeons unfortunately neglected this aspect, but the surgeon should not only learn from teachers, but also have

---

[64] See, for instance, ibid., Capitulum primum de diffinitione cyrugie, fol. t2ra; I.21, fol. t6ra; IV.1, fol. z5ra.

[65] Ibid., II.24, fol. y4ra.

[66] Guglielmo uses the term *auctorizabilis* both in the *Cirurgia* (Capitulum primum de diffinitione cyrugie, fol. t2ra: 'Et scias quod bona remuneratio et salarium optimum auctorizabilem medicum reddunt, et confortatur fides infirmi super eum ...'), and in the *Summa* (Capitulum generale admonitorium, fol. a2rb: 'nam talis inquisitio cum deliberatione reddit medicum auctorizabilem et scientem inter laycos et amicos infirmi...').

experience with armies and practise in all the situations where his skill could be improved.[67] In Guglielmo's view, such advice is still something obvious, needing neither defence nor advocacy. Indeed, Guglielmo himself is at work both after violent riots and fights, and in treating chronic infirmities. He is at work in noble and wealthy houses as well as in prisons, hospitals and convents.[68]

In his interventions the surgeon has a variety of social relations, which are necessary in various ways to improve his knowledge, his success and his fees. The relations with his patients are obviously essential, and Guglielmo devotes a great deal of attention to the way the physician should behave when approaching the patient, also giving a sort of rhetorical and stage-direction-like guidance for the physician's behaviour towards the patient's family and at the patient's bedside. In fact, his relations with the patient imply relations also with the patient's relatives and friends, the women of the house, and laymen (*layci*) in general.

As to these so to speak 'deontological' themes, Guglielmo deals with them in both the *Cirurgia* and the *Summa*. Right at the beginning of the *Cirurgia*, after defining what surgery is, Guglielmo sets out to expound the behaviour suitable for the surgeon as a learned and expert professional.[69] The first precept is that a great deal of care must be taken by the surgeon to acquire as much knowledge as possible of the condition of his patient in order to reach a scientific diagnosis.[70] The second precept is that the patient's full trust must be won by the surgeon. To achieve this aim, the physician should indulge his patient's wishes as long as they are harmless, should hearten and coax him with soothing words (that is, he should 'blanditiis et verbis delectabilibus et suavibus infirmum confortare'),[71] and should promise him health even in a desperate case. Through these expedients, the physician will strengthen his patient's disposition, and this will make the therapy more likely to succeed. However – and this is the third set of precepts – the physician should also take care of his own image and reputation and behave in such a way as to keep them up while dealing with his patients and their relatives and acquaintances. Thus, he should not withhold the real situation of his patient from his friends. He should not deal secretly and questionably with the women of the house. He should abide by the laws and the usages of the place where he happens to be

---

[67] For Henri de Mondeville see his *Chirurgie*, p. 132; see also T. Pesenti, '"*Professores chirurgie*", "*medici ciroici*", e "*barbitonsores*" a Padova nell'età di Leonardo Buffi da Bertipaglia († dopo il 1448)', *Quaderni per la storia dell'Università di Padova*, 11 (1978), 1–38.

[68] See above, p. 163.

[69] See *Cirurgia*, Capitulum primum de diffinitione cyrugie, fol. t2ra: 'Operantibus autem secundum artem et scientam tria sunt necessaria.'

[70] Ibid.: 'Cyrurgicus totaliter se debet prebere infirmo in investigatione compositionis et complexionis membri lesi et esse infirmitatis. Aliter enim deluditur hec scientia, et finem cyrurgicus per operationem suam non sequitur laudabilem.'

[71] Ibid.

working.[72] Above all, he should not treat with too much familiarity (*familiaritas*) the *layci*, that is, the laymen who are always ready to find fault with the professionals.

Besides giving these general instructions about the way a physician should behave in the *Cirurgia*, Guglielmo often mentions the *solemnitas*, the 'gravity', of the physician.[73] By this term Guglielmo is referring to the set of (rhetorical as well as scientific) rules and devices according to which the physician reaches and, even more important, expresses his evaluation of the case he is dealing with. The *solemnitas* is the rhetorical form in which the diagnosis (which, although scientifically neutral, bears an emotional impact, mainly when it is dubious or unfavourable) is made known; thus it becomes a *prognosticatio* which can not harm the physician's reputation, whatever the outcome of the medical intervention. In other words, the *solemnitas* is used as follows. The surgeon is sometimes confronted with very serious cases (for instance, wounds in the head and damage to the brain), where the *iudicium scientiale*, the scientific assessment, is unfavourable. He should not refrain from intervening even in such a situation, claims Guglielmo.[74] However, he should adapt the wording of his evaluation to those he is talking to, and thus he should express his evaluation in different ways to his patient, his patient's relatives and friends, and the laymen, in such a way as to give confidence to his patient, inform his family of the real danger, and prevent the laymen from putting the blame on the operator if the intervention is unsuccessful. This strategy, which culminates in the *solemnitas* and which encompasses scientific elements, rhetorical skills and professional ways of behaving, is definitely not simple. This is why Guglielmo, when recounting some difficult cases he has dealt with, explains the therapeutical and technical data, but does not overlook these rhetorical aspects, as he deems them essential for the professional.

Besides the relations with his patient's environment, the surgeon's activity has to do also with more professional figures: the previous physicians (those whose interventions had not been successful, as Guglielmo

---

[72] For this advice, see ibid., fol. t2rab. These deontological precepts were already present in classical medicine, and were proposed again later in the School of Salerno: see, for instance, Arcimatteo, 'De instructione medici', in S. De Renzi, *Collectio salernitana* (Naples, 1852–9), vol. II, pp. 74–5; vol. V, pp. 333–4, 348–9; see also L. C. MacKinney, 'Medical ethics and etiquettes in the early Middle Ages', *Bulletin of the History of Medicine*, 26 (1952), 1–31; and J. Agrimi and C. Crisciani, *Medicina del corpo e medicina dell'anima* (Milan, 1978), esp. pp. 9–18, 36–9. Guglielmo deals with this advice also, and more widely, in the *Summa*: see 'Capitulum generale admonitorium in quo determinatur de rebus que pertinent ad honorem et laudem cum utilitate et fine bono medicinalis operationis, et erunt admonitiones undecim' (fol. a2ra–va). In these pages we can find sentences and formulae already used in the *Cyrurgia*.

[73] See, for instance, *Cirurgia*, II.5, fol. x5ra; II.6, fol. x5rb; III.17, fol. z2va.

[74] Ibid., II.5, fol. x5ra: 'Et quamvis hoc iudicium sit scientiale, non mihi videtur bonum neque utile ut medicus se desperet nec propter hoc consulo ut a medicamine rationabili desistat ac si posset infirmum per suam cogitativam scientiam liberare …; sed utatur medicus prognosticatione in talibus ne laycis detrahatur.' See also III.17, fol. z2va.

often remarks), other physicians with whom Guglielmo collaborates and whom he consults,[75] unlearned practitioners (ignorant people always ready to criticize),[76] and particularly assistant-pupils and assistant-attendants. The model physician proposed by Guglielmo is described as having complex relations with these attendants.[77] Indeed, they can be considered like instruments – not artificial but human – indispensable to the success of the medical intervention, and therefore Guglielmo gives instructions on their 'use'. But they are also collaborators, whose specific ability is appreciated, and they are pupils, whose training has to be directed and encouraged.

We must now consider a point which concerns both the components we can identify in the text of the *Cirurgia* and the relations through which the surgeon-physician performs his activity. Guglielmo presents a flexible and articulated situation, which is certainly defined by unifying functions – the *ingenium*, the role of writing, the ability of the practitioner – but is not fixed in a static scheme. In this context, a hierarchical order or linkage between epistemological factors in the field of the discipline, or between practitioners in the field of the profession, is not stressed. On the contrary, Guglielmo emphasizes the fruitful exchanges which a *sapiens* and *usualis medicus* is able to effect: the exchanges between the sentences of the authors of the tradition, and the results of his personal experience; between the Ancients and the contemporary *rationabiliter operantes*, the practitioners who operate rationally; between following the rules and taking risks; and finally between the contributions of the physicians more inclined towards theoretical elaborations, and the practitioners closer to practice. None of these factors can be defined as dominant. All of them have their limits and can be subjected to criticism. Any one of them can be useful to those who possess *doctrina* and *usus* and are therefore able to evaluate them. For this reason there is no lack of polemical statements in Guglielmo's texts. The stolid physicians, the positions of the Ancients, the trends of the contemporary scientific community, the mistakes of some – even renowned – *auctores*, the techniques of other practitioners are criticized in turn. However, these criticisms are never seen as drastic exclusions on principle.[78] For this reason, we can find in Guglielmo's pages no sarcastic evaluations of the too-abstract knowledge of the theoretical (*theorici*) physicians,[79] nor can we find – which is most significant – any violent attacks (so widespread and

---

[75] For medical cases in which Guglielmo collaborates with other physicians see, for instance, *Cirurgia*, 1.20, fol. t5vb; II.5, fol. x5rb; II.15, fol. y2rb–va; III.26, fol. z4rb. In the *Summa* (fol. a2va) Guglielmo gives some rules for consultations among professionals.

[76] On the *layci* see *Cirurgia*, Capitulum primum de diffinitione cyrugie, fol. t2ra; 1.58, fol. v5vb; II.3, fol. x4ra; II.5, fol. x5ra. They are mentioned many times also in the *Summa*.

[77] See for instance, *Cirurgia*, 1.44, fol. v3vb; 1.47, fol. v4va; III.9, fol. y6vb; III.14, fol. z1vb; III.26, fol. z4ra.

[78] See also here Siraisi, this volume, pp. 88–109.

[79] However, we can find some doubts and criticisms of the opinions and the procedures of other physicians; see, for instance, *Cirurgia*, II.9, fol. x6ra; II.12, fol. y1rb; III.17, fol. z2rb; III.26, fol. z4ra.

sharp in texts which will appear immediately afterwards) on the manual and empirical practitioners. Since medical knowledge has not yet been structured in a rigid scheme of hierarchically ordered doctrinal and professional levels, clearly Guglielmo neither needs to defend the autonomy of his own competence against the supposedly superior control of theory, nor guarantee its dignity by differentiating it from the casual practices of the empirics, *vulgares* and *layci*.

VI

The *Cirurgia* and the *Summa* represent, in their continuity one with the other, the evolution of the epistemological reflections of Guglielmo on medicine as an art, *ars*, or as an operative *scientia*. This evolution shows itself through the connection between two types of practice: surgery and *practica*. They are unified by the very profession of the author and by the closeness of the doctrinal fields and operative domains of both surgery and *practica* of that period. We are therefore faced with two specialisms, not hierarchically arranged as such, but simply distinguished by their *modi operandi* and by the technical and conceptual apparatus they involve. However, the *practica*, according to Guglielmo, has a more solid disciplinary structure, although surgery should in some cases be considered nobler because it is more efficacious.[80] First of all, the *practica* has at its disposal a broader and more specialized repertory of *auctores*: Hippocrates, Galen, Avicenna, Rhazes, Serapion. Furthermore, their texts are already divided into sections which correspond to specific divisions of the discipline: diet, maintenance of health, blood-letting, causes, signs and diseases, diseases from head to toe, fevers, etc. ('De regimine cibi et potus', 'De conservatione sanitatis', 'De flebotomia', 'De causis', 'De signis', 'De morbis a capite ad calcem', 'De febribus', etc.); this is the same arrangement which will be proposed by the statutes and curricula aimed at regulating teaching according to a precise and gradual sequence of lecturing and teaching (*ordo legendi* and *docendi*).[81] Even more, this tradition of authors appears diversified and not repetitious, as is revealed by the differences in the opinions these authors hold and in the names of the diseases they deal with, and by the range of therapeutic procedures (*viae*) they propose. According to Guglielmo, we are dealing here with specialist views which are comparable: the surgical tradition (Albucasis) can be compared with the medical tradition (for example, Avicenna);[82] in the medical tradition the more philosophically oriented trends (such as Avicenna)[83] can be compared with the more specifically

---

[80] See, for instance, *Summa*, 1.34, fol. c7vb; 1.168, fol. i2va; 1.191, fol. k2va.
[81] See Malagola, *Statuti*, pp. 275–7.
[82] *Summa*, 1.10, fol. b4vb.
[83] Ibid., 1.132, fol. g8rb; 1.144, fol. h3vb: 'Ut volunt philosophi et specialiter Avicenna'.

medical ones (Rhazes, Serapion).[84] Guglielmo records with painstaking detail the precise differences between various points of view and between authorial positions on specific issues. Dealing with these differences requires an approach more in the line of a teacher than in that of a physician-surgeon. Indeed, the differences mentioned above must be interpreted in order to grasp the true intention of the author, the *intentio auctoris*; they are such as to require a conciliatory exegesis if the truest and surest route is to be found.[85] Indeed, such an interpretation and such a conciliation may be obtained through those principles and techniques which are used, or were soon to be used, by the university medical literature of that period. A principle of that kind and which Guglielmo stresses is that, when two authors disagree, the author who is more competent in that particular field is the one to be preferred. Among the techniques used to overcome terminological differences (for example, in nosological definitions and in anatomical nomenclature), Guglielmo includes – albeit with extreme caution – exercises with synonyms.[86] To reconcile the theoretical and therapeutical discrepancies, Guglielmo often resorts to *argumenta* – of reason, of experience, of authority – arranged according to the canonical schemes of the *questio* and supported by Aristotelian logic and natural philosophy. For instance, Guglielmo opens the second book of his *Summa*, devoted to fevers, with a sort of theoretical introduction. Here he distinguishes the genera and species of fevers by their causes. He distinguishes the *medicinales* causes from other causes and defines the nature (*natura*) of those medical causes. In their turn, the medical causes are subdivided into primitive, antecedent and conjoint (*primitivae, antecedentes* and *conjunctas*).[87] Guglielmo deals with this and similar subjects using the logical techniques of scholastic argumentation and within the framework of Aristotelian epistemology.[88]

[84] Ibid., 1.148, fol. h4va: 'voluerunt medici et specialiter Serapio'.
[85] Ibid., II.8 ('de febre tertiana pura interpolata'), fol. 15va: 'diversitas antiquorum tollitur sic. Avicenna cum dixit quod flebotomia erat conveniens respexit multitudinem materie intra venas et extra, que melius removetur per flebotomiam quam per mundificationem. Almansor respexit singularitatem materie que melius removetur nisi sanguinea fuerit per medicinam quam per flebotomiam. In mundificatione materie in principio cum mirabolanis et tamarindis respexit Rasis materiam plus quam dispositionem; Avicenna magis timuit dispositionem quam materiam et propter hoc fuit contentus in exhibitione tamarindorum tantum . . .; et propter hoc quilibet bene dixit, sed Rasis melius.'
[86] Ibid., 1.12, fol. b5ra: 'Omne apostema cerebri vel velaminis calidum vel frigidum communi nomine karabitus appellatur, et ab Almansore appellatur birsen et ab Avicenna sirsen sed apostema pectoris et costarum appellatur ab Avicenna birsen et ab Almansore sirsen; et per hoc videre potes quod in nominibus non est multa vis nisi apud medicos nominales, qui delectantur in debilibus et truffis et non in inquisitione rei et eius causa seu causis.'
[87] See ibid., II.1, fols. k6va–k7ra. For a discussion about genera and species of causes in medicine, see also ibid., 1.120, fol. g1vab. Here it is clear that the divergence of opinions over whether *asclites* is more dangerous than *timpanites* can be solved if the distinction among the causes is taken into account.
[88] But see ibid., II.3, fol. l1vb on the limits of the *quaestio* in medicine: 'Hec species effimere febris questionem habet. Videtur enim quibusdam hominibus quod hec febris non sit accidens sed egritudo per se . . . Si autem vellet aliquis dicere quod non est egritudo per se

The resulting text, the *Summa*, because of the very aspects by which it is distinguished from the *Cirurgia*, is closer on the whole to the *Practicae* which were being almost contemporaneously produced in the university environment, for example that of Guglielmo Corvi. These aspects are essentially three: the role of the *auctores*, the arrangement of the text, the function of reason (*ratio*). The way in which the *Summa* is written is already highly authorial and rich in quotations. In fact, Guglielmo himself affirms that he wished to write following both the experience which had occurred to himself and to his contemporaries and the reports of the ancients: 'secundum quod nostro tempore occurrit pre manibus nobis et penes narrationem antiquorum'.[89] The account of what the ancients wrote, the *narratio antiquorum*, described by Guglielmo as one of the three ways towards the establishment and growth of medical knowledge, is placed on the same level as the other two, which are *ratio* and *experientia*.[90] The written tradition, that is, what all medical philosophers believe ('volunt omnes philosophi medicinales'),[91] has truth value, and serves to authenticate certain procedures and findings.[92] The disciplinary written tradition of the *philosophi* stands now alongside, if not above, success in the profession and the validation by the community of professionals (the wise physicians, the *sapientes medici*) as a criterion of scientificity of the *modi operandi* and as an instrument of verification, which here means to reveal the truth.[93] However, Guglielmo also expresses some caution about the texts of the *auctores*, which are to be checked and corrected bearing in mind the historical periods and geographical regions in which they were written. Since these periods and regions are different from those of their present usage, they cannot be used directly.[94] This critical attitude is made possible by the fact that the contemporary scientific community of the *sapientes operatores*[95] is able to work out a learned doctrinal tradition of its own, and can thus offer a *via* which is *scientialis*,[96] a scientific pathway to knowledge.

A similar shift between the *summa* and the *Cirurgia* is also evident in the

---

febris effimera que sequitur ad apostema, imo est accidens … et sic febris apostematis semper accidens iudicabitur ita quod per similitudinem erit omnis febris accidens … Dicendum quod hec questio non est conferens in arte et operatione medicinali, sed est potius nocens et impediens.'

[89] Ibid., IV.3, fol. p1vb.

[90] Ibid., IV.11, fol. r4rab: 'res particulares et sensibiles cum quibus medici operantur possint cognosci tribus viis, ratione, experimento et narratione antiquorum, secundum quod in suis libris reperiuntur ipse res scripte cum naturis et operationibus suis'.

[91] Ibid., I.182, fol. xi7va; see also I.1, fols. a3vb, b1ra; I.67, fol. d7rb; I.111, fol. f4vb; I.192, fol. k3rb.

[92] See ibid., I.120, fol. g2va: 'et hoc manifeste apud nos fuit verificatum per usum et per dicta philosophorum'.

[93] Ibid., I.151, fol. h5va; II.35, fols. n2ra–n3ra.

[94] Ibid., I.1, fols. a4va, a5rab; I.10, fol. b5ra; I.192, fol. k3rb–va. On this theme, see C. Crisciani, 'History, novelty, and progress in scholastic medicine', *Osiris*, 2nd series, 6 (1990), 118–39.

[95] See *Summa*, I.193, fol. k4ra.

[96] Ibid., I.17, fol. c1ra.

organization of the contents of the *Summa*. In the *Cirurgia*, the starting point is what is single and evident to the senses: *this* wound, *this* sore, *this* fracture. In the *Summa*, by contrast, the essence of the diseases is the starting point; thus the definitions and the species of the diseases are here in the foreground; then the causes are listed, precisely because the definition of the essence and the knowledge of the causes are what make medicine a science, and as such teachable; then the *signa* follow; the therapy comes last. In the *Summa*, that is, the route is from the universal to the particular. This is the reason why theory must come first in the *Summa*. By contrast, in the *Cirurgia* the most theoretical part, anatomy, ends the treatise. Moreover, in the *Summa* the exposition of the diseases is to be found after the chapter on the conservation of health ('De conservatione sanitatis'). This means that in this case also Guglielmo wants to proceed from a more global analysis (that is about the regimen suitable for man in general, when he is healthy) to a more determinate and specific one (that is about the particular diseases which can harm man). Such an arrangement stems from the conviction that theory explains the causes (only they can reveal to reason what may be hidden from the senses) and theory only sets out the rules and the canons which direct the rational procedure, the *opus rationabile*.

Finally, one more element of the shift we find when comparing the *Cirurgia* with the *Summa* is that a superior intellectual function, reason, *ratio*, controls not just the senses but even *ingenium*, the particular practical reason of the physician. It is no accident that the term *ingenium* very seldom appears in the *Summa*, and, when it does, only in its derivatives – *ingenia*, *ingeniare*.[97] The *sapiens* is qualified here mainly as *rationabilis*.[98] Moreover, if *subtilitas*, subtlety, is also here the feature peculiar to the practitioner, it is now submitted to the control of *ratio* and *auctoritas*, reason and authority. In fact reason, which is the *ratio* both of the authors and of the scientific community, is universal,[99] while *ingenium* is particular and pertains to the individual. Moreover, reason is also the universally valid *ratio* of the Philosopher, embedded in Aristotelian natural philosophy. Let us underline here a clear example of the controlling power which is ascribed to philosophical reason in the *Summa*. This example deals with the female role in reproduction and with the Galenic two-seed theory,[100] a crucial problem for both physicians and philosophers. Guglielmo acknowledges in Aristotle, the *auctor* par excellence, the very authority of reason. Aristotle proved with many *rationes* that 'this opinion, although affirmed by the

---

[97] See ibid., 1.18, fol. cıva; 1.151, fol. h5va.

[98] Ibid., 1.1, fol. a7va; see also the 'Capitulum generale admonitorium', fol. a2va, and 1.196, fol. k5ra.

[99] See ibid., 'Capitulum generale admonitorium', fol. a2rb: 'omnes sapientes conveniunt'; 1.111, fol. f4vb: 'volunt medici omnes', 'dicunt omnes antiqui'; 11.35, fol. n3ra: 'voluerunt omnes philosophi'; *passim*.

[100] See H. Rodnite Lemay, 'William of Saliceto on human sexuality', *Viator*, 12 (1981), 165–81.

medical men, following sense, is not necessarily true' ('hec sententia quamvis secundum sensum a medicis affirmetur quoad veritatem non est necessaria'). Therefore, it is necessary to correct the opinion of the physicians on this matter by means of the Aristotelian text. In fact, it is clear to those who understand the truth through the words of the Philosopher ('apparet manifeste intelligentibus veritatem per verba philosophi') that only the male seed is needed for generation. This is the theory that all the *sapientes* must hold. The physicians stick to the sensory evidence; they can judge subtly, *subtiliter iudicare*, but only according to what they can see (*subtiliter videre*). By contrast, the philosophers are seeking for reasons and causes, and therefore only they can reach the truth.[101] Guglielmo could have found in the *Canon* (see I. I, 5.1 and III. XXI, 1.2) these epistemological criteria to reconcile opposite philosophical and medical theories. The *subtile ingenium*, the link between reason and senses, in the *Cirurgia* controls, verifies and rules *rationes* and *auctores*; here in the *Summa* it is instead confined to specialist data and is rooted in the sensory domain. Only by going beyond these too determinate and concrete features can the results of *ingenium* be inserted in a more comprehensive theory. In this way *medicina* as an operative science can become part of the theoretical and wider domain of natural philosophy, *philosophia naturalis*.

VII

The transition to a much more rigid epistemological, didactical and professional order is even more evident if the *Cirurgia* of Guglielmo is compared with the surgical treatises[102] of his pupil Lanfranco.[103] Guy de Chauliac, writing about the authors of his discipline, states that 'Guglielmo da Saliceto was a major figure and wrote two *summa*s both in physic and in surgery' ('Guielmus de Saliceto valens homo fuit, et in physica et in cirurgia duas summas composuit'), while he sneers at Lanfranco, who 'also wrote a book in which he put little he had not taken from Guglielmo, but arranged in a different order' ('etiam librum scripsit, in quo non multa

---

[101] *Summa*, 1.176, fol. i4rab.
[102] Lanfranco of Milan wrote two surgical treatises. The *Cyrurgia parva* was written in Lyons and dedicated to his friend Bernard. The *Practica que dicitur ars completa totius cyrurgie* (or *Cyrurgia magna*) was finished in Paris (1296) and was dedicated to the same friend Bernard and to the King of France, Philip the Fair (see also D. Jacquart, this volume, pp. 186–210). The first printed edition of these two works appeared in Venice in 1498 (with the text of Guy de Chauliac). They were reprinted many times and translated into various languages.
[103] What we know about Lanfranco's life is only what he records in his works: see E. Wickersheimer, *Dictionnaire biographique des médecins en France au moyen âge* (Paris, 1936), vol. II, p. 518. Because of political troubles he was banished from Milan by Matteo Visconti, and worked as a professional in France, living in Lyons for a period. Afterwards (in 1295) he reached Paris, where he was well accepted, particularly by the physician Jean de Passavant (who was a teacher in the faculty of medicine at Paris University at the time).

posuit nisi que a Guillielmo recepit, in alio tamen ordine mutavit').[104] These judgements are very much to the point, even more than Guy meant. Here indeed the 'different order' is not just the order in which the doctrinal contents of surgery are arranged in Lanfranco's text, but it is the more comprehensive order by which medical knowledge is structured by Lanfranco's time.

Here we can only cursorily touch upon some aspects of a comparison which surely needs deeper consideration. Surgery as a discipline is placed by Lanfranco in a medical science which has been structured now into a theoretical part and a practical part, *pars theorica* and *pars practica*, and which is organized in levels, hierarchially ordered from the top of the theory down to the bottom of the surgical intervention.[105] Surgery is fit to be inserted into this field of knowledge only if it is able to define the boundaries (*metae*)[106] – of object, method and scope – which it must not overrun. Moreover, surgery must be connected with, and depend on, the superior levels of the more general science of medicine according to the rules of 'subalternation', *subalternatio*, which are now well defined and compulsory. Furthermore, within the surgical tradition, the various trends – the *viae* – which Guglielmo was following easily, now stand as real and separate sects (*sectae*).[107] While the 'concrete epistemology' of Guglielmo resulted in direct links between reason and experience, here, in Lanfranco's text, we can find more accurate distinctions. Of course, Lanfranco too underlines the operative nature of surgery and holds that surgery implies the work of the hand, *opus manuale*,[108] and indeed consists in manual operation on the human body, 'operari cum manibus in humano corpore'.[109] But he is more aware than Guglielmo of the distinct and foundational role of theoretical medicine, of reason, and of doctrine. This is why in Lanfranco's pages, instead of Guglielmo's oxymorons, two parallel series of concepts are stressed; one series refers to the rational and doctrinal field, the other one to the artificial and operative one. In other words, in the text of Lanfranco we can find by his time standard couples of terms, like for instance: 'ratio **et** experientia', 'auctores **et** experimentum', 'vidi **et** studui', 'doctrina **et** experimenta'.[110] The loose way in which the different periods and stages of the disciplinary tradition of surgery were considered by Guglielmo is changed here into an ordered chronological sequence, where the ancients, the modern and the contemporary authors have different and predetermined weights.[111] The exchanges on a par among different kinds

---

[104] Guy de Chauliac, *Cyrurgia*, fol. 2vb.
[105] See *Cyrurgia magna*, fol. 167vab.
[106] See ibid., fols. 181rb, 196rb; see also *Cyrurgia parva*, fols. 163ra, 164va.
[107] See, for instance, *Cyrurgia magna*, fols. 172va, 174ra, 177ra, 182va.
[108] Ibid., fol. 198va.
[109] Ibid., fol. 167va.
[110] See, for instance, ibid., fols. 172va, 210vb; *Cyrurgia parva*, fol. 166rb.
[111] See, for instance, *Cyrurgia magna*, fols. 172va, 174ra, 182va.

of practitioners, so much appreciated by Guglielmo, give way to sharp and vigorous polemics.

Let us give some examples. In many a case Lanfranco describes his intervention as if he were the decisive person[112] who on his arrival resolved a hopeless situation, which had become hopeless because of the conceited ignorance of the physicians who had been present before he arrived. Indeed these physicians, in their haughtiness, look down on the surgeon, but in the end they, or the patients themselves, have to resort to his competence and skill. For instance, Lanfranco succeeds in giving the right diagnosis in a case of *antrax* while 'one great and famous physician did not know the disease at all' ('unus magnus et famosus physicus ipsam egritudinem minime cognovisset').[113] Also, Lanfranco finds fault with the hasty and hazardous incisions made by those physicians who think they can replace a surgeon.[114] Similarly, he states that the cure of joint pains is not known even by 'bonis et famosis medicis', good and famous physicians.[115] However, no less fault is found by Lanfranco with the laymen (often referred to as *idiotae*)[116] who promise quick recoveries, but are utterly without doctrine. He describes a very serious case in which he gave his advice (*consilium*).[117] But the patient's mother refused it and, after dismissing Lanfranco, turned to a layman, whose boastful promises led the patient almost to death. Then, a *physicus* was called, who gave the same advice that Lanfranco had already given. In another case (where the patient has been struck by a paralysis)[118] the laymen acknowledges his ignorance, and then Lanfranco takes action and obtains a partial success. On most occasions, however, according to Lanfranco the laymen act in a rough and gross way,[119] without care for the variation in their patients (whether old, young, strong, weak, etc.), and without knowledge of the diversity of the therapies required by the different situations. In general, such polemic is typical of someone who has to guarantee the specific scope of his own knowledge, and at the same time stays inside a scheme which is now rigidly systematic. Thus, on the one hand (and looking upwards), Lanfranco, as we have seen, often points out the mistakes of the too theoretical physicians, who have no respect for the surgeon's competence. On the other hand (and looking downwards), he

---

[112] Ibid., fol. 187ra: 'de malo in peius quotidie procedebat. Tunc quasi in casu desperationis fui vocatus, et inveni eam in statu pessimo ...'

[113] Ibid., fol. 186ra; also in another case (fol. 191va) Lanfranco succeeds with a patient who had had many other doctors, but whose illness daily increased: 'multos alios habuerat medicos ... et egritudo quotidie augebatur'.

[114] Ibid., fol. 187rb.

[115] Ibid., fol. 188vb.

[116] See, for instance, *Cyrurgia parva*, fol. 161ra; *Cyrurgia magna*, fol. 172rab.

[117] Ibid.

[118] Ibid., fol. 176vb.

[119] Ibid., fol. 199va: '... quidam audacter aggrediunt nullis consideratis particularibus, quoniam ignorant omnino scientiam medicine. Vidi quosdam qui senes, iuvenes, fortes, debiles uno et eodem modo curare volebant ...'; see also fols. 200vb and 202va.

stresses the distance which lies between the surgeon and the laymen, the *layci*. In Lanfranco's pages the laymen have become empirics, *empirici*, who are to be shunned and condemned because they lack doctrine, do not learn from teachers, make imprudent and mindless choices, and use their very few notions as if they were of absolute value. Even when they happen to be aware of some efficacious remedies, or to have some particular skill,[120] it is the task of the *cyrurgicus rationabilis*[121] to take hold of their notions and to embody them in his own learned competence.

Finally, we can point out another significant difference between Lanfranco's and Guglielmo's positions. On the whole, Lanfranco appears to bring the teaching aspects of the physician's activity into prominence, as distinct from the more operational ones, while Guglielmo described the surgeon-physician at work in a variety of places and social situations, which were at the same time and on the same level both working and teaching places. Indeed, it seems that in Lanfranco's view the value of the stability of the teaching institutions is more important than the practitioner's fruitful wandering and travelling as described by Guglielmo. This does not imply that Lanfranco, both as a man and as a professional, did not have a dynamic life, nor that he was not widely travelled. Nor does it imply that Lanfranco did not stress (as Guglielmo did) his lively activity as a surgeon, even mentioning the variety of places and situations in which he was called to deal with the medical cases of which he was now giving a detailed account.[122] But we want to stress here that he seems to attach great importance to the practice of teaching as carried out within stable institutions. This is the meaning of his well-known praise of Paris,[123] a place rich in peace and studies, where the sciences flourish and scholars are favoured, and where at last Lanfranco also arrived. Indeed, the two movements which Lanfranco points out with most spirited evidence are his own journey from Italy to France and the journey of medical science and tradition from school to school and from sect to sect.[124] And in the end both Lanfranco and medical science arrive at the university of Paris, where

---

[120] Ibid., fols. 201rb, 201va, 206va.

[121] Ibid., fol. 202va.

[122] In the *Cyrurgia magna* Lanfranco records some medical cases which occurred during his time in Milan (fols. 172rab, 174ra, 176vb, 186ra, 187ra) and in Lyons (see, for instance, fol. 191va).

[123] With warm praises of Paris and its 'suavissimum studium et honorabilissimum' Lanfranco begins and ends the *Cyrurgia magna* (Proemium, fols. 166va and 210vb). For other praises of Paris more or less contemporary with that of Lanfranco, where this city is seen mainly as a fount of knowledge, see C. J. Classen, *Die Stadt im Spiegel der Descriptiones und Laudes Urbium* (Hildesheim, Zurich and New York 1986), esp. pp. 60–1, 64; M. Corti, 'Parigi nel medioevo come luogo mentale', in *Studi di cultura francese ed europea in onore di L. Maranini* (Fasano, 1983), pp. 63–72.

[124] For some hints of the various trends of surgical knowledge and its historical evolution, see *Cyrurgia magna*, fols. 170va, 174ra, 176rab, 182va.

there is indeed now a great number of teachers of medicine[125] and where Lanfranco is able to find, in the scientific community gathered there, fertile ground for writing his text.[126] And in his representation of the development of surgery, this is precisely the route which surgery is also taking, according to Lanfranco's perhaps too optimistic wishful thinking.

[125] Lanfranco mentions specifically the 'phisicorum intelligentia' (ibid., fol. 166va) and the 'magistri medicine' (fol. 210vb) in Paris.

[126] Ibid., fol. 210vb: 'perveni Parisius, ubi tantam et talem habui comitivam qualis et quante centesimo non sum dignus. Ibi rogatus a quibusdam dominis et magistris ... necnon a quibusdam valentibus bachalariis ... quod ea que de rationibus cyrurgie legendo dicebam et meum operationis modum et experimenta quibus utebar in scriptis ad communem utilitatem et recordationem perpetuam compilarem, ipsorum petitionem admittens, onus assumpsi.'

3

How to write a Latin book on surgery: organizing principles and authorial devices in Guglielmo da Saliceto and Dino del Garbo

NANCY G. SIRAISI

The large output of books on surgery by authors associated with north Italian cities in the later twelfth and thirteenth centuries is a prominent landmark in the topography of medieval medical history. Much historical attention has been devoted to the series of works that began with Roger Frugard at Parma, and continued with Rolandino of Parma at Bologna, Bruno Longoburgo of Calabria at Padua, Guglielmo da Saliceto at Piacenza and Verona, Teodorico Borgognoni of Lucca at Bologna, and Lanfranco of Milan whom exile brought to Paris. Collectively, the books written by these men provide evidence for the formation of an intellectually and technically ambitious north Italian medical community in which surgery was emerging as a specialized interest of particular importance. Some of these manuals – notably that of Teodorico – have been much praised for their practical insights; and the free use of anecdote by several of the authors provides many glimpses of the world of thirteenth-century surgical practice.[1]

The commentary on the sections on surgery of Book 4 of the *Canon* of Avicenna by Dino del Garbo (d. 1327), who at different times held professorships at the Universities of Bologna, Padua and Siena, may appear at first sight to have little in common with the series of books named

---

[1] For general discussion, M. Tabanelli, *La chirurgia italiana nell'alto medioevo*, 2 vols. (Florence, 1965); Gundolf Keil, 'Mittelalterliche Chirurgie', *Acta Medicae Historiae Patavina*, 30 (1983–4), 45–64, especially 49–52; Pierre Huard and Mirko Drazen Grmek, *Mille ans de chirurgie en occident: Ve–XVe siècles* (Paris, 1966), pp. 18–35. A useful concise account, with references, of the history and findings of scholarship on the surgery of Roger and related texts is provided in Wolfgang Löchel, *Die Zahnmedizin Rogers und der Rogerglossen: Ein Beitrag zur Geschichte der Zahnheilkund im Hoch- und Spätmittelalter*, Würzburger medizin-historische Forschungen, vol. v (Hanover, 1976), pp. 12–66.

above.[2] The format of a scholastic commentary seems antithetical to that of a manual of practice, and the intellectual milieu implied by Giovanni Villani's description of Dino as 'grandissimo dottore in fisica et in più scienze naturali e filosofiche,' as well as by Dino's own learned and highly philosophical commentaries on the Hippocratic *De natura fetus* and the *Canzone d'amore* of Cavalcanti, far removed from that of the working surgeon.[3] Yet Dino alternated university teaching in other cities with practice in his native Florence throughout his career. His social origins and involvement in surgery can be shown to have been very similar to those of other thirteenth-century north Italian writers on the subject; while their manuals, just as much as his commentary, were grounded in the response of literate and latinate *medici* to the influx of information about surgery from the Islamic world.

The task that each of these writers on surgery, including Dino, set himself was to compose a Latin book, drawing on learned tradition, about a specialized technical or craft subject in which he was personally proficient. The organization of the *Chirurgia* of Roger Frugard may have owed much to his learned amanuensis Guido da Arezzo the Younger,[4] but the rest of those named appear to have combined the skills of working surgeon and Latin author. As one might expect, successive authors drew on recent predecessors as well as on learned texts in translation: for example, there is some relation between the work of Teodorico and Bruno.[5] None the less, the professional and personal priorities of each author clearly shaped his choice of presentation. Comparison of the approaches to the task of writing a book on surgery adopted by Guglielmo da Saliceto and Dino del Garbo, who were separated by only one generation and shared personal connections as well as a milieu, is instructive as to both differences and similarities.

In what follows, the focus will be on the rhetorical and pedagogical strategies whereby Guglielmo and Dino sought to bring surgical learning into relation with surgical practice; the chapter of Agrimi and Crisciani earlier in this volume explores epistemological aspects of the relation between theory and practice in surgery in the identical late thirteenth-

---

[2] Bio-bibliographical information about Dino, with references, is compiled in Siraisi, *Taddeo Alderotti and his pupils* (Princeton, NJ, 1981), pp. 55–64.

[3] *Cronica* 10.41; *Scriptum Dini super libro de natura fetus Hypocratis*, printed with Jacobus Forliviensis, *Expositio ... supra capitulum Avicenne De generatione embrionis* (Venice, 1502); Otto Bird, 'The Canzone d'Amore of Cavalcanti according to the Commentary of Dino del Garbo: text and commentary', *Mediaeval Studies*, 2 (1940), 150–203; 3 (1941), 117–60.

[4] The text is edited (and was first correctly identified) in Karl Sudhoff, *Beiträge zur Geschichte der Chirurgie im Mittelalter: Graphische und textliche Untersuchungen in mittelalterlichen Handschriften*, vol. II, pp. 156–236, Studien zur Geschichte der Medizin, 12 (Leipzig, 1918); the redactor's explanation of his role occurs on p. 187; his identity is noted in a manuscript colophon (see p. 153).

[5] Examples of parallel passages from the works of Bruno and Teodorico are printed in Tabanelli, *Chirurgia*, vol. I, pp. 485–9.

century north Italian context and the same specific case of Guglielmo da Saliceto. Full comparative analysis of Guglielmo's *Chirurgia* and Dino's commentary on sections of Book 4 of the *Canon* of Avicenna, known to its copyists and early printers as Dino's *Chirurgia*, lies far beyond the scope of this chapter. Instead, after a preliminary glance at the context of the authors, I shall briefly compare five aspects of these works: announced or apparent reasons for composition; definition of surgery; structure and organization; authorial presence; and the extent and nature of authorial attention to the critical comparison of learned sources with one another and/or with 'experience'.[6]

The dating of both Guglielmo da Saliceto's *Chirurgia* and Dino del Garbo's early career, when he wrote the commentary on the surgical parts of the *Canon*, presents problems. Guglielmo's book exists in two versions, the first of which is dated 1268 and the second, longer one, 1275 or 1276. Dino wrote the first two-thirds of the commentary during a period when he was living in Florence, having been forced to abandon studies in Bologna by the outbreak of war, probably in 1296, but possibly in the 1270s. He left off the commentary in order to go back to his studies, but finally completed it perhaps around 1308. There seems to be no doubt, however, that Dino's father, described by Dino as an expert surgeon, is to be identified with the Bono to whom Guglielmo da Saliceto dedicated his book.[7]

---

[6] I have used Gulielmus de Saliceto, *Cyrurgia*, printed with his *Summa conservationis et curationis* (Venice, 1489; at the New York Academy of Medicine), checking passages quoted or discussed in Bodleian Library, St John's College MS 76, fols. 11ff (table of contents begins fol. 11r, text begins fol. 13r, several pages of illustrations of surgical instruments precede the table of contents), *incipit* 'Hic incipiunt capitula primi libri Gulielmi . . .' a microfilm of which Michael McVaugh was kind enough to lend me; and *Dinus in chirurgia* . . . (Venice, 1536), otherwise known as *Dyni de Florentia expositio super tertia et quarta Fen quarti Canonis Avicenne et super parte quinta*. In what follows, references to Guglielmo da Saliceto's work are by book and chapter; to Dino's by folio.

[7] 'complevimus emendative librum cirugie nostre . . . in civitate Verone in qua faciebamus moram eo quod salarium recipebamus a communi anno currente, M.cc.lxxv. verum est quod ipsum ordinaveramus cursorie ante hoc tempus in Bononia per annos quattuor et de natura sue compositionis et ordinationis facit omnem et faciet intelligentem et studentem in eo optimum cirugicum et bonum medicum': Gulielmus, *Cyrurgia*, colophon (not found in St John's College MS 76). (In this and following quoted passages, capitalization and punctuation have been silently modernized.) This edition (but not St John's College MS 76) also contains the date 1279 in Book I, ch. 20. Tabanelli, *Chirurgia*, vol. II, pp. 500–11 contains an account of Guglielmo's career. Both Tabanelli (pp. 512–21) and Tinerario Zucconi, *Guglielmo da Saliceto e la chirurgia dei suoi tempi* (Piacenza, 1977), pp. 73–9, provide lists of manuscripts of the two versions of the *Chirurgia*, in a number of which the date of completion is mentioned. (Additional manuscripts are identified by Agrimi and Crisciani in their chapter in the present volume.) According to Zucconi (p. 73) the oldest known manuscript – dating from the thirteenth century – of the longer version includes the colophon and gives the date as 1276.

Dinus in chirurgia, fol. 119r–v, provides the autobiographical information summarized here, but no dates. A sharp but inconclusive controversy over the dating of Dino's early career is pursued in Bruno Nardi, 'Noterella polemica sull'averroismo di Guido Cavalcanti', *Rassegna di Filosofia*, 3 (1954), 55; and Guido Favati, 'Guido Cavalcanti, Dino del

Whatever the precise dating of their works, therefore, both Guglielmo and Dino wrote at a late stage of the phase of transmission of medical information from Arabic to Latin culture and its adaptation to Latin forms. It deserves to be emphasized that the new surgery arrived in western Europe as part of the general growth of medical learning beginning in the late eleventh century and associated with the appearance of translations. Sections on surgery in the encyclopedic works of Haly Abbas, Rhazes, and Avicenna, and portions of Galen's *Methodus medendi* were major sources, along with the surgical treatise of Albucasis (itself originally part of a general medical encyclopedia). The assimilation of translated material emanating first from the circle of Constantine the African and subsequently from Spain stimulated and provided the basis for the production of the more or less 'original' works directly composed in Latin. By the time Guglielmo and Dino wrote, the process had been going on for well over a century. Ultimately, most of the technical information derived from the tradition of Greek surgery extending back to the Hippocratic corpus, although the multiplication of texts and genres and their adaptation to current needs, direct knowledge of only fragments of the Hippocratic works on surgery, the neglect of Celsus, and the absence of a direct translation into Latin of the sixth book of Paul of Aegina (a major source for the Arabic authors) must have yielded thirteenth-century readers the sense of a confusing diversity of authoritative sources.[8] The whole process bears comparison with two other major episodes of reception of information about surgery in medieval cultures: the transmission of the Greek tradition to the Islamic world in the ninth to eleventh centuries; and the transformation of the Latin tradition into the large body of vernacular writing on surgery – as on other aspects of practical medicine – that appeared in western Europe during the fourteenth and fifteenth centuries.

The growing availability of technical information in the learned tongue evidently interacted with social factors to enlarge the intellectual and

Garbo, e l'averroismo di Bruno Nardi', *Filologia Romanza*, 2 (1955), 80–1. Dino's move to Siena, where he taught during the academic year 1308–9), is dated by documents in *Chartularium studii senensis*, ed. G. Cecchini and G. Prunai, vol. 1 (Siena, 1942), pp. 91–2. That Dino was in fact the son of the surgeon Bono del Garbo is established on the basis of archival evidence in A. Corsini, 'Nuovo contributo di notizie intorno di maestro Tommaso del Garbo', *Rivista di Storia delle Scienze Mediche e Naturali*, 16 (1925), 268.

[8] On Celsus, L. D. Reynolds, *Texts and transmission: a survey of the Latin classics* (Oxford, 1983), pp. 46–7, and Augusto Beccaria, *I codici di medicina del periodo presalernitano (secoli IX, X, e XI)*, Storia e Letteratura, 53 (Rome, 1956), pp. 25–6, 152–6, 277–9, 312–13; Pearl Kibre, *Hippocrates Latinus: repertorium of Hippocratic writings in the Latin Middle Ages* (New York, 1985), pp. 93–4, 110, 124, 234; Eugene F. Rice, 'Paulus Aegineta', *Catalogus translationum et commentariorum: medieval and Renaissance Latin translations and commentaries*, ed. Paul Oskar Kristeller and F. Edward Cranz, vol. IV (Washington, DC, 1980), pp. 150–67, indicating that complete translations of Paul's work into Latin, including Book 6 on surgery, did not appear until the sixteenth century; Manfred Ullmann, *Die Medizin im Islam* (Leiden, 1970), pp. 86–7, 141–2, 150.

professional opportunities of *medici* possessing skill in surgery. In practical terms, the demand for, and hence the supply of, surgical skill in northern Italy during the twelfth and thirteenth centuries was doubtless enlarged both by the development of a flourishing commercial economy that fostered the growth of all kinds of crafts, trades, and specializations and by the frequency of local warfare. And for ambitious practitioners command of Latin literacy served the eminently practical purposes of simultaneously providing access to technical information and enhancing status. By their existence, Latin treatises by surgeon-authors asserted a relation between learned tradition and current practice; yet the nature of this relation remained ambiguous and open to different forms of expression.

Both Guglielmo da Saliceto and Dino del Garbo received and imparted training at Bologna, but their experiences spanned a period of significant development in the institutionalization of medical studies there. Guglielmo is said to have arrived in Bologna by 1230, a time when the city already attracted practitioner-teachers and students of medicine, including a notable group of surgeons, some of whom were authors. However, there appears to be no evidence of formal institutional academic organization of any kind of medical teaching at that early date. At Bologna, Guglielmo also completed the first version of his *Chirurgia* for the benefit of students in 1268; he is perhaps also to be identified with a Magister Gulielmus who was teaching and practising there in 1269.[9] Most of his career seems, however, to have been spent as a practitioner in other cities, chiefly Piacenza and Verona, where he completed the second, longer version of the *Chirurgia*. Probably in the late 1260s the institutionalization of medical teaching in the university context and academic corporations of arts and medicine began to take shape at Bologna.[10] By the time Dino began his studies, much medical instruction had been drawn within the university milieu, but this was still a very recent occurrence. Precisely for Dino's generation, it would seem, the relation between actual practice, practical instruction by demonstration, the teaching of *practica* from books, and the relation of theory and practice, and the relation between professional competence and academic status must have taken on new dimensions and a new complexity.

REASONS FOR WRITING

The idea of treating surgery in a separate, specialized, textbook was in itself an innovation in western medicine in the twelfth and thirteenth centuries; and authors frequently pointed out, in an *accessus* or elsewhere, some of the

---

[9] Tabanelli, *Chirurgia*, vol. II, pp. 508–9; M. Sarti and M. Fattorini, *De claris archigymnasii bononiensis professoribus*, ed. C. Albicini and C. Malagola (Bologna, 1888), vol. I, part 2, pp. 553–4.

[10] See note 7, above. For a summary of institutional developments at Bologna, see Siraisi, *Taddeo Alderotti*, pp. 18–22.

objectives they hoped to achieve by writing such works. Thus, Guido da Arezzo stressed the value of 'deliberate reasoning', 'certain order', convenience and brevity in his presentation of Roger's teaching. Bruno Longoburgo thought that what was needed was a compilation that would bring together in a single work the opinions of the main authorities: Galen, Rhazes, Haly Abbas, Albucasis and Avicenna. Lanfranco included among his priorities the need to explain differences in nomenclature between Salernitan writers and translated Greek and Arab sources. Teodorico focused on the idea of the mutual authentication of current surgical practice and ancient authority; he treated as especially, and equally, authoritative his own master (and, probably, father), Ugo da Lucca, and Galen 'whom we knew to differ with the aforesaid outstanding man [that is, Ugo] in no respect'.[11]

The goals of Guglielmo da Saliceto's *Chirurgia* need to be considered in conjunction with those of his treatise on hygiene and therapy, the *Summa conservationis et curationis*, since the two works jointly constitute a carefully articulated scheme of medical/surgical instruction. Guglielmo introduced both books by outlining specific pedagogical objectives. The proem to the *Summa* begin with citations from Aristotle's *Metaphysics*, *De sensu and sensato*, and *De somno et vigilia* about the nature of *scientia* and the power of the rational soul to acquire it, and goes on to explain that Guglielmo has reduced to writing those things which he has acquired over a long time 'through rational use in medical operation'. Although written at the request of the prior of Sant'Ambrogio of Piacenza and his *socii* and for common utility, the book was especially intended for Guglielmo's son Leonardino, whom his father wished to introduce 'to the profession of the art of medicine'. Guglielmo explained that the division of the book into parts and chapters was designed to facilitate reference, as was the uniform arrangement of each chapter, proceeding from the name of a particular disease, followed by its 'matter', its symptoms, the treatments 'according to the intention of the philosophers', and ending with those things 'which have been verified by me through use and operation'.[12]

---

[11] Prologues to Books 1 and 2 of the treatise of Roger Frugard (Sudhoff, *Beiträge*, vol. II, pp. 156, 187); proem to Bruno Longoburgo, *Cyrurgia magna*, printed with Guy de Chauliac, *Cyrurgia* (Venice, 1498) fol. 83 (82)r; Lanfranco, *Ars completa totius cyrurgie, tractatus* 3, *doctrina* 1, ch. 6, fol. 182 (181)v in the same volume; ' ... quem a predicto viro eximio in nullo modo novimus discordare', Teodorico, *Cyrurgia*, also in the same volume, proem, fol. 106 (105)r.

[12] 'Et etiam tum propter continuam instantiam domini Ruffini prioris Sancti Ambrosii de Placentia et sociorum eius et amore cuiusdam filii mei qui Leonardinus vocatur quem ad professionem artis medicinalis inducam per posse, tum propter utilitatem quam pronominati et posteriores ex presenti opere poterunt consequi nolui quod reclusum erat in anima et acquisitum ex longo tempore ut post meum non esse evanesceret absque communi utilitate. Dividam hoc opus in quatuor partes et proponam unicuique parti propria capitula, ut quid inquiretur facilius invenire possit. Et cum hoc in unoquoque capitulo uniuscuiusque partis ponam primo egritudinem nominative, secundo materiam, tertio signa significantia super egritudinem et causas. Post hoc ponam curam breviter penes

Guglielmo further informed readers of his *Summa* that it deliberately excluded material on manual operations because he had already written on that subject elsewhere. The reference is to the *Chirurgia*, described in its preface as 'a book about manual operation', and, in a colophon found in variant versions, as compiled for students.[13] The preface and immediately following introductory chapter of the *Chirurgia* join a noteworthy justification of Guglielmo's use in the book of examples drawn from his personal experience as teaching devices (see further below) with a general account of surgery in which the emphasis on reason, *scientia*, and formal pedagogy is as prominent as in the proem of the *Summa*. Denunciation of ignorant surgeons is of course a familiar topos in Latin treatises on surgery; in Guglielmo's version, the culprits practice 'irrationally' because they do not learn how to operate from men endowed with *scientia* but 'from ignorant people who have in no way acquired knowledge of the forms, shapes and dispositions of the bodily parts and the causes of illness, nor can they grasp and determine anything except something sensible, corruptible, and particular, and thus they end their lives in vain on account of ignorance of the essential principles of this art'.[14]

For most of Guglielmo's working life, the normal form of surgical (and medical) education in north Italian cities, including Bologna, was doubtless direct private instruction by individual practitioners of their own *socii*, sons, or apprentices. However, the passage just quoted, with its mention of reason, *scientia*, and principles, insistence on the importance of having teachers endowed with *scientia*, and allusions to Aristotelian definitions of scientific knowledge and cognition, shows that by the middle decades of the century academic ways of organizing and transmitting knowledge could have a powerful attraction for a surgeon with connections to Bologna. Yet Guglielmo also perceived incompatibility between the scholastic model of learning through open exchange of rational arguments that he apparently admired and the claim of the *medicus* to authority based on the special, secret skills and knowledge belonging to a craft. Consequently, he advised his readers that 'it is disgraceful and indecent to decide [*determinare*] by disputing about causes of the illness and the appropriate action in the presence of the patient and of laymen ... it seems better and more appropriate that every enquiry with a colleague or one's *socius* should take place in private'. This was because the laity, who 'always disparage the

---

philosophorum intentionem. Ultimo de his dicam que sunt verificata apud me per usum et operationem': *Summa conservationis*, proem, sig. a2r.

[13] 'librum de operatione manuali'. For the colophon, see Tabanelli, *Chirurgia*, vol. II, pp. 508–9.

[14] 'ab ignorantibus qui in formis membrorum figuris et dispositionibus et causis infirmatum in nullo modo se exercuerunt, neque extra rem sensibilem corruptibilem et particularem possunt aliquid apprehendere vel determinare [St John's College MS 76: extunare?], et sic finiunt vitam suam in vanum propter ignorantiam de principiis necessariis ad hanc artem': Guilelmus, *Cyrurgia*, introductory chapter.

'wise', and presumably did not appreciate the value of academic discussion, would take any differences of opinion among *medici* as a sign that their art was *not* based on reason.[15]

According to Filippo Villani, Dino del Garbo's commentary on the surgical portions of the *Canon* was subsequently used as a textbook in the schools and Dino himself gave university lectures on surgery late in his career.[16] None the less, the commentary did not originate in a set of school lectures. Instead the young Dino was moved to write something on the subject of surgery when he spent a year under the tutelage of his father, 'who in this art was more expert than anyone else',[17] and saw him practise every day. Thus, whereas Guglielmo presented himself as a mature practitioner transmitting the fruits of long experience to his son, Dino stressed that, despite his own youth, he had the benefit of his father's experience. In either case, of course, the idea of the descent of accumulated practical medical and surgical knowledge in a particular family is the same. (In the next generation, Dino's son Tommaso, too, lost no opportunity in calling attention to his descent from the famously learned and successful Dino.)

Even if Dino's exposition did not begin as academic lectures, the idea of casting his work in commentary form may have occurred to him as a result of the single year of medical study he had already spent at the University of Bologna before returning to work with his father in Florence. The study of arts and philosophy that doubtless preceded or accompanied his beginning medical studies at the university would also have familiarized him with commentary as a genre. Dino completed the commentary on portions of Book 4 under discussion here after he had obtained his doctorate in medicine and was a professor at the University of Siena, so that its last section may be linked to his academic instruction. However, he stated emphatically that the final version of the whole included no alterations to the first part written when he was a youth observing his father's practice.[18]

Dino may thus be counted among the pioneers in extending formal commentary to the *Canon*. Later in his career, moreover, he produced commentaries on other portions of the *Canon* relating to practice: the general treatise on principles of disease and therapy in section 4 of Book 1,

---

[15] 'inhonestum est et indecens est coram infirmo et laicis de causis infirmitatis et operationibus disputando determinare ... melius et decentius videtur ut omnis inquisitio cum altero et socio fiat in secreto ... quia laici semper detrahunt sapientibus': *Summa conservationis*, proem, sig. a2r.

[16] 'Hic juvenis adhuc super tertia et quarta parte seu [*sic*] quinti Canonis Avicenne expositiones conscripsit utiles et subtiles tam in practica quam in theorica cyrugie, que in studiis ordinariis magistraliter perleguntur, cum jam grandevus Senis legeret': F. Villani, *Liber de civitatis Florentia famosis civibus*, ed. G. C. Galletti (Florence, 1848), p. 27.

[17] 'qui in hac scientia pre ceteris erat expertus: *Dinus in chirugia*, fol. 119r.

[18] 'Et quia primam partem fecimus cum adhuc eramus iuvenis etate et scientia valde. Sic si aliqua essent imperfecta dicta quam bene rationabiliter excusatio mihi fiet. Volumus non mutare illa dicta quam fecerimus ut nulli appareat esse mirabile si sic in brevi tempore si[t] possibile alicui homini pervenire in scientia ad ea de quibus multis apparet esse mirabile': ibid., fol. 119v.

and Book 2 on medicinal simples.[19] (Hence it appears that both Guglielmo and Dino began by writing on surgery and subsequently extended their authorial range to other aspects of practical medicine.) Dino's initial decision to cast in the form of a commentary a work on surgery that, like several of its immediate predecessors, combined a family tradition of practice with the teachings of learned authorities, endorsed the primacy of analysis and comparison of authoritative texts in all areas of medical instruction. In addition to being implicit in his choice of commentary format, Dino's commitment to the primacy of study of texts was made explicit in remarks on surgical education; in his view, a good surgeon ideally needed both knowledge of the principles of medicine learned from books and supervised training under a skilled practitioner; but, if both could not be obtained, the booklearning was more important, because 'he who knows and visualizes what is in the books with a small amount of practice arrives at that [level of skill] which many of those who do not know the things contained in the books are in no way able to reach'.[20]

Dino's emphasis on the importance of study did not of course preclude an intention to write a book of practical use to working surgeons, as his inclusion of comments about the need for them to be quick and deft and have good instruments makes clear. The choice of commentary format constituted a shift in emphasis rather than any radically new departure in the already long tradition of transmission in Latin of technical information about surgery. For example, it was in Dino's view of great practical importance to guide the student to be selective in his use of the books: 'And I have already drawn attention to every place in this book that refers to an operation in which there is error and [reason to] fear, because it is necessary that you beware of such operations and not attempt them.'[21] Yet the awareness, common to Dino and other Latinate surgeons, of possible hazards in following some procedures handed down by learned tradition in the texts was doubtless itself heightened by textual study, since Albucasis made a similar remark.[22]

DEFINITIONS OF SURGERY

From Greek tradition mediated via Arabo-Latin texts, twelfth- and thir-teenth-century authors derived two types of definition of surgery. The first

---

[19] *Dyni florentini super quarta fen primi Avicenne preclarissima commentaria: que Dilucidatorium totius practice generalis medicinalis scientie nuncupatur*, printed with *Exposition Dini super canones generales de virtutibus medicinarum simplicium secundi Canonis Avicenne* (Venice, 1514).

[20] 'ille qui quod est in libris novit atque imaginatur cum pauca operationis noticia perveniet at illud ad quod multi eorum qui ea que continentur in libris non noverunt nullo modo poterunt pervenire': *Dinus in chirugia*, fol. 1r–v.

[21] 'Et ego iam excitavi in omni loco huius libri in quo venit operatio in qua est error et timor, quare necesse est vobis ut caveatis illud et dimittatis ipsum': ibid., fol. 1v.

[22] Albucasis, *On surgery and instruments*, ed. and trans. M. S. Spink and G. L. Lewis (London, 1973), preface to Book 1, p. 6.

restricted surgery to its literal meaning of manual operation (incision, cautery, suturing, manipulation etc.) and classified it as one of three 'instruments of medicine', the others being diet and medication. The second, broader definition classified as surgery the treatment by any means of certain conditions. These included the traumatic injuries and ulcers grouped in Galenic doctrine under the heading of *solutio continuitatis*, as well as *apostemata* (abscesses and tumours), and various conditions marked by eruptions on the external surface of the body.[23] To these basic definitions according to, respectively, type of procedure or conditions treated, authors influenced by Aristotelian concepts of knowledge added considerations relating to the place of surgery among the arts and sciences and the type of knowledge offered by surgery. Guglielmo da Saliceto adopted a definition of the first type, Dino del Garbo carefully weighed the two and introduced further distinctions, but they were united in insisting that in at least some aspects surgery qualified as *scientia*.

Thus, according to Guglielmo surgery is 'the *scientia* teaching the method of operating manually on the flesh, *nervi*, and bones of human beings'.[24] Surgery is not any particular surgical operation but is a *scientia* contained under medicine; individual operations depend on the *scientia* of surgery just as the particular does on the universal. Guglielmo's definition of surgery, his characterization of the *Chirurgia* as 'about manual operation', his division of subject matter between the *Chirurgia* and the *Summa*, and the way in which he drew his readers' attention to that division all suggest that he wished to differentiate surgery from the rest of practical medicine as clearly as possible, and that his main criterion for distinguishing the two was the type of procedure employed. The consistency and thoroughness with which he endeavoured to make this distinction is illustrated by the fact that fistula and bladder stone are discussed in both the *Chirurgia* and the *Summa*, instructions for operation by incision being provided in the former, and advice on treatment solely by medication in the latter.[25] None the less, Guglielmo did not in fact achieve a complete separation on the basis of procedures, both because the concept of *operatio manualis* included the actual administration or application of medications, and because treatment by incision or cautery was routinely accompanied by external medication, and frequently by dietary advice and potions to be taken internally. Hence, the *Chirurgia* contains many references to treatment by medication to be administered in conjunction with treatment by incision or cautery, and concludes with an entire section (Book 5) classifying and listing such preparations.

---

[23] *Solutio continuitatis* (to use the terminology of Latin Galenism) is, for example, one of the fundamental categories into which types of disease, abnormality, or injury are classified in Galen's *Methodus medendi*.

[24] 'scientia docens modum et qualitatem operandi in carne nervo et osse hominis manibus': *Cyrurgia*, general introductory chapter.

[25] *Summa conservationis*, Book 1, chs. 149 and 183; *Cyrurgia*, Book 1, chs. 46 and 47.

Dino found himself obliged to consider not only how surgery should be defined, but also whether the *Chirurgia* of Avicenna, that is, those sections of Book 4 of the *Canon* covering *apostemata* and traumatic injuries, was properly so called. In dealing with this problem, Dino elaborated the twofold definition of surgery into a triple one. He began by dismissing the definition that classified surgery as simple manual operation – an instrument of practical medicine; surgery in this sense was neither *scientia* in itself nor part of the *scientia* of medicine, so that such a definition was clearly unhelpful in categorizing Avicenna's text. However, there was both a narrow and a broad sense in which surgery could be considered *scientia*. In the proper sense the *scientia* of surgery consisted, for Dino as it had for Guglielmo, in teaching how to operate manually on the body. More broadly, according to Dino, surgery was the *scientia* of teaching all kinds of treatment for any condition in which manual operation might ultimately be required. It was in this broad sense that Avicenna's 'surgery' – which, as Dino pointed out, includes much information about treatment by regimen and medication – deserved the name.[26]

The effect of such a definition was clearly to de-emphasize the distinction between surgery and the rest of practical medicine. Dino's authorial strategy (including his choice of the *Canon* as the focus of his work) may well have been inspired by a desire to emphasize that surgery had a legitimate place as part of 'rational' medicine of the kind transmitted in a university setting. Nevertheless, his approach was by no means unrelated to the realities of contemporary practice, in which conditions considered to fall under the domain of surgery were frequently treated by diet and internal or external medication, and minor surgical procedures (bloodletting, cupping) played a wide role in the treatment of complexional (that is, most internal) disorders. Dino's extensive discussions throughout his exposition – far exceeding anything of the kind found in Guglielmo's *Chirurgia* – of issues relating to complexion theory in treatment by both internal and external medication seem likely to have blurred the boundary yet further.

STRUCTURE AND ORGANIZATION

Guglielmo da Saliceto's work is divided into five books,[27] the contents of the first three being arranged in order from head to toe: (1) diseases from internal causes that are manifest on the exterior of the body (the contents include hydrocephalus in infants, tumours of various kinds, stone in the bladder and hernia); (2) wounds and bruises; (3) fractures and dislocations; (4) anatomy; (5) cauteries, instruments and medications. In broad sequence

[26] *Dinus in chirurgia*, fol. 1r.
[27] In the 1489 edition. The fifth book may occasionally have been divided into fifth and sixth books in other versions.

of subject matter, although not in detail, the first three books recall the organization of the sections of Avicenna's *Canon* devoted to *chirurgia*, although the *Canon* is certainly not the only possible model for this type of arrangement.

By providing a separate fourth book on anatomy Guglielmo advertised his conviction that knowledge of anatomy was essential for successful surgery. Books 1–3 of the *Chirurgia* are, moreover, notable for the care with which regional anatomy is incorporated into surgical instruction; Guglielmo habitually warned students of the need to pay attention to the possibility of damage to adjacent structures when treating wounds or performing surgery at particular body sites. Thus, in discussing wounds of the back of the neck, Guglielmo taught his readers to be alert to the danger of spinal-cord injury, which could result in paralysis; similarly, the subject of wounds of the throat led him to point out the hazard of damage to the trachea.[28] However, the brevity of the separate anatomical section (five chapters, as compared to sixty-seven, twenty-six and twenty-nine in Books 1–3, respectively) and relegation to Book 4 reflect the author's belief that anatomical study was valuable only in so far as it served surgical purposes. Guglielmo introduced Book 4 by announcing that not all the minute divisions of anatomy were sensibly perceptible, and that even if they were it would be both tedious and useless to enumerate them; and that his anatomical discussion would accordingly be confined to pointing out structures particularly likely to be injured in the course of surgical intervention.[29] Unlike Mondino dei Liuzzi in the preface to his *Anatomia* written a generation later, Guglielmo da Saliceto made no attempt to present the study of human anatomy as inherently valuable because it gives knowledge about a noble part of God's creation.

The main outline of Dino's book was of course determined by the organization and content of the sections of the *Canon* on which he commented. These dealt with *apostemata* and *lepra* (4.3); wounds, bruises, ulcers and injuries to *nervi* (4.4); and fracture of the skull (part 4.5.3). The surgical parts of the *Canon* also include tractates on dislocations and fractures in general (4.5.1 and 2), as well as chapters on fractures of other specific parts of the body (remainder of 4.5.3), on which Dino did not comment.[30]

---

[28] *Cyrurgia*, Book 2, chs. 5 and 7.

[29] 'Quamvis permissum sit determinare de anathomia intentio non fuit enumerare omnia membra particulariter quamquam antiqui conati sint membra particulariter dividere et enumerare in membris particularibus, et quamvis sit necessarium confiteri membra simplicia non ratificari [St Johns College MS 76: ramnificari] neque in infinitum dividi cum omne corpus sit figuratum [finitum], tamen [cum] neque eorum rarificationes neque divisiones perfecte sunt sensibus manifeste ... Et etiam cum sit possibile anathomiam seu ultimam membrorum divisionem et eorum numerum ponere in scriptis ex positione tali tantum tedium proveniret quod anima de eius virtute aut non aliquid aut modicum non utile comprehenderet': ibid., Book 4, ch. 1.

[30] 'Clarissimi doctoris Gentili de Florentia super primum et secundum tractatum fen quinte quarti canonis Avicenne, scilicet de dislocationibus et fracturis in quos Dynus non exposuit

Although anatomy is covered in the *Canon*, its treatment is divided between part of the first section of Book 1 and the twenty-one sections on the anatomy, diseases and treatments of various parts of the body from head to foot found in Book 3. Thus, although Dino was just as insistent upon the importance of anatomical knowledge for surgeons as Guglielmo – echoing Albucasis in the flat statement 'anyone who is not in a position to see anatomy does not escape falling into error whereby men are killed'[31] – he included little anatomical exposition and no separate section on anatomy. Nevertheless, Dino allowed himself great freedom, ignoring some surgical topics treated by Avicenna entirely and selecting others for extended discussion; presumably his basis for choosing topics on which to expatiate was either his own interest in the subject or because he found Avicenna's discussion inadequate or problematic. His complete omission of commentary on Avicenna's tractate on dislocations and on most of the tractate on fractures has already been noted; by contrast, his disquisition on cranial fractures is extensive.

Apart from the commentary format itself, the most important structural feature that marks off Dino's *Chirurgia* from earlier Latin works on the subject is the frequent introduction of scholastic *quaestiones*. These are used not only to compare Avicenna's teaching on particular topics with those of other authors, but on occasion also as a means of enquiring into the practical usefulness of Avicenna's recommendations. Dino's use of the *quaestio* is an essential tool in his effort to arrive at an understanding of the proper relationship of learned authorities and current practice in surgery, and will accordingly be discussed further below.

AUTHORIAL PRESENCE

A strong authorial presence is a feature of a number of thirteenth- and fourteenth-century Latin books on surgery. Surgeon-authors both described what they claimed were their own techniques and included anecdotes about themselves, their patients, and their teachers, colleagues and pupils. Of course, the great bulk of surgical writing is not anecdotal, and anecdotes can also occasionally be found in other kinds of medical writing. None the less, personal anecdote or reminiscence seems markedly more prevalent in surgical than other medical books.

---

expositio incipit feliciter': *Dinus in chirurgia*, fol. 119v. The interpolated section of much less elaborate commentary than Dino's on the tractate on dislocations and the introductory chapter of the tractate on fractures continues to fol. 132v; Dino's commentary on the section on skull fractures occupies fols. 132v–142v; commentary on the remainder of the tractate on fractures (from the jawbone to the feet) by Gentilis de Florentia follows from fol. 143r to 147r.

31 'qui non est sufficiens videre anathomiam non evadere quin cadat in errorem quo interficiuntur homines': *Dinus in chirurgia*, fol. 1v; Albucasis, *On surgery and instruments*, p. 2.

One would have to be very ingenuous to take such anecdotes at their face value as simple reportage. No doubt some stories were to an extent actually grounded in the author's personal experience, but it was experience selected or shaped with specific ends in view. One of the most obvious purposes was simply to provide examples of the teller's success. In this respect, the stories seem almost like secular parallels to one kind of narrative told about miraculous cures. With the authority of an example in the gospel itself, such narratives had since antiquity often included the topos of the patient's prior, and useless, consultation of secular medical practitioners before being healed by miraculous means. By contrast, as one might expect, surgeons' stories usually present the specialist as successful in both diagnosis and treatment, through which great danger is skilfully overcome. But like the successes of the saints, surgeons' successes frequently follow or are contrasted with others' failures; not, to be sure, failures of spiritual healers, but failures of rival specialists, of less highly trained empirics, or of the patient's family and friends. Thus Lanfranco recounted how he had treated a fifteen-year-old youth who had cut his arm, with injury to a *nervus* and much loss of blood. Lanfranco wanted to strip the blood vessel and ligate it, but the boy's mother mistrusted this treatment and summoned a 'lay surgeon', under whose care the patient worsened until he was at the point of death. In this crisis, a physician friend of the family took the distraught mother to task for exchanging Lanfranco's expert ministrations for those of an untrained practitioner; the physician then instructed the latter to do what Lanfranco had recommended, with the result that the boy recovered.[32] The anecdote manages to combine an *exemplum* of Lanfranco's success with a technical description of one of his preferred methods of treatment, while simultaneously placing him squarely in professional and intellectual solidarity with the *medicus* against the irrationality of the mother and the ignorance of the empiric.

In addition, such stories could serve not just as general examples of a surgeon's skill, but also as evidence of specific, individual cures that he had performed at particular, identifiable times and places. They would thus be evidence of his ability to adapt general rules to particular cases (in itself a Galenic principle). Such would certainly seem to be the implication of the accompaniment of some of these anecdotes by details about the name, age, sex, occupation and social position of the patient, the circumstances of his or her injury, and the identity of bystanders, and, especially, other medical attendants. Of course, naming patients was also a way of indicating the large number and, if possible, social distinction – or at any rate respectability – of the clients successfully treated by a surgeon. Both purposes may have been behind the well-known list of patients whom John of Arderne (1307–post 1377) claimed to have cured of anal fistulas: of nineteen patients

---

[32] Lanfranco, *Cyrurgia, tractatus* 1, *doctrina* 3, chapter 9, printed with Guy de Chauliac, *Cyrurgia*, fol. 172/(171)r.

named, two were identified as knightly or noble, and eight as members of the clergy (as is apparent from Peter Murray Jones' chapter in the present volume, the writings of John of Arderne have many features in common – both as regards rhetorical strategy and the way in which learned tradition is related to surgical practices – with thirteenth-century surgical treatises from Italy).[33]

Guglielmo da Saliceto made notably extensive use of personal anecdote, and enriched his stories with much circumstantial detail. Some of them seem to have been inspired primarily by competitiveness and self-advertisement, and perhaps involved exaggeration of the severity of the patient's injury. One case in point may be Guglielmo's description of his success in treating Giovanni da Pavia's abdominal wound (although it is not impossible that a recovery of the type alleged took place). When Giovanni was wounded in the belly the practitioner first summoned, Guglielmo's friend Master Ottobono da Pavia, saw the intestines hanging out of the wound and said, 'He's a dead man.' None the less, Ottobono tried and failed to put the gut back in place. Then he and the patient's friends rushed to the Palazzo Comunale to fetch Guglielmo himself. When Guglielmo saw the condition of the patient he was extremely anxious, especially since, according to him, the intestines themselves were injured and faecal matter was escaping. As an emergency measure, there being no time to send for medications, Guglielmo washed the intestines in heated wine and succeeded in restoring them in place. The wound was sutured, Ottobono undertook post-operative care, and subsequently 'after his cure the patient married and had children and lived for a long time'. Without the accompanying personal details, the anecdote had direct antecedents in the technical literature: Albucasis had also described how he successfully treated an abdominal wound from which the gut was protruding by simply washing the intestines (in his case in honey-water – washing the intestines in wine in preference to water was recommended by Avicenna), and had noted that wounds that actually perforated the intestine could in some cases be cured.[34] In this instance, the technical literature offered Guglielmo da Saliceto both a suggestion, or endorsement, for a method of treatment, and also a rhetorical model for describing what had been done.

Yet Guglielmo da Saliceto also stands out among surgical authors by reason of his deliberate and systematic use of anecdotal case histories for pedagogical purposes. In this respect, his use of accounts of his own cases in the *Chirurgia* merits comparison with the contemporary development of the practice of compiling medical *consilia* for purposes of study. As noted

[33] *Treatises of fistula in ano, haemorrhoids, and clysters by John Arderne from an early fifteenth-century manuscript translation*, ed. D'Arcy Power, Early English Text Society, no. 139 (London, 1910; reprint 1968), pp. 1–3.

[34] '"Mortuus est" ... et habuit infirmus post curationem uxorem et filios et vixit longo tempore': *Cyrurgia*, Book 2, ch. 15; *On surgery and instruments*, pp. 542, 548–9; *Canon*, 4. 4. 1. 7, in *Dinus in chirurgia*, fol. 72r.

above, Guglielmo announced in the preface of the *Chirurgia* his intention frequently to draw for instructional purposes on *exempla* from his own experience; and, in the body of his text, selected (and no doubt adapted) cases are carefully deployed to illustrate principles and information derived from the learned, textual tradition. Guglielmo's use of personal narrative thus provided one solution to the problem of integrating formal, text-based instruction and craft training.

His method is exemplified by his choice of three cases to illustrate the point that wounds to the head or neck could result in paralysis if the spinal cord or brain was injured, but that such paralysis was not necessarily permanent or fatal. In the first, Lazzarino of Cremona received a sword wound to the head so severe that at first Guglielmo prognosticated death; the patient survived, but three days later became paralysed and incontinent. Thanks to the healing power of nature and Guglielmo's treatment, however, he ultimately recovered completely and lived another twenty years. The second case was that of a patient wounded by an arrow in the neck who also became paralysed, incontinent, and, as a result, deeply depressed. Having been given up for dead, he made a partial recovery under Guglielmo's treatment; this patient survived for ten years, but could walk only with the aid of crutches. The third such victim whom Guglielmo had seen, Gabriele da Pirolo, was less fortunate: the *medicus* who treated him was unable to prevent his arrow wound from being followed in less than a month by rigour, fever and death.[35] Guglielmo thus claimed only the more or less successful outcomes for himself, referring the total failure of treatment to an unnamed colleague or rival. None the less, his readiness to admit to initially mistaken prognosis in the first case and only partial success in the second is exceptional; it provided a good measure of the seriousness of his pedagogical intent, as well as inspiring confidence that his narratives, however much edited, bear some relation to his actual experience. The foregoing example also shows that Guglielmo occasionally used his anecdotal case histories as a tool for the critical evaluation and amplification of learned tradition. Wounds to the brain – and by extension the spinal cord – occurred on a list of always, or almost always, fatal injuries first found in the Hippocratic *Aphorisms* and repeated by various subsequent authors, including Avicenna.[36]

Following the normal conventions of commentary, Dino almost entirely omitted personal reminiscence or anecdote from his *Chirurgia*. The solitary exception is the explanation of how the work came to be written. Yet Dino was far from wanting to exclude his own experience from his work. On the contrary, he insisted, as we have seen, that the book was grounded in his father's and his own surgical practice; moreover, he included frequent discussions of or allusions to current surgical techniques,

[35] *Cyrurgia*, Book 2, chapter 5.
[36] *Aphorisms*, 6.18; *Canon*, 4.4.1.1

including endorsement of dry healing of wounds and various denunciations of 'stupid surgeons'.[37] How close he was to surgical practice is indicated by a passage in which he tried to tell his readers how to suture a straight cut. According to Dino, sutures should be placed not too deep and not too near the surface, the depth varying according to the depth of the wound; the stitches should be not too tight (painful and likely to produce inflammation) and not too loose (ineffective); the thread ought to be untwisted silk, because twisted silk is too strong and cuts the flesh, but too weak a thread will break.[38] This explanation seems to read like the result of someone trying to find words to describe a procedure he is used to demonstrating directly. ('*This* is the right kind of thread; watch how I do it; now you try.') Moreover, Dino's instructions do not appear simply to echo the technical literature, although he was fully familiar with detailed descriptions of various methods of suturing provided by the principal authorities. Elsewhere in his commentary, he reviewed and classified a number of the methods of suturing abdominal wounds described by Avicenna, Galen and Albucasis, and unhesitatingly expressed his personal preference for one particular method, thus giving further evidence of independence of judgement that was perhaps based on personal experience.[39]

One motive for Dino's choice of the commentary genre may therefore have been precisely a desire to sever discussion of surgical procedures not from experience as such, but from personal reminiscences and individual examples. From the standpoint of one aspiring to return to the world of the universities and the environment of Aristotelian natural philosophy, such a step would enhance the intellectual status of surgery both by emphasizing its claims to generality or universality and hence to *scientia*; it would also eliminate overt evidence of self-advertisement or commercial competition with rivals.

Dino's treatment of the standard list of fatal wounds hence contrasts sharply with Guglielmo's. Like Guglielmo, he drew on both personal knowledge and learned texts in order to provide a comprehensive and practically useful description of such wounds and their symptoms. But in Dino's case, personal knowledge – certainly suggested, for example, in his detailed descriptions of symptoms (even if some of these symptoms are also described in other texts) – is neither privileged nor emphasized. Instead, the

---

[37] 'Quidam nam stolidi medici dicunt utiliorem fore vulneribis pultibus mollitivis ... Sed hoc quod ipsi dicunt falsissimum est et erroneum, quod maxime apparet per Galenum in *Tegni* et etiam in *De ingenio sanitatis*, quia omne vulnus, in quantum vulnus exiccari oportet': *Dinus in chirurgia*, fol. 61r.

[38] Ibid., fol. 63r. The description does not appear to be based on the much more complex and detailed discussion of three different methods of suturing provided by Albucasis (*On surgery and instruments*, pp. 540–6).

[39] *Dinus in Chirurgia* fol. 72v, with Avicenna, *Canon*, 4.4.1.7, at fol. 72r–v. See also Albucasis, *On surgery and instruments*, pp. 542–6.

focus is on the citation of other authorities and on rational argument to amplify and clarify Avicenna's text. Thus, Dino drew on Galen's commentary on the relevant Hippocratic aphorism to explain the reason why wounds to certain organs should be mortal, and on Aristotle's *Parts of animals* for the importance of the heart to the entire body's functioning. He found reasons to explain the apparent inconsistency between the statement of the textual authorities that wounds to the bladder were fatal, but, 'as we see' surgical incisions made in the bladder to remove stones could heal. Perhaps this was because the incision was made in the neck of the bladder, or possibly because the operation was done mostly in children (whose most moist flesh healed readily). As for surgeon's stories, Dino expressed his own opinion of some of them with the remark, 'And from this it is evident that the claim of certain surgeons to have seen part of the brain coming out of the wound of a patient who subsequently survived is incredible.' Perhaps, Dino opined, in the presence of a skull fracture unskilled surgeons had mistaken pus or 'a certain sticky humidity which is joined to the parts of the brain' for brain tissue.[40]

CRITICAL COMPARISONS AMONG AUTHORITIES AND BETWEEN TEXTUAL AUTHORITY AND 'EXPERIENCE'

Guglielmo da Saliceto occasionally directly criticized *antiqui* in medicine in the light of his own experience; for example, he expressed his disapproval of an implied recommendation to perform surgical operations on newborn infants, and his disbelief that tooth extraction could be achieved by medication alone.[41] As we have seen, moreover, he sometimes classified examples from his own experience as a way of refining, explaining, or commenting upon traditional teaching. Furthermore, in addition to displaying a general awareness of scholastic method in his introductory statements, he occasionally made rudimentary use of a *quaestio* as a tool of analysis in his own writing; thus, a chapter on cautery opens with a *dubium* as to whether cautery is useful for all complexional illnesses (the answer is yes).[42] Despite these few instances, however, systematic criticism, analysis, or comparison of sources was certainly not the purpose of the *Chirurgia*.

Rather, the focus of the book is predominantly on direct instruction in diagnosis and manual treatment of surgical conditions (with appropriate supplementary medication). In the prefatory statement justifying his use of *exempla* that has already been alluded to, Guglielmo explained his own

---

[40] 'Et ex hoc apparet quod incredibile est id quod dicunt quidam cyrugici se vidisse iam de vulnere exire quandam partem cerebri et tamen infirmum evadere ... expellitur aliquando per vulnus quedam humiditas viscosa que est coadunata in partibus cerebri que humiditas assimilatur substantie cerebri credunt illi cyrugici': *Dinus in chirurgia*, fols. 59r–60r, with quoted passages on fol. 59v.

[41] *Cyrurgia*, Book 1, ch. 1; *Summa conservationis*, Book 1, ch. 68, sig. [d7r].

[42] Ibid., Book 5, ch. 1.

view of the relation between 'experience' in a vague general or communal sense, his attested personal experiences, and authoritative sources in authenticating these instructions:

the correction of this art is not properly achieved except through use and operation. For the correction [or confirmation] of every art depending on operation is not achieved except for this way and manner, and on account of this it is correct in this teaching to proceed according to those things which had been manifested to me by use and operation over a long time and, for the most part, to use examples to move swiftly through the areas of knowledge in which I have laboured with my own hands.[43]

Guglielmo's careful phrasing gives 'use and operation' – that is, practical experience, preferably one's own – an essential function in confirming, and sometimes elaborating, refining, or on particular points correcting the principles and methodology belonging to the art of surgery. Such a formulation does not, of course, imply that significant innovation or major departures from tradition are expected to ensue. Guglielmo, like other surgeon-authors, assumed that the *ars* of surgery had been fully and, with some exceptions, accurately laid out in the learned sources – given the relatively unchanging nature of the actual technical limitations on the development of surgery, there was some justification for this attitude.[44] And he like other authors found in written sources models for written descriptions of surgical procedures, considered as pieces of technical literature. Whether or not the procedures were always usable, the descriptions certainly were.

Hence, as Guglielmo's wording in this passage also makes clear, he was not claiming to have personally performed all the procedures or employed all the medications described in his book. The range of Guglielmo's experience may have influenced the selection of topics to be included in the *Chirurgia*, but is highly unlikely to have been the sole deciding factor in the process of combination, compression, omission and addition through which the *Chirurgia*, like other thirteenth-century books on surgery, was evidently largely constructed from standard authorities and recent Latin works. Thus, despite Guglielmo's strong and genuinely impressive insistence on the need to subject traditional surgical doctrine to the test of experience, he and his readers probably assumed that, except in a few specific instances, such doctrines would successfully pass this test, even

---

[43] 'rectificatio huius artis non sit proprie nisi per usum et operationem. Nam rectificatio [St John's College MS 76: certificatio] omnis artis pendentis ab operatione non rectificatur [certificatur] nisi hac via et modo et propter hoc rectum est in hac doctrina [parte] procedere secundum ea que mihi per usum et operationes [operacione] longo tempore manifestata fuerunt et per exempla ut plurimum currere in sermonibus in quibus propriis manibus laboravi'; ibid., proem.

[44] See Chiara Crisciani, "History, novelty, and progress in scholastic medicine', *Osiris*, 2nd series, 6 (1990), 118–39.

when no actual trial had been performed within the scope of their personal knowledge.

Throughout his commentary, Dino habitually submitted Avicenna's recommendations to critical examination in the light of other authoritative texts, and frequently also weighed Avicenna's teaching against current surgical practice and vice versa. He routinely compared Avicenna's statements with those of Galen – usually but not always from *De ingenio sanitatis* (*Methodus medendi*) – and Albucasis on the same subject. In many instances, this practice yielded mainly fuller theoretical explanation of causes, as in the discussion of fatal wounds already summarized. But in other cases, such as the passage – also mentioned above – in which Dino compared the authorities' recommendations for suturing, the same method provided a framework within which to describe and evaluate different manual techniques. In yet other instances, he used Galen and Albucasis to supply Avicenna's omissions. For example, the part of the *Canon* that he was expounding failed to discuss wounds of the chest cavity. 'In order to complete the teaching of surgery', Dino added a chapter on the subject based on Galen and Albucasis (and Avicenna's own remarks elsewhere in the *Canon*), even though he admitted that such addition was irrelevant to commentary on the text in hand.[45]

Dino carried out much of his analysis by means of scholastic *quaestiones*. Often enough, these yielded chiefly long theoretical disquisitions on the complexional value of medications. In some instances, however, Dino turned the *quaestio* into an effective tool of criticism and enquiry about pragmatic matters of manual technique in surgery. Space permits only the example of two interrelated *quaestiones* from his discussion of skull fractures. Can a skull fracture ever be successfully treated with suturing of the skin, medication, and a plaster alone? And, can a skull fracture ever be cured without making an incision and finding and removing fragments of bone?[46]

The problem, according to Dino, was that all the famous authors insist on the necessity of incision, elevation of any depressed bone, and removal of fragments. However, 'it is widely believed' that many are cured by plasters alone, without the other procedures; empirics say they do it, and 'we indeed believe that we have seen the result that they are able to bring about with [plasters]'. Furthermore, Dino recognized that the purpose of

---

[45] 'Cum dictum fuerit prius quod vulnerum penetrantium quedam sunt penetrantia in concavitatem membrorum nutritivorum ut que fiunt in partibus ventris ab umbilico infra et parum supra; quedam sunt penetrantia in concavitate membrorum spiritualium que fiunt in partibus pectoris vel toracis aut dorsi. Cum Avicenna non determinet nisi de primis vulneribus penetrantibus ... idcirco nos quamquam non spectet ad propositum Avicenne ad completionem tamen doctrinam cirugie de his vulneribus et cura ipsorum aliquid capitulum breve extractum ex dictis Avicenne in 3° et Albucasis et Galeni *De ingenio* constituemus': *Dinus in chirurgia*, fol. 73v.

[46] Ibid., fols. 136v–139r.

the procedure of 'elevation and detection' was solely to ensure that no bone fragments were left and that fluid did not collect between the bone and the *dura mater*. In a case in which there was no reason to fear these things, there would be no need to undertake a procedure which in itself involved additional hazard, since it could cause *apostemata* in the membrane. Furthermore, he alleged that some plasters had the power to draw humidity, and virulent poisons, and even bone fragments to the surface.

Weighing all these considerations, Dino came to the conclusion that he was prepared to say, 'audaciously', that he did not think it impossible that skull fractures might occasionally be cured by means of plasters, even without elevation of bone and manual removal of fragments. However, in most cases a plaster alone would not be sufficient, and it was always 'safer' to follow the recommendation of the authorities.[47] He then went on to describe in some detail the circumstances that might permit the judicious surgeon to attempt to cure with a plaster alone: the patient should have good humours (that is, good general health), the break in the skin should be large enough to allow any moisture that formed to run off, and the fracture should not involve scraping of the bone or *dura mater*. Only rarely, however, would all these conditions occur together.

As for the empirics, since they believe that it is possible always to cure by using plasters alone, but do not know how to distinguish one kind of wound from another, they apply plasters indiscriminately in all cases; as a result they occasionally cure and frequently kill.[48] The *rationalis medicus*, in Dino's view, ought rather to adhere to the safer method recommended by the authors. Dino explained the common belief in the frequency and ease of cure by plasters alone as a result of the readiness with which, if something occurs sometimes, the vulgar spread abroad that it happens in every case (particularly, one may add, when the subject is a supposedly painless cure for a painful or dangerous condition). But the empirics also deceive people, because they proclaim that any kind of head wound is a skull fracture and then claim credit for curing it with plasters.[49]

The common professional activities (teaching, writing, treating patients) and the common heritage of technical literature and practised techniques

---

[47] 'Dicendum est ad hoc quod credimus cognoscere que sunt emplastra ex quibus etiam componuntur et cum quibus isti empirici dicunt se curare talia vulnera que sunt cum fractura cranei absque alio modo curationis et credimus etiam vidisse effectus quos cum eis agere possunt. Et ideo ex ratione motus, et etiam ex his aliis que experientia vidi, dico audacter ad istam dubitationem quod non credimus impossibile esse ... licet autem talis modus curationis sit possibiliis tamen dico quod in pluribus non sufficit, et dico etiam quod tutior est modus curationis quem docent auctores': ibid., fol. 138v.

[48] 'Isti empirici qui cum talibus emplastris procedunt aliquando curaverunt, semper credentes posse curare propterea quia nesciunt distinguere dispositiones vulnerum, indifferenter administrantes talia emplastra in quocunque vulnere, multos interficiunt': ibid., fol. 138v.

[49] 'Dicendum quod ad famam quam dant laici et vulgares qui non cognoscunt ea que sunt artis medicine sufficit quod solum illud quandoque accidit. Nam vulgares quando aliquid

shared by Guglielmo da Saliceto and Dino del Garbo gave their books on surgery many traits in common. Both books are products of the knowledge and practice of literate working surgeons in north Italian cities of the second half of the thirteenth century. Both were the work of authors influenced by contemporary trends – both institutional and intellectual – in academic education. The major difference between the practical manual and the scholastic commentary may indeed be the difference in form.

But that difference is by no means trivial or insignificant. Even before he himself was fully integrated into an academic community, Dino chose the quintessential academic format of exposition. The work on surgery that he chose to expound gave extensive treatment to the medical treatment of *apostemata*, *lepra*, and ulcers, that is, those aspects of surgery hardest to distinguish from general 'practical medicine'; and he weighted the content of his commentary further in the same direction with long discussions of *complexio* in relation to *apostemata* and their medication. While claiming to supplement Avicenna so as to supply complete teaching on surgery, he omitted the – surely essential – topic of fractures of the long bones. And he seems to have deliberately sought out problems or conflicts between authorities that lent themselves to investigation by means of scholastic *quaestiones*. These decisions and preferences of Dino's mark a significant turning point in one man's career. With this commentary, Dino successfully inserted himself into the university world of prestigious academic authorship. His strategy also vividly illustrates the pull of the institutionalized academic milieu during the last years of the thirteenth century. The promise of ordered wisdom and enhanced intellectual status exercised a powerful attraction for ambitious medical men. From Dino's standpoint, a move to the Italian university milieu must have seemed a wholly desirable step not only for himself but for surgery as a discipline. He could not have foreseen the most striking development in the history of literate surgery in the fourteenth and fifteenth centuries: its lively dissemination outside the universities, outside Italy, and in vernacular as well as Latin cultural settings.

vident semel accidere, quia rationem ignorant postea diffamant quod illud semper accidat ... Adiuvat autem ad deceptionem laicorum iudicii et vulgarium propterea quia decipiuntur ab istis empiricis. Nam isti empirici quia sagaces sunt in decipiendo quodlibet vulnus capitis quantumque sit leve dicunt et faciunt credere vulgaribus quod sit cum fractura cranei, et dato quod non sit': ibid., fol. 139r.

A final feature of Dino's commentary, at least in its early printed version, that may be mentioned is a handful of allusions to Book 6 of the work of Paul of Aegina (not directly known in the West until the sixteenth century – see note 8 above). This author is several times named in Avicenna's text, but the references in Dino's commentary do not merely echo Avicenna. Such remarks as 'Paulus nam in suo 6 libro *De fractura cranei* hanc opinionem maxime imporbat [*sic*], dicit nam ad litteram talia verba' and 'Et intellige quod omnia ista verba que ponentur etiam usque ad finem capituli sunt verba Pauli ad litteram sicut apparet in capitulo quod fecit de hac cura expresse' suggest rather the comparison of the two texts: *Dinus in chirurgia*, fols. 134r, 140v. These references cluster in the section on skull fractures. So far, I have not identified the intermediary source.

4

Derivation and revulsion: the theory and practice of medieval phlebotomy

PEDRO GIL-SOTRES

Therapeutic blood-letting or phlebotomy is the evacuation of blood by means of opening a vein, so as to reduce the volume of blood contained in the body. This universal and ancient practice was used empirically by primitive cultures. Greek medicine endowed it with theoretical principles, based at first on humoralism taken from a developing Galenism. In this system it was understood that the body contained four fluids or *humores*: blood, phlegm, yellow bile and black bile. Blood-letting was used in order to correct disorders of the humoral quantity.[1]

The importance of the life-giving liquid which it aimed to remove and the particular layout of the venous network throughout the human body made this therapeutic practice the principal treatment for a large number of illnesses. Galen and Arabic Galenism defined the indications for, and the contra-indications against phlebotomy in considerable detail. As for medieval Latin Galenism, its development depended on translations, produced in the south of Italy and Toledo, of certain texts written by Galen and Arab physicians.

As far as the methods used to carry out phlebotomy were concerned, from antiquity onwards two distinct methods of diverting blood from a particular part of the body were distinguished, namely *derivation* and *revulsion*. In derivation, blood was let at a point close to the affected area; in the case of revulsion, at the most remote point possible. Both methods had precise indications for use in the case of different illnesses and were widely employed by medieval physicians. However, historical awareness of this fact was lost in the course of the sixteenth century. Those involved in the

---

[1] For a study of blood-letting in Galen and in the earlier Greek literature, see P. Brain, *Galen on bloodletting* (Cambridge, 1986). An analysis of phlebotomy in medieval Latin Galenism can be found in my introduction to *Tractatus de consideracionibus operis medicine sive de flebotomia*, edited by L. Demaitre, pp. 9–120, which is vol. IV of *Arnaldi de Villanova opera medica omnia* (Barcelona, 1988). References to the same practice are to be found in L. E. Voigts and M. R. McVaugh, 'A Latin technical phlebotomy and its Middle English translation', *Transactions of the American Philosophical Society*, 74, part 2 (1984), 1–69.

so-called 'blood-letting controversy' demonstrated total ignorance of the theory and practice of medieval phlebotomy, at least as regards the use of derivation. The world of medical humanism misinterpreted the reality of medieval medicine, because of ignorance both of the theoretical assumptions that it had taken as its starting point and of its practical accomplishments. The distorted image of medieval medicine that was thus presented has been reinforced by certain recent historical works, which have interpreted medieval phlebotomy from the standpoint of Renaissance physicians.[2] One of the practical consequences of the Renaissance debate on *pleuritis* ('pains in the chest or side') was the rejection of the practice of revulsion at the start of illness as habitual technique, it being stated that that was the only thing that medieval physicians did. The study of this controversy has led some historians to claim that medieval physicians were ignorant of the technique of derivation, and that they basically made use only of revulsion in their medical advice.[3] According to this interpretation of the facts, revulsion must have been the commonest practice among Arab physicians, and Latin physicians continued this practice until it was definitively rejected in the sixteenth century. However, a direct reading of both the Greek and Arab medical sources which medieval physicians had access to, as well as of the original Latin medical literature, in which the doctrine and practice of phlebotomy as followed by medieval Galenism is expounded, offers a different interpretation.

This chapter presents firstly a framework for the theoretical and practical aspects of the practice of blood-letting in the Middle Ages; secondly, it will be shown that the derivative method was in fact frequently used by medieval physicians (and the way in which they acquired such knowledge will also be discussed); thirdly, the way in which the practice of blood-letting was actually performed will be described.

MEDIEVAL PHLEBOTOMY: BETWEEN SURGERY AND MEDICATION

In the Middle Ages the study of the therapeutics of blood-letting was centred upon three different types of text, which correspond to three clearly defined chronological stages. In the first place, there exists a series of very short early medieval texts known as *Epistulae de flebotomia*. These are works of a practical nature and lack theoretical discussions. They frequently

---

[2] The historians of the blood-letting controversy, J. B. de C. M. Saunders and C. D. O'Malley, *Andreas Vesalius Bruxellensis: the bloodletting letter of 1539. An annotated translation and study of the evolution of Vesalius' scientific development* (New York, 1946), maintain this point of view, as does H. Schipperges, *Der Garten der Gesundheit: Medizin im Mittelalter* (Munich and Zurich, 1985), Spanish trans. (Barcelona, 1987), p. 101.

[3] 'the Arab practice in which bleeding was generally, if not exclusively, revulsive at a site chosen as remote as possible from the seat of the affection. The Arab practice was the standard from the mediaeval period until the sixteenth century ... ': Saunders and O'Malley, *Andreas Vesalius ... the bloodletting letter*, p. 15.

appear in association with astrological works of a popular nature, and, to judge by the number of surviving copies, they must have been widely used throughout the Middle Ages.[4] There are also a large number of similar texts of Salernitan origin, attributed to one or another of the masters of the Salerno school of medicine.[5] To these should be added the so-called calendars (*calendaria*) translated from Arabic into Latin, which incorporated indications of the best times for letting blood.[6]

A second group of works consists of paragraphs devoted to therapeutic blood-letting in more general medical treatises. They contain a greater amount of theoretical discussion than the first group of works and were clearly dependent on the chapter devoted to phlebotomy in Avicenna's *Canon*. On occasions, they had an independent manuscript life and figured in codices as anonymous works.[7]

Finally, a third form of literature dealing with phlebotomy began to develop during the late thirteenth century. These were monographs dedicated to blood-letting drawn up by writers belonging to scholastic academic circles. They were composed by two masters at the Montpellier faculty of medicine, where great interest was being expressed in this subject around this date. They were Arnau de Vilanova's *Tractatus de considerationibus operis medicine*[8] and Bernard de Gordon's *De flebotomia*.[9]

[4] For the manuscripts see P. Kibre, *Hippocrates Latinus: repertorium of Hippocratic writings in the Latin Middle Ages* (New York, 1985), pp. 154–5. Similar examples are to be found in the collections of early medieval manuscripts. See E. Wickersheimer, *Les manuscrits Latins de médecine du haut moyen âge dans les bibliothèques de France* (Paris, 1966); A. Beccaria, *I codici di medicina del periodo presalernitano (secoli IX, X e XI)* (Rome, 1956).

[5] Published in the form of doctoral theses directed by K. Sudhoff: A. Morgenstern, *Das Aderlassgedicht des Johannes von Aquila und seine Stellung in der Aderlasslehre des Mittelalters, samt dem Abdruck der lateinischen Übersetzung der Schrift Peri flebotomia Ypocratis nach den Handschriften in Brüssel und Dresden* (Leipzig, 1917); R. Czarnecki, *Ein Aderlasstraktat angeblich des Roger von Salerno samt einem lateinischen und einem griechischen Texte zur 'Phlebotomia Hippocratis'* (Leipzig, 1919); H. Erchenbrecher, *Der Salernitaner Arzt Archimatthaeus und ein bis heute unbekannter Aderlasstraktat unter seinem Namen Cod. Berol. lat. 4° N° 375* (Leipzig, 1919); R. Buerschaper, *Ein bisher unbekannter Aderlasstraktat des Salernitaner Arztes Maurus 'De flebotomia'* (Leipzig, 1919); H. Seyfert, *Die Flebotomia Richardi Anglici* (Leipzig, 1895).

[6] See J. Martínez and L. García-Ballester, 'Las *Epistulae de flebotomia* y los *Calendaria* en el galenismo práctico de los siglos XIII y XIV en la Corona de Aragón', in *Coloquio Internacional Galeno: Obra, pensamiento e influencia* (Madrid, 1991); pp. 281–9.

[7] This happened, for example, in the case of the extensive exposition produced by Jean de St Amand in the *Expositio supra Antidotarium Nicolai*. The manuscript transmission of this fragment suggested the existence of an independent work, entitled *De flebotomia*, attributed to Jean de St Amand, and which was edited as a doctoral dissertation by G. Kurt, 'Johannes de Sancto Amando und ein Aderlasstraktat unter seinem Namen' (University of Leipzig, 1922).

[8] The bibliography on Arnau is very extensive. For his biography, J. A. Paniagua, *El Maestro Arnau de Vilanova médico* (Valencia, 1969) is useful. There is a critical edition of the *Tractatus de consideracionibus operis medicine sive de flebotomia*, prepared by L. Demaitre in vol. IV of *Arnaldi de Villanova Opera medica omnia* (Barcelona, 1988).

[9] For his biography see L. Demaitre, *Doctor Bernard de Gordon: professor and practitioner* (Toronto, 1980). The *De flebotomia* is the first part of a more extensive treatise entitled *De conservatione vitae humanae*, printed on only one occasion in the *Opus lilium medicine*

If we now turn to the contents of the literature on phlebotomy we can similarly distinguish three different stages, which depended on the developments of Arabic-to-Latin and Greek-to-Latin translation. The first period began in the early Middle Ages and continued until the thirteenth century. It is characterized by successive versions of the pseudo-Hippocratic text, *Epistola Ypocratis de flebotomia*; a considerable number of practical tracts were derived from this. In these, phlebotomy is considered exclusively as a surgical operation. The final point of this stage was reached with the works derived from Salerno and the consequent introduction of Constantine's *Pantegni* into the medical world.

The second period opens with the appearance of the *Canon* in scholastic contexts and covers the second half of the thirteenth century and the first quarter of the fourteenth century. In this stage of medieval scholasticism ideas on phlebotomy were enriched by the incorporation of the Toledan translations of Galen and by the assimilation of what was to become the key for their interpretation: Avicenna's *Canon*. The end of this period was marked by the significant Greek-to-Latin translation by Niccolò da Reggio of the last book of Galen specially dedicated to phlebotomy: the *De curandi ratione per venae sectionem*.[10]

The third phase, which commenced with this translation, continued without break down to the sixteenth century. The end of this phase was marked by the controversy between physicians concerning the treatment of *pleuritis*. This can be said to have started with Pierre Brissot's work, *Apologetica disceptatio*, published in Paris in 1525.[11]

These periods reflect a significant evolution in the therapeutic status accorded to phlebotomy. Both the early medieval tracts and the works derived from the Salerno area defined blood-letting as 'a correct incision of the veins', a statement to which its immediate effect was often added: 'with an effusion of blood'.[12] What constitutes the common denominator of this family of texts is thus the interpretation of phlebotomy as an exclusively *surgical* practice, performed by the opening of a vein and allowing the blood that springs forth from the wound to flow.

The surgical nature of therapeutic blood-letting became widely accepted in medieval schools of medicine on the basis of the *Pantegni*. The following

---

(Lyons, 1574), pp. 667–727. For the manuscripts, the list supplied by Demaitre can be consulted.

[10] See L. Thorndike, 'Translation of works of Galen from the Greek by Niccolò da Reggio (*c.* 1308–1345)', *Byzantina Metabyzantina*, 1 (1946), 213–35; see the translation into English in Brain, *Galen on bloodletting*, pp. 67–99. For the chronology of Galen's works on venesection, see Brain's book and the bibliography used in the discussion on pp. 100–11 there.

[11] P. Brissot, *Apologetica disceptatio qua docetur per quae loca sanguis mitti debeat* ... (Paris, 1525).

[12] This occurs, for example, in the tract falsely attributed to Arnau de Vilanova: 'Flebotomia est veneranda vene incisio cum effusione sanguinis', MS Gerona, 75, fol. 8ra, and in many other short treatises. See P. Gil-Sotres, *Scripta minora de flebotomia en la tradición médica del siglo XIII* (Santander and Pamplona, 1986), pp. 32–4.

passage can be read in the ninth book of the second part – *practica* – of this work:

Surgery is carried out on the veins, on the flesh and on the bones. In the case of non-throbbing veins, it is called phlebotomy; in the case of throbbing veins [arteries], it is known as sectioning or incision.[13]

Such a definition – the only one of blood-letting in the whole work – is closely connected with the less explicit one proposed for surgery in Joannitius' *Isagoge*, an educational text whose great practical importance in the teaching of medicine is well known:

Surgery falls into two classes; surgery on the flesh and on the bones. In the case of the flesh through cutting, sewing and cauterizing; in the case of the bone through consolidating, joining and setting.[14]

The surgical nature of phlebotomy is also demonstrated in the writings of later authors. Thus, Ricardus Anglicus,[15] in his treatise on phlebotomy, made a very similar observation:

Sometimes surgery is carried out on the flesh; on other occasions on the bone and on others on the veins. The form of surgery carried out on the vein has a twofold nature, since one type is that on throbbing veins and the other is that performed on non-throbbing veins.[16]

The surgeon Henri de Mondeville,[17] when referring to the *Isagoge*, expounded this surgical characteristic of blood-letting in more detail:

The types of surgery, as Joannitius points out, are two in number: one in which the surgeon acts on the hard parts of the body such as the bones; the other in which he operates on the soft parts, such as the flesh. And a third may be added when those parts are operated on which are of intermediate consistency, between the hard and soft ones, such as cartilage, nerves, veins and arteries.[18]

---

[13] 'Chirurgia igitur aut fit in venis aut in carne aut in osse. In venis quidem non pulsantibus appellatur phlebotomia. In venis pulsantibus sectio aut incisio nuncupatur': *Pantegni, Practice,* lib. IX, c. I, in *Omnia opera Isaac* (Lyons, 1515), vol. I, fol. 119r.

[14] 'Chirurgia duplex est in carne et in osse. In carne ut incidere, suere, coquere; in osse ut solidare aut innectare aut reddere': *Isagoge,* as printed in *Articella* (Venice, 1523).

[15] The current state of studies on this writer can be seen in the *Supplément* volume by D. Jacquart (Geneva, 1979), pp. 256–7, to E. Wickersheimer, *Dictionnaire biographique des médecins en France au moyen âge* (Paris, 1936; reprinted Geneva, 1979).

[16] 'Cyrurgia enim alia fit in carne alia in osse alia in venis. Illa autem quae fit in venis duplex est, quia alia est quae in venis pulsatilibus alia quae fit in venis non pulsatilibus': *De flebotomia;* printed in Seyfert, *Die flebotomia Richardi Anglici,* p. I.

[17] On whom see Wickersheimer, *Dictionnaire biographique,* pp. 282–3, and Jacquart, *Supplément,* pp. 117–18.

[18] 'Species cyrurgiae sic dicit Ioahnnitius in fine, sunt duae: una cum qua cyrurgicus operatur in membris duris ut in ossibus; alia cum qua operatur in mollibus ut in carne. Et potest superaddi tertia species, cum qua operatur in membris mediis inter duritiem et mollitiem, ut in cartilaginibus, nervis, venis et arteriis': J. L. Pagel (ed.), *Die Chirurgie des Heinrich von Mondeville (Hermondaville) nach Berliner, Erfurter und Pariser Codices zum ersten Mal herausgegeben* (Berlin, 1892), pp. 62–3.

This original view, which considered blood-letting as a strictly surgical activity, was drastically altered by the appearance in university circles of the *Canon*. Avicenna, far from maintaining the surgical aspect as the main defining factor of phlebotomy, proposed the following formulation: 'phlebotomy is the universal evacuation that discharges in abundance'.[19] This definition emphasizes a strictly *medical* concept – that of evacuation – and makes no reference whatsoever to the surgical operation by means of which it is carried out. In this way, phlebotomy became comparable with the other purgative remedies. Ample proof of this can be found in the fact that henceforth study of the question was included in those textbooks devoted to the analysis of medicine, as with Jean de St Amand's commentary on the popular work *Antidotarium Nicolai*, and the *De simplicibus*, written by Arnau de Vilanova. The change in orientation brought about by Avicenna through his definition of phlebotomy was accompanied by a further significant change: this is the place he assigned in the *Canon* as a whole to the study of therapeutic blood-letting. The *Pantegni* had included phlebotomy in the *practical* part of the work. Avicenna, on the other hand, transferred it to the first book, whose title 'On the general things of medical science'[20] signifies *theory*.

The new position that phlebotomy was to hold with respect to the various therapeutic practices in this period depended, in short, on two works whose influence on university circles was enormous. On the one hand, there was the *Pantegni* by Haly Abbas (al-Majusi), translated and abridged by Constantine in the south of Italy in the late eleventh century; and on the other, Avicenna's *Canon*, translated by Gerard of Cremona in Toledo about a hundred years afterwards. On the basis of the knowledge of phlebotomy contained in these two treatises two separate currents were established which were to impose a different pattern on this practice.

The transition from one stage to the other is exemplified by the treatise on the healing of fevers by means of phlebotomy drawn up in the years 1239 and 1240 by Henry of Winchester, chancellor of the University of Montpellier, and the author of the earliest extant written work produced by a professor at its faculty of medicine.[21] The sources of this work were limited to the *Articella* and the *corpus* translated by Constantine. It should be emphasized that Henry of Winchester did not make any reference to Avicenna's *Canon*, nor to other texts making up the medical *Corpus*

---

[19] 'Flebotomia est evacuatio universalis que multitudinem evacuat': *Canon*, lib. 1, fen 4, c. 20 (Venice, 1527), fol. 59va.
[20] 'Liber primus est de rebus universalibus sciencie medicine': *Canon*, lib. 1, fen 4, c. 20, fol. 1.
[21] On this author see M. R. McVaugh, 'An early discussion of medicinal degrees at Montpellier by Henry of Winchester', *Bulletin of the History of Medicine*, 49 (1975), 57–71, esp. 57–8, and the bibliography cited therein. Henry writes on fevers and blood-letting in the work *Tractatus de egritudinibus fleubotomandis*, edited by Voigts and McVaugh in 'A Latin technical phlebotomy'.

Toletanum; however, he did discuss significant disagreements between the *antiqui* and the *moderni*[22] which had to be properly interpreted. In particular, when considering the treatment of the fever known as *causon*, the ancients proposed that phlebotomy should be withheld, given the characteristics of this putrid fever, whereas the 'moderns' – among them Henry of Winchester – were keenly in favour of its application. Henry makes clear exactly who the 'ancients' were:

> Those writers who deal with the *causon* do not recommend the use of phlebotomy, as is clear from the *Viaticum* and in Constantine's *Book of fevers* ... the moderns, in contrast, recommend blood-letting in small amounts...[23]

The *antiqui*, therefore, were those who followed the approaches contained in the writings translated by Constantine. Opposing them, then, who were the 'moderns'?

Gualterius Angilonis, a writer apparently contemporary with Henry of Winchester, included phlebotomy in his *Summa medicinalis* among the measures recommended to cure the fever known as *causon*: 'Carry out the phlebotomy on the cardiac vein if the bile is in the veins of the heart, or on the basilic vein if it is in those of the liver.'[24] Gualterius Angilonis was familiar with the *Canon* and made extensive use of it, resorting to its authority in many passages of his book. It must be accepted, therefore, that in the first half of the thirteenth century certain medical authors underwent a development with respect to phlebotomy, the starting point for which was the arrival of the *Canon* in university circles.

Yet this state of affairs did not mean the complete disappearance of the surgical understanding of blood-letting. One example of this is to be found in the treatise on blood-letting attributed to Ricardus Anglicus, perhaps composed in the first half of the thirteenth century,[25] which exhibits several features which might be taken to suggest that it was a transitional work. The text is clearly oriented towards the medical practitioner rather than emphasizing the theoretical aspects of this therapeutic act; this explains the importance given to the semiology of the blood that is drained off. The author appears to have known, and even used, Henry of Winchester's

---

[22] 'Antiqui minuebant patientes synocham usque ad syncopim ... Nos autem, timentes secundum vulgi opinionem, tantum pluribus vicibus detrahimus quantum ipsi semel ... ': *Tractatus de egritudinibus fleubotomandis* (ed. Voigts and McVaugh, 'A Latin technical phlebotomy'), pp. 40–2.

[23] 'Notandum quod auctores tractantes de causone precipiunt non fieri minutionem, ut patet in Viatico, Libro febrium Constantini ... Moderni vero in causone precipiunt minui in parva quantitate ... ': ibid, pp. 48–9.

[24] 'Fiat flebotomia de vena cardyaca, si colera sit in venis cordis, aut de basilica si fuerit in epate': *Summa medicinalis*; in P. Diepgen (ed.), *Gualteri Angilonis Summa medicinalis* (Leipzig, 1911), p. 208. On this writer see Wickersheimer, *Dictionnaire biographique* pp. 170–3; and Jacquart, *Supplément*, pp. 80–1.

[25] Printed by Seyfert, *Die flebotomia*.

work.[26] The description he supplies of the veins on which phlebotomy is practised could have come from the *Canon* or from Rhazes' *Liber ad Almansorem*; it does not seem to have had any connection with that used in the works emanating from Salerno. Nevertheless, it maintains the status of phlebotomy at the same level as the Salernitan writers, restricting it within the same limited horizons of a simple surgical operation carried out on the veins.[27]

The change we can detect in the Montpellier authors mentioned above is found also in Jean de St Amand, a master linked with the faculty of medicine of Paris in the second half of the thirteenth century.[28] In a lengthy reference to phlebotomy that he included in his *Expositio supra Antidotarium Nicolai*, he demonstrates that he was in possession of theoretical knowledge of a far higher standard than that of previous writers. There can be no doubt that this was because he had extensive knowledge of what García-Ballester has called the 'new Galen'[29] and of the key to interpreting it: Avicenna's *Canon*.

Galen is the author most frequently cited by Jean de St Amand, as he makes reference to his authority on no fewer than forty-two occasions in order to support the doctrine that he expounds. The majority of these references – seventeen, to be precise – are to the *Methodus medendi*, in the version called *Megategni* and which was attributed to Constantine. Galen's commentaries on the Hippocratic aphorisms are the second most frequently cited work, with thirteen explicit references, while Galen's commentary on Hippocrates' book of prognosis has a single mention. This exhausts the Galenic texts derived from Arabic-Latin translations from the south of Italy. The remainder of the references are to writings by Galen translated from Arabic into Latin in Toledo: the *De simplicibus medicinis*, the commentary on the *Regimen acutorum morborum*, and the *De crisi*, are specifically mentioned once each; the *Tegni*, with the commentaries of Haly Ridwan, is mentioned twice. The others are general references to Galen, which it has not been possible to identify more precisely.

The author who is next most often cited is Avicenna, with thirty-three direct references, the greater part of which are to the chapter of the *Canon* on phlebotomy. Jean de St Amand's familiarity with Avicenna's principal medical work enabled him to count on first-class support for interpreting and understanding the works of Galen which were known to him. Throughout the text continual efforts are made to reconcile the two

---

26 The direction to use blood-letting in the case of fevers offers significant parallels with Henry of Winchester's text. See Seyfert, *Die flebotomia*, p. 7; and Voigts and McVaugh, 'A Latin technical phlebotomy', pp. 48–9.

27 See note 16.

28 See Danielle Jacquart, Chapter 6 in this volume.

29 See L. García-Ballester, 'Arnau de Vilanova (*c.* 1240–1311) y la reforma de los estudios médicos en Montpellier (1309): el Hipócrates latino y la introducción del nuevo Galeno', *Dynamis*, 2 (1982), 97–158.

authors' opinions at those points where they disagree, although on occasions this leads to the literal meaning of what they had written being stretched.

The fragment on phlebotomy of Jean de St Amand's *Expositio supra antidotarium Nicolai* reflects the use of other Arabic sources. In the first place is Rhazes with his *Liber ad Almansorem*, which merited six references; then Haly Abbas, with two references to his *De urinis* and one to the *Liber dietarum*; and Haly Ridwan, with one to his commentary on the *Tegni*. The references in this text are completed by five references to the Hippocratic *Aphorisms*, one mention of Joannitius, another of a certain Alexander – who can be identified as the physician from Alexandria, Alexander of Tralles – and three references to works by Aristotle: two to the *Libri de animalibus* and one to the *Regimen principum* or *Secretum secretorum*, which, although apocryphal, was widely diffused in the Middle Ages. It is obvious that these were novelties in the intellectual make-up of someone like Jean de St Amand, who was associated with university circles in Paris and who, in the course of the 1270s and 1280s, had come into contact with the full impact of the new Galenic texts and those of Arab writers such as Avicenna, Rhazes and Haly Ridwan. This enabled him to go beyond an approach based on the texts of the so-called *Articella*, supported by the *Pantegni*. Nor was it purely fortuitous that he included Aristotle's *libri naturales*, especially those grouped under the title of *De animalibus*.

With this collection of sources St Amand confronted the problems that arose from such a common and widespread practice as phlebotomy, the practical application of which on the population in general was in the hands of barbers (*barbitonsores*) with little or no professional training. He did so, as was usual given the methodology of the period, in the form of *quaestiones*, in which he put together the opinions both of the new texts and of the old ones that came from Salerno. His work is an important landmark in the process of change in the study of phlebotomy and constitutes the link joining the knowledge provided by physicians in the twelfth century and the first half of the thirteenth century to the developments and analysis carried out by the masters of Montpellier at the turn of the thirteenth and fourteenth centuries.

At the end of the thirteenth century, the different positions drew closer together. University-trained physicians built bridges which enabled them to bring together both characteristics of phlebotomy. This is what happened in Montpellier, where a growing interest can be observed in the problems produced by the evacuation of blood. Evidence of this is the fact that, between the closing years of the thirteenth century and the opening of the fourteenth century, two works referring to this question were produced: the *Tractatus de considerationibus operis medicine* by Arnau de Vilanova, written around the year 1295, and the *De flebotomia*, composed by Bernard de Gordon in 1308. Both works recognized, following the *Canon*, that phlebotomy was a form of evacuation, but they also emphasized its surgical nature.

The formula proposed by Arnau de Vilanova was original and reflected the tendency to unite the two currents that we have been discussing:

This is, then, the definition of phlebotomy, an incision in a vein that evacuates the blood and the humours that flow in the veins together with it. In other words, it is the evacuation of the blood and humours flowing together with it in the veins, carried out by means of incision of the veins.[30]

The position of Bernard de Gordon, expressed in the *De flebotomia*, was similar to that maintained by Arnau. The synthesis is here expressed by placing the two definitions one after the other: first that found in the *Canon* and, immediately afterwards, a variant of that offered by the *Pantegni*:

Phlebotomy is the universal evacuation that discharges the humours abundantly; this definition is the same as that expounded by Avicenna in fen IV of Book I. By phlebotomy we understand the opening of a vein carried out with the phlebotome or with the lancet.[31]

This express recognition of the existence of the two factors that made up phlebotomy did not, however, mean that both were present on equal terms. (This fact, as will be seen, had clear practical and social repercussions.) Thus, when these two writers analysed the effects of blood-letting on the human body, they were to say: 'It is obvious that the effect of phlebotomy, by itself, is evacuation';[32] and 'the first and principal reason why phlebotomy is performed is that of evacuation'.[33]

The fact that phlebotomy provoked the evacuation of all the humours made it similar to purgative medicines. Later medieval physicians emphasized its therapeutic role by taking the action of purgatives as a point of comparison: 'Phlebotomy is also a universal medicine for all those ills caused by excess; therefore it purges the whole body.'[34]

I believe that the fact that both these Montpellier masters joined the two characteristics of phlebotomy in their definitions was not only an intellectual resolution of two traditions of medical texts. It was also an expression of the somewhat ambiguous position that phlebotomy had at the level

---

[30] 'Est ergo diffinicio quod flebotomia est incisio vene evacuans sanguinem et humores cum sanguine decurrentes in venis. Vel est evacuacio sanguinis et humorum cum sanguine decurrencium in venis facta per incisionem venarum, quod idem est': *Tractatus de consideracionibus operis medicine* (ed. Demaitre), p. 144.

[31] 'Flebotomia est evacuacio universalis multitudinem humorum evacuans. Hec est descripcio Avicenne fen 4, liber I. Per flebotomiam intelligimus apercionem vene factam cum flebotomo sive cum lanceola': *De flebotomia*, MS Cues, 308, fol. 27rb.

[32] 'Planum est autem ut diximus quia effectus flebotomie per se est evacuacio . . . ', Arnau de Vilanova, *Tractatus de consideracionibus operis medicine* (ed. Demaitre), p. 178.

[33] 'Intencio autem flebotomie primo et principaliter est propter evacuacionem': Bernard de Gordon, *De flebotomia*, MS Cues, 308, fol. 27vb.

[34] 'Flebotomia autem est universalis medicina omnis passionis ex plenitudine. Flebotomia igitur purgat totum corpus': ibid., fol. 27va.

of everyday, practical activity. In spite of the wide theoretical discussion provided by university masters and despite their efforts to extend their tools of intellectual analysis to this technique, in fact it was generally carried out by health 'professionals' who were closer to the masses. I am referring to the barbers or *barbitonsores* who, in the thirteenth and fourteenth centuries, made up the basic, primary level of a health-care system that was already quite complex and widespread. This does not mean that those physicians and surgeons with direct or indirect university training renounced the practice of blood-letting with their own hands, but it was perhaps in the practical performance of phlebotomy that medieval social differences amongst medical practitioners were most in evidence. There can be no doubt that the opinion of Avicenna on phlebotomy as a universal medical treatment, as expressed in his *Canon*, strengthened and gave prestige to the practice of blood-letting in the course of the thirteenth and fourteenth centuries, and in effect it became the most usual therapeutic direction given by physicians, to the extent that it was explicitly included in the contracts that municipal councils drew up with physicians (*phisici*) and surgeons (*chirurgici*).[35] The widespread application and high frequency of phlebotomy must have caused numerous personal misadventures and unpleasant social events (the smell of rotting blood spilled in the street; the unpleasant sight of the receptacles in which blood was collected; the practice of phlebotomy by barbers in the street in full view of the public, and so on), and even led to intervention by the civil authorities.[36]

Such events prompted physicians to lay down therapeutic indications for phlebotomy, especially as regards the length of time during which it was to be performed, a matter of particular significance throughout the Middle Ages, as we shall see.[37] But references to such interventions reveal much about the social dimension of blood-letting, such as: the social spread of phlebotomy; the dominant role of the *barbitonsores* as regards its execution; the risks arising from it being poorly applied; even the doctrinal foundations upon which this simple technique rested; and the professional rivalry existing between the different groups of health 'professionals' (barbers, physicians and surgeons).[38] From the point of view of a university-trained surgeon like Henri de Mondeville, the situation in the first decade of the fourteenth century was that:

---

[35] An an example, see the text of the contract between the town of Castelló d'Empúries (Catalonia) and Master Bernat de Berriacho (29 November 1309), reproduced by M. McVaugh, 'Bernat de Berriacho (*fl.* 1301–43) and the *ordinacio* of Bishop Ponç de Gualba', *Arxiu de Textos Catalans Antics*, 9 (1990), 250–2.

[36] Arxiu Històric Municipal de Barcelona (AHMB), Consell de Cent, I-8, fol. 115v (27 February 1324 ?); Arxiu de la Corona d'Aragó, C, reg. 627, fol. 74v (22 October 1352). The same prohibitions also affected the blood-letting carried out by veterinary surgeons on beasts of burden, for example, AHMB, Consell de Cent, v-1, fol. 46r (27 February 1353); fol. 105 (11 January 1356), among others.

[37] On indication, see F. Kudlien and R. J. Durling, '"Endeixis" as a scientific term', in F. Kudlien and R. J. Durling (eds.), *Galen's method of healing* (Leiden, 1991), pp. 103–13.

[38] See Martínez Gázquez and García-Ballester, 'Las *Epistulae de flebotomia*', pp. 281–9.

Hardly anyone asks the surgeon for advice before being bled, except those who are suffering from surgical troubles; for the rich, the nobles and the prelates follow the advice of physicians, and the common people are sufficiently content with the barbers.[39]

Such prescription of phlebotomy by the barbers was not of the so-called preservative kind – that is to say, the variety that was performed on healthy individuals in spring or at the beginning of summer so as to avoid the appearance of illnesses caused by repletion – but true *therapeutic* blood-letting. It is significant, for example, that in 1322 the King of the Crown of Aragon, Alphonso the Benign, forbade the barbers of Valencia to bleed without the intervention of a physician on Egyptian days, on dog days and those on which the moon was in conjunction,[40] clear proof of the fact that, except on those days, barbers were indeed able to prescribe blood-letting, as well as carry it out. In fact, the relationship between phlebotomy and the time for which it was to last were subjects to which medieval Galenism paid particular attention and about which the population as a whole was especially sensitive. Indeed the question of the time bleeding should last gained so much importance that it finally became a limiting factor of the therapeutic technique itself: an error in timing could bring about the patient's death. It would seem that the wide spread of the Arab-Latin tradition of calendars (*calendaria*), which contained a simple, practical form of Galenism, was related to this concern. This was a very popular literary genre, which circulated in translations into Romance languages (for example Catalan), most probably by the thirteenth century and definitely in the fourteenth century. Barbers appear to have had access to this form of literature. In it, the mortal consequences of not observing the *tempora debita* (the due time) in phlebotomy were stressed. Curiously enough, the royal document addressed to the barbers of Valencia made use of terminology and arguments derived from these *calendaria*, a form of literature that brought Galenism down to the last link in a chain that offered medical attention to the population at large.[41]

The change in the barbers' function from being mere practitioners, and the adoption by them of the leading role in deciding whether phlebotomy was appropriate or not, must have taken place from the second half of the

---

[39] 'Quia pauci quaerunt a cyrurgicis consilium de fleubotomia facienda, nisi qui morbum cyrurgicum patiuntur, quoniam divites, nobiles et prelati in hoc casu acquiescunt consilio medicorum, et vulgares barberiis ut plurimum se committunt': *Chirurgia* (ed. Pagel), p. 366.

[40] 'Nullus barbitonsor de cetero audeat vel presumat civitate Valencie vel eius suburbiis, quecumque minuere sive flebotomare primis triginta diebus canicolaribus et etiam in illis diebus qui dicuntur egipciaci nec in plenilunio aut in contorn [*sic*] seu coniunccione Lune, nisi id necessitas evidens exigat aut de consilio medicorum': published by L. García-Balles-ter and M. R. McVaugh, 'Nota sobre el control de la actividad médica y quirúrgica de los barberos (*barbers, barbitonsores*) en los *Furs* de Valencia de 1329', *Homenatge al Doctor Sebastià García Martínez* (Valencia, 1989), p. 88.

[41] See Martínez Gázquez and García-Ballester, 'Las *Epistulae de flebotomia*'.

thirteenth century onwards. Various pieces of evidence allow us to deduce that throughout this period a gradual change came about as far as responsibility in the practice of phlebotomy was concerned: it changed from being a practice performed by members of the higher health professions and passed to those of lower rank. The words of two surgeons, Lanfranco de Milan (d. before 1306) and Henri de Mondeville (d. *c.* 1325) seem to point to this conclusion. The former blamed his colleagues for having lost the pre-eminent role in giving indications for phlebotomy to be carried out: 'Because of our pride, phlebotomy is today a trade that has been left to the hands of the barbers, whereas for the ancients it was a practice for physicians.'[42] Similarly, though offering an explanation that comes closer to the real cause of change, Henri de Mondeville said:

Physicians abandoned blood-letting to surgeons a long time ago, because they say it is an unworthy practice for them ... afterwards, the surgeons left this operation to barbers for two reasons: because it is a practice that provides little income and because there is little prestige attached to it and it is unimportant and only arises incidentally.[43]

These motives explain why physicians abandoned their responsibilities for phlebotomy. Partly it was because it was an *operatio manualis* that lowered their status to that of the unlearned surgeons, but also because of the small financial reward and limited prestige that performing it generated. The reasons why better-trained surgeons ceased to do it were similar. In this way it can be seen how, in the period under consideration, even though the therapeutic status of phlebotomy was raised, its practical application became more and more closely associated with the hands of the barbers. Phlebotomy, in spite of now being considered a form of evacuation (its medical status), continued to be considered, because of professional concerns, as the most routine *operatio manualis*.

DERIVATION AND REVULSION IN MEDIEVAL MEDICAL PRACTICE

The basic action of phlebotomy was successfully to evacuate the blood and the other humours that were mixed with it in the veins. This effect warranted it being described as a universal evacuant, as it was by Avicenna in the *Canon*,[44] for it had three simultaneous functions. In the first place, the effect of phlebotomy was the elimination from the veins of the mixture of

---

[42] 'Propter nostram superbiam phlebotomiae officium hodie barbitonsoribus fit relictum quod antiquitus erat medicorum opus': *Practica Magistri Lanfranci de Mediolano* (Venice, 1546), fol. 249r.

[43] 'Medici tamen ab antiquo operationem istam cyrurgicis reliquerunt propter indecentiam sicut dicunt, et forte aliud latet. Et ulterius istam operationem cyrurgici usque ad barberios repulerunt propter duos: primum quia est operatio pauci lucri; secundo quoniam ibi est magisterium paucum et leve et casuale': *Chirurgia* (ed. Pagel), pp. 363–4.

[44] 'Flebotomia est evacuatio universalis que multitudinem evacuat': *Canon*, lib. 1, fen 4, c. 20, fol. 73v.

humours contained in the blood. However, in addition, blood-letting achieved the evacuation of the blood itself, and was the only way of removing this humour from the body, perhaps, they thought, because of nature's resistance to losing the life-giving humour. Finally, and as a consequence of the particular disposition of the network of veins, therapeutic blood-letting made the evacuation of pathological matter from any organ of the body possible.

The main use of phlebotomy was to be found in those situations that exhibited plethora, that is to say those that were characterized by a considerable quantitative increase in the humours. However, its effect varied according to which blood vessel was opened, for opening a vein in proximity to the seat of the lesion did not produce the same effect as opening a distant vein. For, in the first case, the evacuating effect of phlebotomy was direct and almost exclusive; it eliminated the excess of humours or unhealthy matter that was responsible for the illness. But, in the second case, the alterations brought about in the volume of the humours as a whole had to be added to the first simple evacuative effect, as the humours were all set in motion by the opening of a route towards the exterior. For this reason, from antiquity onwards, physicians had distinguished two ways of carrying out phlebotomy, according to the distance between the point of incision and the focal point of the illness, known respectively as *derivation* and *revulsion*, and which in medieval writings were described by the terms 'attractive' and 'diversive'.

The concepts that corresponded to the terms derivation and revulsion appear to be closely related, in both ancient and medieval sources. That is to say, the characteristics that are used to define the one are always specified using the other as the starting point. Revulsion (*antispasis*) and derivation (*parokheteusis*) may be respectively translated by 'turn towards the other side, reject' and 'derive, put to one side'. Both terms are to be found in the Hippocratic writings, but the former appears quite frequently, whereas the latter appears in only two of the works in the collection: *Epidemics* and *On the humours*.[45]

The mention that occurs in the book of the *Epidemics* describes the way both practices had their effect:

Derivation towards the head or towards the sides, there where the humour tends to be, otherwise, revulsion: in disorders of the upper part, towards the lower; towards the upper part in those disorders that are lower.[46]

---

[45] See M. H. Marganne, 'Sur l'origine Hippocratique des concepts de révulsion et dérivation', *L'Antiquité Classique*, 49 (1980), 115–30, and Brain, *Galen on bloodletting*, pp. 113–21.

[46] References to writings from the *Corpus Hippocraticum* are always made, unless otherwise stated, according to the edition of E. Littré, *Œuvres complètes d'Hippocrate* (Paris, 1839–61). The volume is indicated by means of Roman numerals, while page numbers are shown by Arabic figures. In this case v, 284.

From this passage it can be deduced that derivation was a form of evacuation carried out according to the normal tendencies of the flow of the humours, whereas revulsion was associated with an idea of opposition or the diametrically opposite direction.

The different importance given to each of these two terms in the Hippocratic works raises certain difficulties. Was it due to the fact that derivative practices were less common than revulsive ones? Or was the omission of derivation as a technical term simply owing to the obvious nature of the action being carried out? The latter seems to be the correct explanation: derivative practices were so commonplace that they could be mentioned without technical details.[47] Nevertheless, it would seem that venesection did not occupy a place of importance in any of the Hippocratic works, nor did they offer a rational explanation of its use, or give precise instructions on where to use it.[48]

Galen, in contrast, made abundant use of phlebotomy, offered a rational explanation of it, supplied a wealth of information for its practice and systematized the indications for its use.[49] At various points in his works, Galen expounded the difference between the two methods, although references to revulsion are far more numerous than to derivation. In his commentary on *Epidemics*, the Hippocratic passage quoted above is glossed thus:

Moreover, if in any evacuation we are to bring about that kind of vomiting, he [Hippocrates] calls it 'revulsion'; exactly as we induce vomitings [by revulsion] by applying irritants to the uterus or the bladder or the fundament.[50]

In this passage he seems to let it be understood that revulsion functions by diverting the humours from the affected parts and directing them towards healthy areas. If derivation was a procedure in some way opposite to revulsion, then it must be concluded that carrying it out consisted of directing the flow of the humours from the healthy parts to the diseased ones. Taking this quotation as a starting point, some historians have gone so far as to state that the difference between the two types of evacuation lay in this.[51]

However, and as will be seen below, the difference between derivation and revulsion, rather than being associated with the healthy and infected parts, was related to the distance between the focal point of the lesion and

---

[47] See Marganne, 'Sur l'origine', p. 129.
[48] Brain, *Galen on bloodletting*, pp. 119–22.
[49] Ibid., pp. 122–57.
[50] 'At si in aliqua id genus evacuatione vomitum citaverimus, revulsionem hanc nominat, ut si vomitus etiam retraxerimus, ad uterum aut vesicam aut sedem incitantes': Galen's second commentary on the sixth book of the *Epidemics*. References to Galen's works are made by means of the edition prepared by C. G. Kühn, *Claudii Galeni opera omnia* (Leipzig, 1821–33), indicated by the initial K. The volume is indicated by Roman numerals, while Arabic figures show the page number. In this case: K XVIIA, 905–6.
[51] See Saunders and O'Malley, *Andreas Vesalius*, p. 13.

the point where the vein was cut. This idea is to be found clearly expressed at other places in Galen's works:

Derivation is carried out at neighbouring parts: as when that which is evacuated by the palate is led through the nostrils by derivation. And revulsion happens in the contrary way, as in a downward expulsion; just as that which flows through the fundament we derive through the uterus, and we revulse upwards.[52]

The relationship between derivation and revulsion and the varying distance from the affected point may be better appreciated from a further passage:

For example, we revulse the uterus if we bleed a vein in the elbow or if we place the cupping glasses below the breasts ... In contrast, derivation is carried out if we incise the veins of the legs or ankles or place the cupping glasses on the thighs.[53]

In this passage, referring to the treatment of amenorrhoea, Galen makes use of a single apparently injured organ as an example. Hence it is quite clear that the suitability of the different veins for bleeding depended only on the distance between them and the sick part of the body.

What line was followed by medieval Galenism when it came to practising blood-letting? Latin physicians, following the precepts of Arab Galenism, used both derivation and revulsion. But what happened was that they used a different terminology, and hence has arisen the difficulty in identifying their practice of the two kinds of phlebotomy.

Most of those Latin authors who dealt with phlebotomy between the late twelfth century and the first half of the fourteenth century – all those prior to the Latin translations made by Niccolò da Reggio from the Greek between 1308 and 1345 – were ignorant of Galen's principal book on the subject of blood-letting: the *De curandi ratione per venae sectionem*. Guy de Chauliac (*c.* 1290–*c.* 1367–70), in his *Chirurgia magna*, drawn up about 1361, seems to have been the first to consult it.[54] Many of them, however, clearly point out the existence of two forms of blood-letting, with quite precise indications for the use of each. The earliest of these, Henry of Winchester, in his *Tractatus de egritudinibus fleubotomandis*, distinguishes two types of phlebotomy; that carried out by *antispasis* and that performed by *metacente-*

---

[52] 'Derivatio ad vicinos locos fit, quum id quod per palatum vacuatur per nares derivatur; revulsio autem ad contraria, quum ad inferna revellitur. Rursus quod per sedem profluit, id per vulvam derivamus, sursum vero revellimus': *De methodo medendi*, lib. v, c. 3 (K x, 315).

[53] 'Ex utero verbi gratia revelles, si cubiti venam secueris aut sub mammis cucurbitulas admoveris ... Derivabis autem si quae in poplite sunt aut malleolis venas diviseris cucurbitulas femori admoveris ...': *Ad Glauconem de methodo medendi*, lib. II, c. 4 (K xI, 91).

[54] See M. S. Ogden, 'The Galenic works cited in Guy de Chauliac's *Chirurgia magna*', *Journal of the History of Medicine*, 28 (1973), 24–33, item 16. Arnau de Vilanova in his *Tractatus de consideracionibus* cites a *De flebotomia*, which must be identified with the *De curandi ratione per venae sectionem* (see note 115 below). However, such a general reference seems to have been made via an intermediate text, as occurs with other references to Galen's works to be found in works by Arnau. See García-Ballester, 'Arnau de Vilanova', pp. 154–6.

sis. The former is without doubt revulsion, and the terminology that he used is also to be found in the *Pantegni*, in which phlebotomy by means of *antispasis* is mentioned.[55]

For Henry of Winchester revulsive phlebotomy was defined thus: 'By *antispasis* is understood the situation in which phlebotomy is carried out on the opposite part.'[56] Other Latin writers spoke of the revulsive variety of phlebotomy, employing a wide variety of terms, the meanings of which were broadly similar: *distrahere,*[57] *trahere,*[58] *divertere,*[59] all of which were verbs that indicated the possibility of diverting the flow of the humours in a direction opposite to that in which they tended to go naturally. The aim of this practice was to avoid the concentration of humoral matter and, consequently, a possible putrefaction that might lead to an abscess. In his *Tractatus de consideracionibus operis medicine*, Arnau de Vilanova expounded this attribute of therapeutic bleeding:

Phlebotomy leads the humours to the point through which evacuation takes place; thus, in this respect, it is known to be useful in bodies in which it is necessary to lead the blood towards a different or opposite point, as occurs in bodies which are suffering from an intense plethora, in those in which an abscess is beginning to grow, or in those in which the blood is flowing in a particular part where it is feared that it might be very harmful, as happens in the case of those who spit blood because of a lung wound.[60]

Here the two therapeutic possibilities of revulsion are mentioned: (a) the diversion of the flow of humours which, by moving towards a particular point, tend to form an accumulation or deposit – a common situation in the case of hot abscesses of the thorax; and (b) the interruption of the natural flow of the humours (as in menstruation or haemorrhoidal flow) or of a pathological flow (such as epistaxis or haemoptysis).

[55] 'Oportet in initio si dolor ad furculas salierit basilica per antispasim phlebotomari ut materia ad opposita divertatur': *Pantegni, Practice*, lib. VI, c. 11, fol. 105rb. At a late date, in Johannes de Ketham's *Fasciculus medicinalis* very similar terms are used, and phlebotomy by means of *methatesis* and another form by *antifrasis* are mentioned.

[56] 'Per antispasim quando e contraria parte fit minutio; et dicitur antispasis quasi contraria decontractio', Voigts and McVaugh, *Tractatus de egritudinibus fleubotomandis*, p. 36.

[57] Thus Bernard de Gordon says: 'fit evacuacio et distractio': *De flebotomia*, MS Cues 308, fol. 27vb.

[58] Jean de St Amand states: 'Ut humores trahantur ad locum contrarium': *Expositio s. Antidotarium Nicolai*, MS Vat. Ap. Lat. 1205, fol. 74r.

[59] Maynus de Mayneriis says: 'fit ad divertendum et hoc si paciente fluxum sanguinis narium fit phlebotomia de saphenis': *Regimen sanitatis*, c. 37, in *Praxis medicinalis*, p. 52. Guy de Chauliac employed the same expression: 'Sex enim sunt intenciones propter quas fit utilis flebotomia. Prima est ad evacuandum, secundam ad divertendum . . . ': MS Bristol, Avon County Library, 10, fol. 231rb.

[60] 'Iterum eciam flebotomia trahit ad partem per quam evacuat, et ideo ex hac consideracione cognoscitur esse utilis corporibus in quibus necessarium est trahere sanguinem ad diversam vel oppositam partem, qualia sunt corpora maxime plectorica in quibus incipit generari apostema aut corpora in quibus fluit sanguis per aliquam partem ex quo timetur maxime nocumentum sicut in spuentibus sanguinem propter vulnus pulmonis': *Tractatus de consideracionibus operis medicine* (ed. Demaitre), pp. 146–7.

The choice of vein from which revulsion was to be carried out was a question of great interest. In his *De curandi ratione per venae sectionem*, Galen considered this problem and, with the support of the Hippocratic tradition, insisted that revulsion should be performed *kat'ixin*, that is to say 'on the same side as the lesion'.[61] As we have indicated, this work of Galen was not known prior to its translation from the Greek into Latin by Niccolò da Reggio. Thus earlier physicians (among them Arnau de Vilanova and Bernard de Gordon), had no access to it and had to use the 'corporeal diameters'.[62] The first to use these measurements was Arnau de Vilanova. We do not know the reasons for his choice, for we have not been able to locate a similar usage either in the Latin versions of Galen that he had access to or in any of the Arab authors that he was familiar with. But we can reconstruct what the corporeal diameters were. They essentially defined what was 'opposite' when revulsion was being practised. Up and down were opposite in vertical direction, front to back in horizontal direction. Left and right were equally opposites, as were inside and outside. In applying revulsion it was considered advisable in the majority of cases to follow the rule that prohibited using more than one 'opposite'; in other words, not to seek a distance produced by the combination of two diameters, such as, for example: up and right, if the focal point is to be found down and on the left. This is how this is explained by Maynus de Mayneriis in his *Regimen sanitatis*:

As far as revulsion is concerned, bear in mind that it should not be carried out more than one diameter away: from the right side to the left or from below towards the upper part, or the other way round. Phlebotomy should not be performed at a distance of two diameters unless plethora is intense.[63]

Although revulsion appears clearly in the medieval sources, it is not so easy to identify derivation. This is due to the fact that the way in which it was referred to in texts on phlebotomy was highly inconsistent. It has already been noted that Henry of Winchester used the expression *metacentesis* to indicate it, a term which he defined thus:

By *metacentesis`* is meant when blood is withdrawn on the same side as where the illness is to be found. For example, if there is *pleuresis* on the left-hand side,

---

[61] *De curandi ratione per venae sectionem*, K xi, 295–6; translated by Brain, *Galen on bloodletting*, p. 89.

[62] Arnau de Vilanova mentions this method of referring to the corporal dimensions in the *Speculum medicine*: 'Medici per quantitatem intelligunt hic, non genus predicamenti. Nam illud continet sub se numerorum et a tali quantitate non dividitur numeros, sed sumitur hec quantitas per mensura continui sed omnes dyametros que vocantur magnitudines. Iuxta modum quomodo quando solet quantum est istud corpus et respondetur bicubitum, tricubitum in longitudinale, unius autem cubiti in latitudini et palmi unius in spissitudine et sic de aliis': *Speculum medicine*, c. 83; *Opera* (Lyons, 1504), fol. 28rb.

[63] 'Et nota iuxta diversionem quod numquam est facienda diversio nisi per unam diametrum, puta a dextra in sinistra vel a deorsum sursum aut econtra; secundum enim duas diametros non est facienda phlebotomia nisi ubi esset maxima plenitudo': *Regimen sanitatis*, c. 37, in *Praxis medicinalis* (Lyons, 1586), p. 52.

blood-letting should be carried out from the left arm. *Metacentesis* means the same as 'lineal extraction'.[64]

The term *metacentesis* is translated as incision carried out on the body in order to evacuate blood, and it is documented for the first time in the Latin translation of the works of Oribasius, produced in the sixth century.[65] In medical texts on blood-letting, it can only be traced in the work of Henry of Winchester. In the writings of other medieval authors, derivation is expressed by the term *atrahere*,[66] which refers to the action of attracting the blood or the humours towards that part through which they are to be evacuated. There can be no doubt that this is the same derivative action as that mentioned by Galen, for the example used in order to demonstrate this action is identical: the treatment of amenorrhoea. The explanation supposes that when the suppression of menstrual flow has occurred, the treatment to be chosen is that of performing blood-letting on the *saphena* vein, as a result of which the periods will be restored. The proximity of the *saphena* to the organ which was supposedly disturbed and, above all, the fact that this vein collects the blood from those parts located below the liver[67] indicates that the form of phlebotomy being performed here was derivation. This last point becomes even clearer if we take into account the direct effect of drawing blood from this vein, as indicated by Avicenna: 'When the blood of the upper parts is made to go towards the lower ones, it provokes an intense menstrual flow and opens the orifices of haemorrhoids.'[68] The same indication can be found in another Arabic text that was widely used among medieval physicians, Rhazes' *Ad Almansorem*, and so it must be considered to have been widely practised.[69]

The choice of performing derivative or revulsive phlebotomy was decided in the practice of medieval physicians by a series of factors of

---

[64] 'Per metacentesim dicitur fieri quando ex eadem parte in qua est egritudo extrahitur sanguis, verbi gratia, si pleuresis sit in parte sinistra fiat minutio ex sinistro brachio. Metacentesis sonat tantum quantum linearis detractio': Voigts and McVaugh, *Tractatus de egritudinibus fleubotomandis*, p. 36.

[65] See *Thesaurus linguae latinae* (Leipzig, 1936–), VIII, col. 868.

[66] This is the case, for example, in the work of Jean de St Amand: 'Secunda causa indirecta quare fit est ut trahatur materia ad partem illam per quam debet evacuari materia. Unde retencione menstruum et emorroydarum debet aperiri saphena et secundum Galienum et secundum Avicennam ut trahatur materia sanguinis inferius', *Expositio supra Antidotarium Nicolai*, MS Vat. Ap. Palat. Lat. 1205, fol. 73v., and in Bernard de Gordon: 'Tercia consideracio quare fit flebotomia est quoniam atrahit, et ideo quando volumus revocare menstrua tunc trahimus sanguinem versus inferiora', *De flebotomia*, MS Cues 308, fol. 28ra.

[67] 'Ut evacuetur sanguis ex membris que sunt sub epate': Avicenna, *Canon*, lib. I, fen 4, c. 20, fol. 76rb.

[68] 'Et ut sanguis a partibus superioribus ad inferiores declinetur, quare menstrua vehementer provocat et emorroydarum orificia aperit': ibid.

[69] 'Venae vero que in poplitis curvatura subtus reperiuntur et vena que saphena vocatur phlebotomande sunt cum sanguis ad inferiorum corporis partem est trahendus et cum aegritudines huic accidentes parti sunt cronice, et in matrice ac renibus est dolor et cum menstruorum desideratur provocatio': *Ad Almansorem*, lib. VII, c. 21 (Basle, 1544), p. 174.

different importance. Knowledge of these will enable us to establish the existence of derivative practices in later medieval medicine.

The first of these is that indicated by the different temperament of the blood in each of the two halves of the body.[70] The physical explanation behind this presupposes the existence of a warmer temperament in the liver, the point of the second digestion, in comparison with the cold temper of the spleen, the home of the cold, dry humour. By allying this explanation with atmospheric 'temperament' during the seasons of the year, the medieval doctors evolved a doctrine which frequently appears in medieval treatises on phlebotomy: in spring and summer, it is preferable to perform phlebotomy on the right-hand side, since at that time of the year the warm humours, which are centred upon the liver, are predominant. By contrast, in autumn and winter it is advisable to bleed from the left-hand side, owing to the predominance of the cold humours.

The form of phlebotomy that was carried out in order to evacuate an overabundance of humours, so as to avoid them being deposited at one point and producing illness, was always of the derivative variety, as the only criterion used to prescribe it supposed the localization of the excess humoral mass. This type of blood-letting is what some sources call preservative or elective (*electa*);[71] other sources state that it was practised on healthy persons,[72] indicating that it should be prescribed without any illness being present, since it has a preventive function. There can be no doubt that, in medieval practice, the greater part of the blood-letting that took place must have been aimed at preventing the blood, in great abundance in spring, from producing disorders in the body. The reasons for the increase in blood at this time of the year were quite clear; since the qualities of spring were identical to those corresponding to blood as a cardinal humour, the production of blood was facilitated and its proportion in the mixture of the humours thus went up. But there was a further reason. Throughout the winter, and because of the cold, the second digestion was unable to generate enough of the humour blood, while, on the other hand, it produced large quantities of phlegm, which was considered to be nothing other than unconcocted blood. This cold, moist humour was stored in the joints and

---

[70] See P. Gil-Sotres, 'Sangre y patología en la medicina bajomedieval: el substrato material de la flebotomía', *Asclepio*, 38 (1986), 72–104, at 84–6.

[71] The classification of phlebotomy that is put forward in the *Canon* distinguishes between elective and necessary blood-letting. The former was preventive and was used to prevent the appearance of illnesses, and was usually performed above all in spring and autumn. The latter was made necessary by the presence of an illness. See *Canon*, lib. I, fen 4, c. 20.

[72] 'In sanis dico quod in tempore calido ut in vere et in estate magis abundant humores calidi in corpore et propter hoc ex illa parte ex qua abundant magis humores calidi debet fieri flebotomia haec autem est pars dextra. In tempore autem frigido abundant magis humores frigidi et propter hoc ex parte illa in qua abundant magis isti humores est flebotomandum haec autem est pars sinistra': J. L. Pagel (ed.), *Die Concordanciae des Johannes de Sancto Amando nach einer Berliner und zwei Erfurter Handschriften zum ersten Mal herausgegeben nebst einem Nachtrage über die Concordanciae des Petrus de Sancto Floro* (Berlin, 1894), p. 125.

on the arrival of spring, because of the increase in warmth, it was transformed into blood. The combined effect of these two rationales was what
made bleeding from a vein on the right-hand side of the body advisable
when springtime arrived, in order to reduce the volume of blood. Such
advice was repeated in medieval monastic customaries, among various
kinds of sources,[73] but it was also included in medical texts.

Similarly, the statements of Maynus de Mayneriis, when he mentioned
that the left- or right-hand side was to be chosen in accordance with age
and constitution,[74] should be understood in the same light. The predominance of thick, cold humours, typical of autumn and winter, of old
age and of cold constitutions, is relieved by blood-letting on the left-hand
side. The presence of warm, subtle blood would advise, by contrast,
employing evacuation on the right-hand side. This rule, which came to be
preserved in certain well-known lines of the *Regimen sanitatis salernitanum*,[75]
was still referring to preventive bleeding, since the presence of an illness
meant the suspension of such criteria in order to make way for the
consideration of other aspects: fundamentally those arising from the localization of the problem, the existence or otherwise of plethora and the
development of the illness.

As regards the first of these criteria, it is logical to think that physicians
associated the healing effect of phlebotomy with its proximity to the focal
point of the illness. If it was primarily a question of evacuating an
accumulation of a substance, it was clear that a blood vessel had to be
sought that could evacuate the blood from this part of the body. If we turn
to the indications for making the incision in the various veins and their
relationships with particular illnesses,[76] we shall see that on numerous
occasions it was recommended that a vessel located in the vicinity of the
point of lesion – the characteristic that defined derivative blood-letting –
should be used. The cephalic vein was indicated as the most suitable vein for
curing disorders located in the area of the skull or face, because it could
evacuate that area.[77] The left and right basilic veins allowed blood to be

[73] A wide sample of this type of practice can be found in L. Gougaud, 'La pratique de la
   phlébothomie dans les cloîtres', *Revue Mabillon*, 13 (1924), 1–13.
[74] 'Prima consideratio est quod in parte frigidiori temporis, scilicet in hyemi vel iuxta debet
   fieri phlebotomia de parte sinistra, et in parte opposita in estate dextra partis, et universaliter si ex regimine vel complexione naturali aut aetate, nos percipiamus sanguinem esse
   grossum et melancholicum est phlebotomandum ex sinistra parte. Et per oppositum si
   percipiamus sanguinem esse subtilem et calidum et cholericum ex parte dextra est
   phlebotomandum': *Regimen sanitatis*, c. 37, in *Praxis medicinalis*, p. 52.
[75] 'Aestas ver dextras, hyems autumnusque sinistras': *Regimen sanitatis salernitanum*, in S. De
   Renzi (ed.), *Collectio salernitana*, 5 vols. (Naples, 1852–9), vol. v, p. 503.
[76] In this respect, my introduction to the *Tractatus de consideracionibus operis medicine*, in vol. IV
   of *Arnaldi de Villanova Opera medica omnia*, especially pp. 95–105, might be consulted.
[77] 'Ista autem vena copiosius evacuat sanguinem a partibus que sunt supra furculam pectoris
   superiorem quam alie due principales, et ideo plus illis prodest in passionibus illarum
   parcium; et cum a capite sanguinem potencius evacuet quam alie due, ideo eciam respectu

evacuated from the spleen and liver respectively, and they were the veins used in the illnesses centred upon these organs. In all these cases, and in many others, the action sought by means of phlebotomy was always derivative. Examples of this type are abundant in those parts of medical treatises devoted to specific illnesses.

The next factor that concerned later medieval physicians was the existence of plethora. If the volume of the humours had risen, but they maintained the right and proper proportions within the humoral mass as a whole, revulsive phlebotomy was always to be performed. As has already been noted, in order to make the choice of vein the opposite side of one of the corporal diameters was sought, or several of them if plethora in the body was particularly high.[78] Otherwise – that is to say, if one humour was predominant – prior to bleeding it was necessary to reduce the humour by means of specific purges, thereby correcting the balance of the mixture.

Another criterion used to determine on which side phlebotomy was to be carried out, and thus determining the decision between derivation and revulsion, was that deduced from the state of the disordered matter. Two situations were distinguished. The first corresponded to the moment when the matter was flowing (*fluens*), and in this case revulsion had to be carried out. In contrast, if the matter was already localized (*materia fluxa*), the evacuation had to be performed on the same side, in other words, by means of derivation.[79]

Both the state of the matter and the existence of or absence of an abscess had an immediate connection with the *tempus morbi*, in other words, with the different phases of the illness. The physician would consider the side on which the incision was to be performed on the basis of the stage of the illness. At the beginning, he would practise revulsion, while in the static phase and during its decline he would employ derivation. In the same way, in acute illnesses revulsion was prescribed, whereas in chronic ones the practice of derivation was recommended.[80]

In order to complete the list of all the eventualities that the healer might face, a further case needs to be added. If the substance that brought on the symptoms was poisonous and produced 'by the bite of a dangerous animal, such as a snake or a scorpion'[81] or if it was uncontrolled and violent – 'furious' as Henry of Winchester described it – as in the case of anthrax,[82]

---

illarum capitalis vel cephalica meruit nominari': *Tractatus de consideracionibus operis medicine*, p. 155.

[78] See note 63.

[79] Arnau de Vilanova, *Compendium regimenti acutorum, Praxis medicinalis*, p. 181.

[80] 'Si inveterata fuerit egritudo, debet fieri per metacentesim, si recens per antispasim': Voigts and McVaugh, *Tractatus de egritudinibus fleubotomandis*, p. 36.

[81] 'Preterea si quis punctus fuerit a venenoso animali, ut a serpente vel scorpione, fiat per metacentesim si indigeat flebotomia': ibid.

[82] 'Additur ad predictam consideracionem quod si materia fuerit furiosa, sicut in antrace, licet corpus sit plectoricum, debet fieri per metacentesim ne materia furiosa trahatur ad membra nobilia': ibid. And 'Si membrum cretica non gravetur collectione vel materia

then, even though plethora was present, blood-letting was to be derivative to prevent the substance from being carried to other parts of the body, thereby causing greater harm in them.

There is, then, ample evidence for the existence of the two forms of phlebotomy in medieval medical practice. The difficulties involved in identifying derivative practices, owing to the terminology used by these writers, and the hostile and pejorative attitude of Renaissance physicians towards the Middle Ages might go far towards explaining the incorrect interpretation that has hitherto been made of their professional activity and the continued ignorance of the theoretical reasons which served as their justification.

MEDIEVAL TREATMENT OF PLEURITIS OR 'PAINS IN THE CHEST OR SIDE'

It has already been pointed out that medieval Latin physicians prior to Guy de Chauliac (1361) did not have access to Galen's principal work devoted to phlebotomy, the *De curandi ratione per venae sectionem*, and this was the reason why knowledge of the theoretical foundations of therapeutic blood-letting had to be acquired through other works. The largely unsystematic nature of Galen's lengthy works make it necessary to gather together the scattered information about phlebotomy that Galen had left. It cannot be doubted that the key text for providing access to Galen's doctrine on phlebotomy was the *De ingenio sanitatis* (also known as *De methodo medendi*), which supplied the greater part of the information necessary to establish his instructions about blood-letting.[83] Other information on Galen's views on blood-letting was to be found in his *Ad Glauconem de methodo medendi*, and his commentary on the *Aphorisms* of Hippocrates. However, another Galenic work of importance in connection with the subject under study also existed. I am referring here to the *Commentum super regimentum acutorum morborum Hippocratis*.

The medieval tradition of the Hippocratic *Regimen acutorum morborum* and that of the *Commentum* written by Galen are poorly known to us. The oldest manuscripts of the original Hippocratic text, possibly translated by Constantine, are datable to no earlier than the twelfth century. From 1260,

venenosa, flebotomandus est eger per venas longinquiores oppositionis unius dyametri, vel multarum si fuerit corpus plectoricum. Morbo vero confirmato et fluxu cessante per venas propinquiores.': Arnau de Vilanova, *Medicationis parabolae* (ed. Paniagua), IV, rule 46, p. 63.

83 The *De ingenio sanitatis* is the most frequently cited book of Galen in Bernard de Gordon's *De flebotomia*, with thirty-four explicit references. Similarly, in Arnau de Vilanova's *Tractatus de consideracionibus operis medicine*, it is cited seven times, the highest number for any of Galen's works. In the fragment on phlebotomy of the *Expositio super Antidotarium Nicolai* by Jean de St Amand, there are seventeen explicit references, although in this case under the title of *Megategni*, which makes it the most cited text of Galen in this case as well.

it often appears in association with the commentary produced by Galen,[84] the translation of which is attributed to Constantine and to Gerard of Cremona.[85]

During the thirteenth century both works appeared in contexts closely linked with university teaching, and are sometimes found in the manuscripts which include the *Articella* texts.[86] From the second half of that century, they became obligatory reading within the medical curriculum. An anonymous commentary is dated 1257,[87] and three further commentaries by well-known writers must have been composed at a not very much later date; these were the *Abbreviatio* that Jean de St Amand included in the *Revocativum memoriae*,[88] and the commentaries of Petrus Hispanus[89] and of Taddeo Alderotti.[90] From the year 1270 the text figures in the programme of obligatory reading at the University of Paris,[91] which explains the existence of numerous Parisian commentaries. If we look more closely at Montpellier, the Hippocratic *Regimen acutorum morborum* is recorded in the list of texts that had to be commented upon in the faculty of medicine, according to what was laid down in Pope Clement V's Bull of 1309,[92] but by then it must have formed part of the material expounded in the lecture halls for many years. Magister Cardinalis wrote a commentary on this same work,[93]

---

[84] See P. Kibre, *Hippocrates Latinus*, pp. 7–18.

[85] See K. Sudhoff, 'Die kurze "Vita" und Verzeichnis der Arbeiten Gerhards von Cremona, von seinen Schülern und Studiengenossen kurz nach dem Tode des Meisters (1178) zu Toledo verabfasst', *Archiv für Geschichte der Medizin*, 8 (1914), 72–82, at 78; R. Durling, 'A chronological census of Renaissance editions and translations of Galen', *Journal of the Warburg and Courtauld Institutes*, 24 (1961), 230–305, n. 160.

[86] See P. O. Kristeller, *Studi sulla scuola medica salernitana* (Naples, 1986), pp. 109–15.

[87] The *incipit* is as follows: 'Rationes super libro de regimine acutorum. Materia istius libri de regimine acutorum est docere modum curationis illarum acutarum egritudinum.' See Kibre, *Hippocrates Latinus*, p. 19.

[88] *Incipit*: 'In libro acutorum determinatur de cura febrium acutarum et regimine earum.' See Kibre, *Hippocrates Latinus*, p. 23; L. Thorndike and P. Kibre, *A catalogue of incipits of mediaeval scientific writings in Latin*, 2nd edn (London, 1963), col. 689. It was published as a doctoral dissertation by F. Petzold, 'Von des Lebens Ordnung in akuten Krankheiten nebst dem Schluss des "Revocativum Memoriae" des Johann von St Amand' (University of Berlin, 1894).

[89] *Incipit*: 'Quoniam ut ait philosophus in libro analecticorum omnis doctrina . . . ' See Kibre, *Hippocrates Latinus*, p. 24; Wickersheimer, *Dictionnaire biographique*, pp. 638–40; G. Beaujouan, 'Manuscrits médicaux du Moyen Age conservés en Espagne', *Mélanges de la Casa de Velázquez*, 8 (1972), 195; Thorndike and Kibre, *Catalogue*, col. 1307.

[90] Printed in *Expositiones in Arduum aphorismorum Ipocratis Opus . . .* (Venice, 1527).

[91] H. Denifle and A. Chatelain (eds.), *Chartularium Universitatis Parisiensis*, vol. I, Paris, 1889, p. 517.

[92] See A. Germain (ed.), *Cartulaire de l'Université de Montpellier*, Montpellier, 1890, vol. I, p. 220.

[93] The title is as follows: *Scripta supra Regimentum acutorum Hippocratis*, and its *incipit*: 'Quoniam ut Avicenna in primo canonis . . .' See Thorndike and Kibre, *Catalogue*, col. 1308; Wickersheimer, *Dictionnaire biographique*, pp. 94–5; Jacquart, *Supplément*, p. 53.

and, at a later date, Arnau de Vilanova[94] and Bernard de Gordon were to do the same, the latter's work being dated 1294.[95]

In the second book of the *Regimen acutorum morborum* the Hippocratic writer, when dealing with the treatment of pleuritis (*pleuresis*), slips in a very brief observation about phlebotomy. The conciseness of this reference and its general nature would have meant it passing unnoticed had not Galen made use of this point to develop in his own commentary a lengthy description of the veins of the trunk and the arms. In this way, a passage that was almost anodyne became a focal point of overwhelming interest for a scholarly community which lacked direct access to the great books of anatomy written by Galen. Even so, we should not lose sight of the fact that phlebotomy, both in Galen's view and for the medieval Galenists, did not depend so much on the anatomical structure of the network of veins itself (although this also had its role to play, as will be seen shortly) as on ideas about how veins worked, about blood and its movement along the veins. It should be sufficient to recall, for example, that their ideas about the movement of blood were very different from modern ones. Not only did they consider that blood moved in the veins in the opposite direction to what we believe today, but also that it did so at a very slow rate.[96]

The coincidence, in the same Galenic text, both of anatomical details and also of observations concerning phlebotomy, gave university professors of the second half of the thirteenth century new arguments with which to justify phlebotomy on the same or the opposite side. As will be seen below, Bernard de Gordon supported his statement to the effect that in the case of *pleuresis* it was a matter of indifference whether bleeding took place from one arm or the other on the basis of Galen's words, since the veins that feed the side of the pleura start at the same level of the vena cava. Arnau de Vilanova demonstrated similar interest in this same fragment of the Galenic text, basing his analysis of the way phlebotomy acted on this anatomical account.[97]

The passage on phlebotomy included by the Hippocratic writer was, as has been noted, singularly brief:

[94] Edited in the Renaissance, it occupies fol. 207 of the *editio princeps*, and fol. 208 in the parallel editions of Lyons. Its title is *Compendium regimenti acutorum*, and the *incipit*, 'Nota quod quinque sunt consideraciones ...' We have been able to locate the following manuscript copies: Erfurt, F. Ampl., F 264, thirteenth century, fols. 8v–9ra (incomplete); Venice, Marciana ZL DXXXVIII, fourteenth century, fols. 3r–3v; Paris, BN Lat. 7031, fifteenth century, fols. 18r–23v; Munich, Bayerische Staatsbibl. CLM 7576, fifteenth century, fols. 85r–86v; Seville, B. Colombina, 5-1-45, fifteenth century, fols. 42r–43v; Lübeck, Stadtbibl. med. 4°, 10, fifteenth century, fols. 191–2v; Wolfenbüttel, Herzog August B., 2841, fifteenth century, fols. 80v–81v; Vatican, B. Apost., Palat. Lat. 1211, fifteenth century, fols. 27ra–27va; Palat. Lat. 1229, fifteenth century, fols. 251r–252v; Palat. Lat. 1180, fifteenth century, fols. 113r–114r.
[95] See Demaitre, *Doctor Bernard de Gordon*, p. 39.
[96] Brain, *Galen on bloodletting*, pp. 154–7.
[97] See note 117.

And when the pain extends towards the clavicle, or heaviness in the armpit or towards the breast or the diaphragm occurs, then it is well to let blood from the vein that is called basilic.[98]

As can be seen, this reference to the basilic vein does not specify whether the blood-letting should be carried out on the same side as the affected part or on the opposite side. Galen was to pour all his erudition into this text, expanding and defining the words of the Hippocratic writer:

When the pain extends towards the upper limbs, it is well to bleed from the veins that are in the angle of the arm; veins through which it is possible to draw from the blood which is in the unhealthy organ in large quantities and quickly in the opposite direction to that in which it tends.[99]

Thereafter he provides a lengthy explanation of the anatomy of the veins, with a description of the azygous system and of the area it irrigates, establishing a relationship between the pain that appears in pleuritis ('pains in the side or chest') and the tracing of the blood that is to be evacuated.

The option followed by Galen in the treatment of *pleuresis* was to favour revulsive phlebotomy, since he was inclined towards performing evacuation on the vein on the side opposite to the seat of the illness. Galen's efforts to find an anatomical justification to support the instruction to bleed on the opposite side do not seem to have produced positive results, if we take into account the later development of the question. But resting on his authority, the consistent aim of Arab Galenism was to endeavour to guide the disturbed matter to the opposite side.

In the *Canon*, Avicenna proposed that the following treatment should be chosen in the case of abscesses of the thorax:

At the beginning phlebotomy should be carried out on the opposite side and more quickly from the saphenous vein opposed in longitude, and after this from the basilic opposite in latitude ... Then, after several days, once again from the appropriate side in latitude.[100]

That is to say, he interpreted Galen's words 'on the opposite side' by bringing into play the sagittal plane, which includes the view that the saphenous vein is the greatest degree of opposition. However, other representatives of Arab Galenism provided different interpretations of the Galenic text. Haly Abbas offered the following treatment:

---

[98] 'Et quando pervenit dolor ad furculam aut accidit in asse id gravitas aut versus mamillam aut diafragmate, tunc oportet ut flobothomes venam que nominatur basilica'. *Regimen acutorum Hippocratis cum commento Galeni*, in *Articella* (Venice, 1523), fol. 10v.

[99] 'Quando ergo extenditur dolor versus membra alta, tunc oportet ut minuamus ex venis que sunt in curvatura manus, venam per quam possibile est attrahere ex sanguine qui est in membro infirmo ad contrarium partis ad quam declinat quantitatem multam cum velocitate': ibid.

[100] 'Sed in principio ex latere diverso et magis festina de saphena opposita in longitudine et post ipsam de basilica opposita in latitudine ... Deinde post aliquot dies ex latere conveniente in latitudine': *Canon*, lib. III, fen 10, trac. V, c. 1, fol. 254ra.

It is well to phlebotomize at the beginning, if the pain is radiating out towards the clavicle, from the basilic vein by *antispasis*, so that the matter may be taken to the opposite side. If, on the other hand, the matter remains unmoving, bleeding is to take place according to which side is affected.[101]

And Rhazes, in Book I of his *Liber divisionum*, said this of the treatment of *pleuresis*: 'Its cure requires phlebotomy on the basilic vein of the opposite side; later bleeding is to be repeated on the same side as the pain, on the third day.'[102]

The three great Arab physicians thus divided the treatment of *pleuresis* into two stages: at the beginning of treatment they firmly favoured bleeding on the opposite side, with the opposed point being determined either by the sagittal or the transversal axis; they left the recommendation to bleed on the same side for a later moment: three days for Rhazes; when the matter fell still in the case of Haly Abbas.

These ideas were expressed in a similar way by medieval Latin physicians. Thus Jean de St Amand, in his *Abbreviatio* of Galen's commentary, which he included in his *Revocativum memoriae*, was not intimidated by the complications involved in determining the veins to be used:

In the second chapter, which begins 'when the pain radiates towards the shoulder blades', Galen determines the way to cure pleuritis by means of phlebotomy, stating that if the pain radiates towards the shoulder blades and there exists heaviness over the diaphragm, blood-letting is to take place. If you ask from which vein, Hippocrates answers from the basilic . . . Galen, wishing to define the reason why in pleurisy phlebotomy is carried out from the basilic, expounds the anatomy of the veins and what he says is obvious.[103]

But in his *Concordancie* he offers what seems to be his own vision of the treatment of abscesses when there is plethora:

In the cure of abscesses, when the body is suffering from plethora, it is well to do four things; first, evacuate all the body; secondly, attract the matter to the opposite side; thirdly, push the matter back towards another point; fourthly, evaporate the residues that may remain at that point by means of hot aperients at a distance. But

---

[101] 'Oportet in initio si dolor furculas salierit basilicam per antispasim phlebotomari ut materia ad opposita divertatur. Si vero materia quiescat phlebotomari secundum infirmum locum': *Pantegni, Practice*, lib. VI, c. 11, fol. 105r.

[102] 'Et cura eius est phlebotomia basilice ex latere opposito, deinde iteratio phlebotomie ex latere doloris in die tertia . . . ': *Liber divisionum*, lib. I, c. 54 (Basle, 1544), p. 375.

[103] 'In 2° capitulo quod incipit quando ergo dolor ad spatulas ascendendo jam saltus compleverit etc. determinat de cura pleuresis per flebotomiam dicens quod si dolor ascendat usque ad spatulas et sit gravitas super diafragma flebotomia est facienda; si quaeras de qua vena respondet Hippocrates de basilica; si quaeras quantum respondet Hippocrates tantum ut sanguis mutetur in splendidum ruborem aut ex rubore in nigredinem. Galenus volens ponere causam quare fiat in pleuresi flebotomia de basilica ponit anatomiam venarum et patet quod dicit intuenti': *Revocativum memoriae, liber acutorum* (ed. Petzold), p. 19.

understand that this must be done before pus is produced, that is, at the beginning of the disease or in the phase of development.[104]

As can be seen, St Amand maintained the criterion of opposition when it came to performing blood-letting, but he specified something else concerning the phase in which such opposition was correct: 'before pus is produced'.

More problems arise from the analysis of the attitude of Bernard de Gordon, who at three different places in his medical output offers different versions of the same treatment. These works are the *Commentum super regimentum acutorum morborum Hippocratis*,[105] the *Compendium* of the same work addressed to Johannes de Confluente,[106] and the chapter devoted to the treatment of *pleuresis* in the *Lilium medicine*.[107]

In the *Commentum* Bernard established the following specifications in the treatment of *pleuresis*:

Pleuresis develops either with or without bodily plethora. If it develops with plethora, the pain may radiate towards the upper part or downwards. If it radiates upwards the illness may be confirmed or not.[108]

It was pointed out by St Amand that a 'confirmed illness' (*egritudo confirmata*) had the greatest need of an indication of the phase in which intervention should take place. It must (he said) be performed at the moment when the matter changes from being *in fieri* or flowing (*fluens*) to being the matter *in facto esse* or fluid (*fluxa*). The expression 'confirmed illness' expresses the moment when the illness has become established, a situation which is manifested to the physician by the appearance of disturbed, totally transformed matter. Bernard de Gordon went on to say:

If the pain radiates upwards, and plethora exists and the illness is not confirmed, phlebotomy should be from the basilic vein, either right or left. For pleurisy in another part, there is no difference.[109]

---

[104] 'In cura apostematis corpore repleto oportet ut fiant quattuor: Primum, evacuatio totius corporis. Secundum, attractio ad partem oppositam. Tertium, repulsio materiei ad locum alium. Quartum, evaporatio residui quod in loco remanet per calida aperientia distantia sed intellige ista, antequam fiat sanies, scilicet, in principio vel augmento': *Concordanciae* (ed. Pagel), p. 20.

[105] For the manuscripts and editions of this book, see Demaitre, *Doctor Bernard de Gordon*, pp. 191–2.

[106] See ibid., p. 175. Demaitre does not make any reference to the copy I have made use of: MS Cues 308, fols. 105rb–106ra, perhaps because its text continues after, but without any break, that of the *Regimen acutorum*, to which he does, however, refer.

[107] For the manuscripts and editions, see ibid., pp. 185–8.

[108] 'Nunc autem pleuresis est cum plenitudo corporis aut sine. Si cum plenitudine, aut dolor ascendit aut descendit. Si ascendit aut egritudo est confirmata aut non': *Compendium regiminis acutorum*, MS Cues 308, fol. 103vb.

[109] 'Si dolor ascendit et corpus est plectoricum et egritudo non est confirmata fiat flebotomia de basilica utrum autem dextra aut de sinistra. Pleuresi existente in altera parte tantum non est differentia': ibid.

The reason that Bernard considered the incision of the basilic vein to be beneficial, independent of the point where the lesion was located, is anatomical-physiological in nature. Taking as his starting point Galen's commentary on the Hippocratic *Regimen acutorum morborum*, he maintained that the veins that 'feed' the upper ribs spring from the vena cava at the same level. This means that the inflamed point will be the same distance from the trunk of the vena cava, whether it is located on the left or on the right, since the veins that join both parts are identical: that they will provoke the same movement of the humours.[110]

In the *Compendium*, which often accompanies the *Commentum* in the manuscript sources, and the suspicious similarity of which to Arnau de Vilanova's comparable text I have pointed out elsewhere,[111] the treatment recommended for *pleuresis* is different: 'If the matter is flowing, phlebotomy is to be carried out from the basilic vein on the same side. If the matter is fluid, then it is best to do so from the median vein on the same side.'[112] This clearly disagrees with what is stated in the *Commentum* and with the medieval tradition, since what is proposed in both cases is derivative practices against the common application of revulsion in the early stages. However, when he produced the *Lilium medicine* in 1305, he returned to the fold of Latin physicians who were followers of Avicenna. In that work when giving details on the treatment of *pleuresis*, he was to say:

In pleuresis, if plethora is present and the strength is intact, at first carry out the phlebotomy, following Avicenna, from the saphenous vein on the same side; later, if plethora persists, from the basilic on the opposite side, and later, perform from the basilic on the same side.[113]

And in the *Recapitulatio* that closes the text he says:

It remains, then, that at the beginning, if plethora is present, phlebotomy should be carried out from the basilic on the opposite side or from the saphenous vein on the same side; later perform it on the same side.[114]

---

[110] 'Si igitur vena magna ad modum putei per medium pectori ascendit dextra et sinistra basilica equaliter et nulla basilicarum haurit ex minera, si ex puteo medii pectoris tunc restat quod corpore plectorico dolore ascendente egritudine nondum confirmata equale est pleuresi existente in altera parte si fiat de dextra vel sinistra': *Commentum super regimentum acutorum*, MS Cues 308, fols. 103vb–104ra.

[111] See P. Gil-Sotres, 'Sangre y patología en la medicina bajomedieval: la obra de flebotomía de Arnau de Vilanova', Ph.D. thesis (Universidad de Navarra, Pamplona, 1984), pp. 227–36.

[112] 'Hic si materia sit in fluxu de basilica eiusdem partis. Si materia sit fluxa tunc competit de mediana eiusdem partis': *Compendium*, MS Cues 308, fol. 105va.

[113] 'In pleuresi igitur corpore pleno et virtute forti fiat primo flebotomia secundum Avicennam de safena eiusdem lateris; deinde si plenitudo adest de basilica oppositi lateris, deinde de basilica eiusdem lateris': *Lilium medicine*, lib. IV, c. 9.

[114] 'Restat igitur quod in principio corpore plectorico existente debet fieri flebotomia de basilica oppositi lateris aut de saphena eiusdem partis, postea fiat de eadem parte': ibid.

Let us now consider what Arnau de Vilanova's attitude towards this subject was. In the *Tractatus de consideracionibus operis medicine* he stated, as has already been noted, that he had adopted an original position when faced with this problem:

That the aforementioned veins have, as has been said, a different capacity for evacuating the organs of the body can be proved by anatomical dissection, in which the origin or ramification and course of the veins becomes evident. I have already written in detail on this point in the exposition of Galen's commentary on the second part of 'Regimen in acute diseases'. There I have shown in what way, in phlebotomy, the opposition of the part has to be taken into account according to the true and solid arguments of Hippocrates and Galen there, and also in the book 'On phlebotomy'; I have found that no one among the Latins has understood them on this matter.[115]

Unfortunately, not all the text of Arnau's commentary of the *Regimen acutorum morborum* survives.[116] In other, better preserved, texts Arnau shows himself to be another follower of the common doctrine. In the so-called *Compendium regimenti acutorum morborum* he maintains that, in the case of abscesses of the thorax, phlebotomy should be practised only when plethora is in existence. In this case, if the matter is flowing (*fluens*), revulsion is to be carried out, while if it has already settled (*in facto esse*), the correct procedure would be to perform derivation.[117] The doctrine

---

[115] 'Quod autem supradicte vene tam differenter ut dictum est habeant potenciam evacuandi membra corporis probatur ex anathomiis in quibus origo seu ramificacio et transitus ipsarum ostenditur. Nos autem perfecte scripsimus illud in secunda parte regimenti acutorum super exposicione commenti Galieni, ubi eciam ostendimus qualiter in flebotomiis opposicio partis sumenda sit secundum vera et solida fundamenta Ypocratis et Galieni ibidem et eciam in libro de flebotomia, circa quod eos intellexisse neminem latinorum invenimus': *Tractatus de consideracionibus operis medicine* (ed. Demaitre), p. 157. See note 54 above.

[116] In addition to the *Compendium regiminis acutorum*, which figures in the Renaissance editions, there exist three further unpublished commentaries on the 'Regimen for acute diseases' attributed to Arnau de Vilanova. One, entitled *Regimen acutorum*, is anonymous, and begins: 'Intencio Ypocratis in libro regimenti acutorum est . . . '; it was copied in the fourteenth century (Erfurt B. Ampl. Q 368, fols. 88–93r) and is a commentary on the Hippocratic text and not on its Galenic gloss. Another has the title *Lectura venerabili Arnoldi de Nova Villa super regimentis acutorum* (Paris, B. Arsenal 709, fifteenth century, fols. 2r–4v), of which only a fragment is preserved, and which is a gloss on Galen's commentary on the Hippocratic text. And finally, a commentary under the name of Francisco de Cenellis, in the colophon of which the following detail is given by Amplonius von Berka: 'Finitus est tractatus de regimine acutorum febricitancium excerptus ab inmensa profunditate et prolixitate subtili doctoris Arnoldus de Villanova' (Erfurt, B. Ampl. Q 224, fifteenth century, fols. 102v–109r), which follows the *Compendium regiminis acutorum* almost literally.

[117] 'Flebotomia autem competit in apostematibus, sed distinguendo aut corpus est plectoricum aut non, si not sit plectoricum non competit. Si sit plectoricum et dolor ascendit ad spatulam distinguo, aut materia est fluxa aut fluens, si fluens fiat flebotomia ex parte opposita primo de basilica postea de mediana. Si materia sit fluxa facimus flebotomiam ex eadem parte primo de basilica postea de mediana': *Compendium regimenti acutorum, praxis medicinalis* (Lyons, 1586), p. 181.

gathered together in the aphorisms called *Medicationis parabolae*[118] is similar: revulsion at the start of the illness, if plethora is present; derivation in the static phases and those of decline, once the flow has ceased. Therefore, provided no other commentary comes to light, and in view of the fact that the date of composition of the *Medicationis parabolae* is late, I consider that the words of the *Tractatus de consideracionibus* should not be taken into account.

Finally, when Taddeo Alderotti put before his students the *quaestio*: 'On what side should phlebotomy be carried out, on the same side or on the opposite one?',[119] he made the choice of the side on which blood-letting was to take place subject to two variables: the intensity of plethora, and the movement of the humours. Thus, at the beginning of the illness, when plethora was greater and there was an intense mobility of the humours, he recommended revulsion; and when plethora was diminishing and the disturbed humours settled in the affected part, he recommended revulsion.[120]

As we have now had opportunity to demonstrate, the treatment used by medieval physicians in the case of *pleuresis* or 'pains in the side or chest' demonstrates the existence of derivative practices with which they resolutely acted on the mobility of the humours. The name that this form of blood-letting received was different from that given to it in classical antiquity and in the Renaissance, which might explain why it was not always recognized as such by certain Renaissance physicians or by those historians who have approached the field of medieval medicine via the version offered by the Renaissance physicians.

THE PRACTICE OF BLOOD-LETTING IN THE MIDDLE AGES

In order to get closer to what was – or might have been – the practice of blood-letting we shall concentrate on the recommendations formulated by the writers – in particular the masters of Montpellier – of what we call the second period, the transition from the thirteenth to the fourteenth centuries. In every case, the description of blood-letting commences by referring to two elements: the 'illumination' of the place where it was to be carried out[121] and the qualities that the person who was to perform it should be in possession of. And here it was specified that he should have a

---

[118] See note 82 above. *Medicationis parabolae* (ed. Paniagua), IV, 46: 'Infra primum dyatritum rarissime fluxus cessat et plectoria frequenter occurrit; quapropter, ut plurimum, in eo longinquior oppositio servit flebotomie', ibid. IV, 47.

[119] 'Ex quo latere debetur fieri flobotomia, utrum ex eodem latere vel diverso': *Thaddei Florentini expositiones ... in praeclarum regiminis acutorum Ipocratis opus ...* (Venice, 1527), fol. 278va.

[120] 'Ad quod dicit quod hic satis potest intelligi per quantitatem plectorie et per motum humorum; nam existente plectoria multa et humoribus existentibus in motu competit ex latere contrario; sed plectoria existente pauca et humorum quiete tunc competit ex latere eodem': ibid.

[121] 'Quod locus sit luminosus: *De flebotomia*, MS Cues 308, fol. 28rb.

certain minimum amount of training: what was necessary in order to be able to distinguish the anatomical connecting structures: veins, arteries and nerves.[122] Such a detail constitutes yet another piece of evidence that these physicians were writing about poorly qualified individuals with only rudimentary medical knowledge, and that it was necessary to ensure that they possessed enough skill and dexterity. The insistence on this knowledge also indicates the frequency of accidents resulting from these anatomical parts being confused, one of them being the acute pain and paralysis resulting from the nerve being touched.[123] In this respect it was also specified that those practising phlebotomy should have good eyesight and a steady hand,[124] the elderly thereby being excluded.

The preparations for carrying out blood-letting, the preparation of the phlebotomes and the sight of the vessel which was to collect the blood might produce a nervous state and a feeling of uncertainty in the patient, which had to be counteracted by the practitioner. This is the reason why it is stated that his appearance, conversation and behaviour should avoid seriousness and formal severity, the advice being that he should smile and by his own attitude encourage the individual who was to be bled.[125]

Once blood-letting was prescribed by the physician and the vein that was to be opened decided on, the first step for the practitioner to take was to identify the vessel concerned among its surrounding anatomical features. In order to do so, he might make use of a wide variety of techniques whose purpose was to make the vein stand out. The swelling or the filling of the vein was achieved by means of dilating the vessels, increasing their capacity at the point where the incision was to be made. Such an action was accomplished by putting one of the following techniques into practice.

In the first place, this might be achieved by 'using slightly warm things and active humidifiers',[126] such as by bathing the limb in warm water an hour beforehand. Arnau de Vilanova recommended using this system when narrow vessels, such as the saphena vein or salvatella veins were to be incised,[127] so that they could be more easily seen. Another procedure consisted of accumulating blood at the point of the incision by means of

---

[122] 'Quod sciat discernere inter venam et arteriam': ibid.

[123] ' ... unde sciendum quod ex erronea percussione causatur acutissimus dolor quando nervus aut corda pungitur', Arnau de Vilanova, *De consideracionibus operis medicine* (ed. Demaitre), p. 247.

[124] 'Eligendus est autem phlebotomator iuvenis et expertus boni visus': *Regimen sanitatis*, c. 37, in *Praxis medicinalis*, p. 53.

[125] 'Flebotomator debet flebotomare vultu hilari et jocundo et debet animare flebotomandum', *Chirurgia* (ed. Pagel), p. 371.

[126] ' ... oportet uti leviter calefacientibus et humectantibus actu', *Tractatus de consideracionibus operis medicine* (ed. Demaitre), p. 225.

[127] ' ... quando volumus aperire venas pedis sicut saphenas et manus sicut salvatellas que stricte sunt, iubemus predicta membra per horam ante flebotomiam in aqua temperate calida balneare ... ', ibid., pp. 225–6.

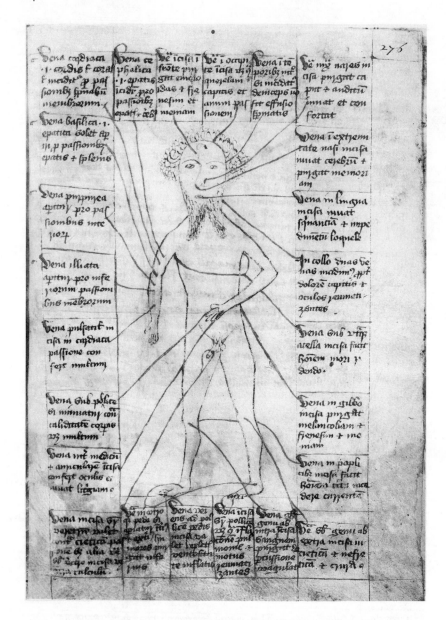

Figure 4 A phlebotomy figure from a French *Miscellanea Medica* of the early fourteenth century. For explanation see foot of p. 145.

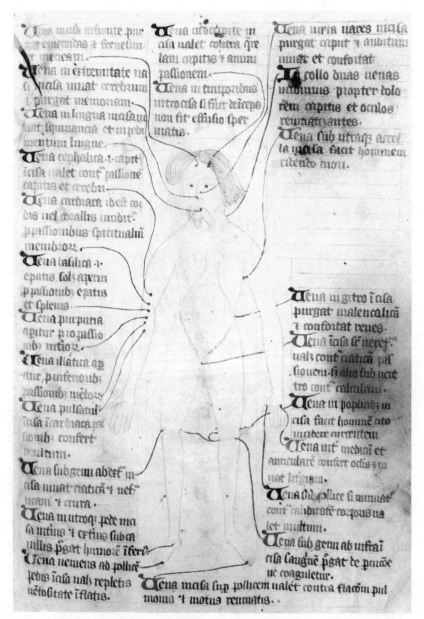

Figure 5 A phlebotomy figure probably of the late thirteenth century. For explanation see foot of p. 145.

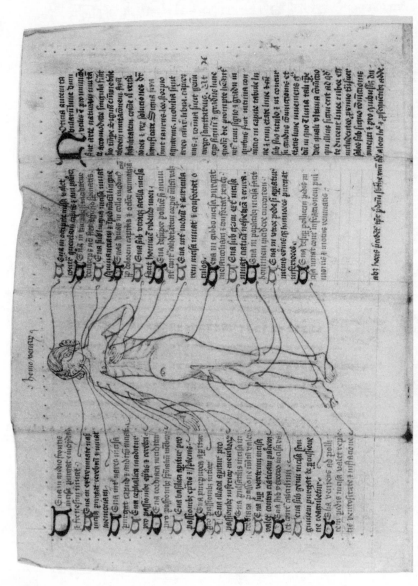

Figure 6 A 'vein man', *homo venarum*, from a fifteenth-century calendar. For explanation see foot of p. 145.

vigorous massage in the area where the vein was located.[128] The same effect could be achieved by exposing the limb to the heat of a fire, as described by medieval monastic customaries, which recommend monks to go to the kitchen before being bled.[129] However, Arnau de Vilanova criticized this practice, pointing out that the heat of a fire only attracted the more subtle parts of the mixture that made up blood, so that there existed the risk that the evacuation might affect only the most valuable components of the blood, above all when the incision was made immediately after exposing the part of the body to the fire. It could only be recommended to counteract the thickening of the skin and the humours provoked by surrounding air conditions in cold weather.[130]

Another way of making the vessel more visible consisted of using a ligature on the limb. In this case a bandage was placed above the point of the incision; this had to be neither very wide, so that it was quite tight, nor very narrow, so that it should help the accumulation of blood.[131] The

---

[128] 'Propter hoc igitur ad attrahendum iusserunt sapientes fricari partem in qua vena queritur': ibid., p. 226.

[129] See L. Gougaud, 'La pratique de la phlébotomie dans les cloîtres', *Revue Mabillon*, 13 (1924), 8.

[130] 'Quidam autem dixerunt quod deberet calefieri ad ignem: quia tamen calor ignis non attrahit nisi quod subtile est non consulimus quod hoc fiat si immediate post debeat vena incidi; aliquociens utile est hoc facere in tempore frigido ad removendum a cute duriciem causatam a frigiditate exteriori ... ', *Tractatus de consideracionibus operis medicine* (ed. Demaitre), p. 226.

[131] 'Ligetur autem cum fascia nec multum lata ut melius stringi valeat, nec multum stricta ut amplius impellere valeat': ibid., p. 227.

Though the first two of these 'vein men' are from the period with which this volume is concerned while the third is from the fifteenth century, the text is in all cases the same. It consists of twenty-four sentences indicating the therapeutic purpose of opening the vein to which the sentence is attached by an indication line. Seven of the veins are named but none are represented in the diagrams.

These figures are not part of the learned physicians' discussion of phlebotomy but relate more to the practice of medicine outside the classroom. Nevertheless, they represent aspects of practice that the learned physicians were trying to rationalize. Thus, a number of the therapeutic designs of opening a vein can be seen to be acting across a bodily 'diameter': the vein in the forehead was opened to 'purge haemorrhoids', and opening that in the temples prevented a flow of semen. The incision of other veins had an effect close to the site of the cut, for the veins of the nose were bled to purge the brain, that of the tongue to remove infirmities of that organ. But there is no mention of 'diameters', revulsion or derivation. The major principle is that veins are connected to different parts and purge them when opened. Thus, of the named veins the cephalica is the vein of the head, the basilica of the liver, the cardiaca of the heart and spiritual organs, the illatica and purpuria of the lower and internal organs. One artery, at the elbow, was opened to benefit the heart.

compressive action of the bandage resulted in the wall of the vessel being altered, thereby producing an accumulation of blood at that point.[132] The point where the ligature was to be applied depended on the locality of the vein which it was planned to open; for those in the angle of the elbow, pressure was applied half way up the arm, above the joint; for the veins in the hands, it was tied at the end of the ulna; and for those in the feet, at the end of the tibia.[133] A procedure for making the jugular veins stand out is described by Arnau de Vilanova with a great wealth of detail:

When we wish to open the veins of the neck, next to the clavicle, that is to say the jugular veins, the neck is squeezed with a narrow strap so that the vein can be seen more easily. It is also useful to hold the breath, after breathing in deeply, and to make the vein more evident one should lean the head towards the other side; in this way skin which before looked wrinkled is stretched and becomes thinner, and for this reason the vein appears more clearly.[134]

Another type of strategy carried out with the aim of making the vein more obvious is not described in the medieval treatises, but is known to us through medieval iconography. In the miniatures that illustrate some medical codices, the person undergoing phlebotomy can be seen gripping a stick with his hand. In this way, by means of muscular contraction, the blood accumulated in the vein, increasing its capacity and facilitating its visibility.

By all these techniques the vein that had to be incised was made to manifest itself to the practitioner as a long body projecting from the surface of the skin, the colour of which was more livid than that of the surrounding parts.[135] But it might also happen that, in spite of all the steps taken, the vessel could not be clearly distinguished. In this case, it was necessary to resort to another type of technique, supported, on this occasion, by the sense of touch.

The description provided by Arnau de Vilanova of this procedure is highly detailed and it is worth reproducing in its entirety:

---

[132] 'Stringatur ergo membrum taliter ut per compressionem venarum factam in loco stricte sanguis ad locum signatum veniat': ibid.

[133] 'Hac igitur intencione stringimus ante incisionem cum fasciola medium adiutorii quando volumus aperire venas que sunt in plicatura brachii. Pro venis autem manus stringimus extremitatem ulne que terminatur in radicem manus; pro venis quoque pedis stringitur extremitas tibie que terminatur ad iuncturam pedis': ibid.

[134] 'Quando autem volumus aperire venas colli videlicet guidegi circa furculam cum stricta corrigia stringimus collum ut manifestetur vena; prodest eciam ad hoc retencio aeris attracti copiose. Ad hoc eciam ut manifestior fit vena debet inclinari caput in partem contrariam: propter hoc enim cutis que prius rugata permanebat tenditur et attenuatur, quamobrem et vena manifestius apparet': ibid., p. 228.

[135] 'Supradictis igitur ligacionibus, fricacionibus et ceteris perfecte observatis, videndum est utrum vena distincte appareat visui secundum colorem et figuram, utpote quod visu distincte comprehendatur corpus oblongum pretendens lividum colorem comparacionem aliarum parcium': ibid.

The surface where the vein is sought has to be touched gently with the index finger, endeavouring to feel if the finger comes across a body in the form of a column that can be displaced from one side to the other. If this is so, when it is pressed, it should give way to the touch like a full wineskin, which will distinguish it from a nerve or a tendon – and when it is released gently, the finger should sense the vein filling up in the same way as a full wineskin.[136]

A simple system of checking enables one to make sure that it was indeed a matter of a vein, and not of an artery, tendon or nerve:

For greater certainty, first the point must be pressed with the middle finger; then, and without moving that finger, the index finger should be applied and with it a point next to the middle finger should be gently pressed, moving progressively in that direction. Then one should carefully assess whether towards the middle finger anything begins to be noticed swelling up, through the movement of some matter contained within it, and if the column fills up with blood. This is something which does not happen in the case of a nerve or a tendon. If this procedure is carried out the point should be carefully noted, because that is where the vein is.[137]

The careful palpation of the area where the vessel was to be found allowed veins to be distinguished from arteries because of the presence of the beat corresponding to the pulse, although it should not be forgotten that, if a ligature was used, the disappearance of the pulse could be the cause of serious mistakes. For this reason, when it was desired to bleed a blood vessel in whose immediate vicinity arteries were located, it was necessary to take other precautions. This happened when it was planned to incise the basilic vein, near which an important artery runs. In such a case, first of all the artery had to be located by means of palpation; next, the arm had to be bound up and one had to check to ascertain whether a small tumour had formed because of the flexing of the elbow at the point where the artery had been beating. If this happened, the point had to be changed, or a branch of the vein which presented no such risks had to be used.[138]

---

[136] ' ... et ideo cum indice tangenda est suaviter pars ubi queritur vena et considerandum utrum digito occurrat corpus mobile lateraliter secundum figuram columpne, ita quod cedat tactui cum primitur sicut uter plenus ad differenciam nervi et corde, et cum suaviter elevetur digitus sentitur vena turgescere ad modum pleni utris': ibid., pp. 228–9.

[137] 'Ut eciam amplior certitudo habeatur debet primo cum medio digito premi locus, deinde illo digito immoto applicetur index et suaviter cum eo prematur locus propinquus medio digito elabendo versus eum; considereturque tunc diligenter utrum versus medium digitum senciatur aliquid manifeste turgescere per motum rei contente interius, ac si corpus columpnare repleretur quod non fit in nervo et corda: quod si sic fiat, notetur diligentissime locus quoniam ibi vena est': ibid.

[138] 'Cum ergo medicus vult aperire venas que sunt in brachio, maxime basilicam sub qua magna locatur arteria, tangat primo locum cum digito, et ubi senserit arteriam pulsare notet; deinde liget brachium et videat cum ligaverit brachium utrum tumor ad modum lentis aut ciceris appareat in loco signato videlicet ubi pulsabat arteria; et si sic, non tangatur quia arteria est que inflatur propter sanguinem impulsum; et melius certificabitur si relaxato ligamine deleatur et iterum reparato appareat. Causa autem propter quam sub tali forma apparet est quia ibi arteria facit quasi extremitatem propterea quia separatur a vena profundando se que curvacio incipit in curvatura brachii, et quanti amplius versus manum tendit tanto amplius profundatur arteria': ibid., pp. 229–30.

Once the vein which it was wished to incise had been located, it was cut with the phlebotome or lancet. For this purpose the practitioner had to have a wide enough range of implements and be able to draw upon different models of instrument. Avicenna said so explicitly: 'It is preferable that the physician should have many phlebotomes, of which some should have a hook [*pilum habentes*] and others should be normal.'[139] This special phlebotome, ending in a point in the form of a hook or a saw, was also described by Arnau de Vilanova,[140] who recommended its use for the opening of narrow, superficial veins, situated at points where there was a risk of harming the underlying parts. For Henri de Mondeville the reper-toire of phlebotomes that the practitioner should possess was also wide:

He should have many clean and shiny phlebotomes of a good standard; sharp ones, sharper ones, and very sharp ones; narrow ones, wide ones; large ones, medium ones and small ones, so that with one or another he is able to operate as the situation demands.[141]

Inventories of the possessions of fourteenth-century barbers, collected in notarial records after their death, confirm the abundance and diversity of the surgical instruments used by these professionals, even by those in the small towns of inland Catalonia, such as Vic or Manresa.[142]

The phlebotome was to be well sharpened to avoid difficulties when the moment came to incise the vein and, above all, because of the risk of an abscess-like lesion being produced in the region of the wound. This piece of advice, with one or more modifications, was included by all the writers who dealt with the subject of phlebotomy, so that we must interpret their insistence as indicating the importance that physicians laid on this.

In order to proceed to make the incision, the phlebotome was held firmly in the middle between the thumb and the next two fingers.[143] In this way, holding it at a slight angle and proceeding gently, it was made to penetrate the vein, care being taken not to break it or damage the opposite wall.[144] Concern about gentleness in the handling of the lancet is also found in the work of Maynus de Mayneriis: 'Veins should be opened as gently as

---

[139] 'Oportet preterea ut minutor flebotomos habeat multos, quorum quidam sint pilum habentes et quidam pilo carentes': *Canon*, lib. I, fen 4, c. 20, fol. 76ra.

[140] ' ... aperiet superficiliater venam cum flebotomo habente pilum seu dentem acutum et incisivum in aliqua sui parte iuxta cuspidem ad modum serre ... ', *Tractatus de consider-acionibus operis medicine* (ed. Demaitre), p. 235.

[141] 'Debet etiam habere plures flebotomos de bono calibe lucidos et politos, acutos, acutiores et acutissimos, strictos, latos, magnos, medios atque parvos, ut modo cum uno, modo cum alio, sicut propositum exigit operetur': *Chirurgia* (ed. Pagel), p. 371.

[142] L. García-Ballester and M. R. McVaugh, work in progress on medicine and medical practitioners in the fourteenth-century Crown of Aragon.

[143] ' ... accipiendus est flebotomus in medio sic ut non vacillet et ut firmius teneatur cum pollice et duobus sequentibus digitis': *Tractatus de consideracionibus operis medicine* (ed. Demaitre), p. 235.

[144] 'Profundetur ergo flebotomus in vena suaviter non prosidiose ne rumpatur, non directe ne inferior vene superficies tangatur sed oblique ... ': ibid.

possible; so, when they are hard, they must be incised with greater firmness than when they are soft.'[145]

The depth and size of the cut which had to be made depended on the objective sought when phlebotomy was prescribed, on the state of the humours and on the type of vein that was to be opened. The presence of condensed, thick humours, either because of the cold or as a result of some physiological or pathological process, required a wider and deeper cut than if the humours were fluid. However, a wide wound which let the blood flow at a steady rate, and which carried out the evacuation in a short time, was more weakening to the patient. The accelerated loss of the vital spirits that were transported by the blood hampered the heart, the organ that would replace them. Phlebotomy like this led rapidly to a syncope (fainting) or to the loss of strength, unless the individual were especially robust. A small opening, even limited to a simple puncture through which the blood flowed drop by drop, prevented the loss of the spirits, but had the drawback of allowing only the subtle blood to leave;[146] unfortunately, this was the kind which possessed the best qualities.[147]

In the same way, the ambient temperature had to be borne in mind. In cold weather the humours were thickened and far more viscous, so that the incision had to be wider. In summer, on the other hand, the heat made the bodily fluids more subtle and lighter, with the result that a small incision was enough to make them flow out.[148] In addition, and in connection with the temperament of the body, there were different constitutions according to the time of life: children had a mixture of humours tending towards heat and moisture since they possessed their *quantum* of innate heat and radical moisture in its entirety. At the other extreme, old people were of a dry, cold constitution, since they had exhausted both their innate heat and their original moisture.

There were, then, four factors which pointed to the choice of a wide or narrow incision; in the first place, the state of strength of the body; secondly, the consistency of the humours; thirdly, the time of year, which was usually limited to knowing whether the weather was cold or warm;

---

[145] 'Vena aperiri quanto suavius est possibile, unde quanto vena est durior tanto aperienda est cum minori suavitate, et quanto mollior cum suaviori': *Regimen sanitatis*, c. 37, in *Praxis medicinalis*, p. 53.

[146] 'Considerato igitur quid est stricta incisio invenitur quod ipsa prebet exitum solum humori vel sanguini subtili, impedit autem exitum grossi; e contrario autem de larga et ampla incisione. Iterum illa utilis est ad conservacionem spirituum et per consequens virtutis, ista vero e converso': *Tractatus de consideracionibus operis medicine* (ed. Demaitre), p. 233.

[147] See P. Gil-Sotres, 'Sangre y patología en la medicina bajomedieval: el substrato material de la flebotomía', *Asclepio*, 38 (1986), 72–104, at 87.

[148] ' ... et ideo ex hac intencione iusserunt sapientes largas incisiones in hyeme facere. In corporibus autem subtilis sanguinis et spiritus utilior est stricta: et hac intencione iubetur fieri talis in pueris et in estate': *Tractatus de consideracionibus operis medicine* (ed. Demaitre), p. 233.

fourthly, the age of the individual undergoing phlebotomy. Most aspects of these factors were clearly expressed by Avicenna.[149] The size of the incision also varied in particular circumstances, especially for certain illnesses. For example, in the treatment of some illnesses, it was advisable to avoid the loss of thick blood, since this helped in the healing of wounds.[150] When revulsion was carried out, the wound had to be smaller than when derivation was performed, no doubt to avoid the movement of the humours leading to prejudicial consequences.

Another point to be borne in mind when practising the incision was the direction of the cut made with the phlebotome. Depending on whether it was carried out following the longitudinal or transverse axis, the effects for the evacuation of blood and the healing of the wound were different. Moreover, it was recommended that the risk of damaging the adjacent parts of the body involved should be adequately assessed. For these reasons, it was recommended that the incision should be made transversally in the case of the veins of the neck, which were highly mobile and easy to lose control over,[151] and in the case of those of the feet, where the closeness of certain other anatomical features made a longitudinal incision hazardous. In these cases, and in others in which there was a danger of the lancet slipping, it was very useful to employ that special phlebotome that had a projection in the shape of a hook at the end. When the vascular bed was free of arteries, nerves and tendons, as occurs in the case of the bed of the salvatella vein, a longitudinal incision was suggested.[152] When the veins that it was sought to open were small or very narrow, the incision had to be transverse to facilitate the outflow of blood and to avoid the closing of the wound through the apposition of the edges. Guy de Chauliac, following Albucasis, systematized the forms that incisions were supposed to have in accordance with the type of vein, and recommended a longitudinal opening in the so-called common veins, that is to say, the three largest veins of the angle of the elbow – the cephalic vein, the basilic and the median vein – keeping transverse incision for the so-called particular veins.[153] Finally, the form of the wound made in phlebotomy affected the process of healing. When, for therapeutic reasons, a rapid or delayed closure of the vein was sought, it had to be taken into account that

---

[149] See *Canon*, lib. I, fen 4, c. 20, fol. 60ra.

[150] '... quamobrem iubent sapientes subtilem aut strictam facere incisionem in curacione vulnerum pulmonis et pectoris, quoniam grossus sanguis ad consolidacionem utilior est subtili': *Tractatus de consideracionibus operis medicine* (ed. Demaitre), p. 233.

[151] 'Vene autem sic mobiles sunt vene colli, et ideo in eis secundum latum fit incisio': *Tractatus de consideracionibus operis medicine* (ed. Demaitre), p. 234.

[152] 'In salvatella vero cum sita sit quasi in valle securior est incisio secundum longum facta quam aliter: non enim timetur mobilitas eius lateraliter': ibid.

[153] 'Abulcassis vero triplicem tradit modum incidendi venas: comunes per longitudinem; venas particulares per transversum; arterias per ligaturam et cauterium': *Chirurgia magna* (Lyons, 1585), p. 363.

an incision along the longitudinal axis healed more easily than one follow-ing the transversal axis.[154]

Once the site of incision had been pinpointed, the practitioner had to make sure that the blood flowed in the correct amount to solve the problem that had generated the need for blood-letting. In this respect, the medieval physicians of this period were not particularly interested in making a quantitative assessment of the blood that could be extracted by phlebotomy, by using measurements of capacity or weight. The criteria that they employed were by contrast basically clinical: the appearance that the liquid that sprang from the wound presented, the relief that evacuation offered, and the state of the patient's strength.

Medieval medicine developed an extensive catalogue of signs based on the observation of blood extracted by phlebotomy. Such an enthusiast of clinical practice as the physician Bernard de Gordon justified the attention paid to the blood that was drawn off:

> In the mass of blood the virtues [*virtus*], the complexion and the operation of both the similar and the official parts shines forth. It is thus evident that from the disposition of the blood we can come to knowledge of the disposition of the whole body.[155]

The argument that this writer was offering was quite straightforward: if by means of the examination of urine and faeces – mere waste products – the physician was able to diagnose the state of the internal organs, then the semiology of the blood must be far more meaningful.[156] A special form of literature was developed to study the analysis of the appearance of blood, and the meaning of this for diagnostic purposes,[157] and large amounts of space in the texts on phlebotomy were dedicated to the same subject.[158] In a previous section, the contracts between municipal councils and medical practitioners were alluded to. It is not by mere chance that the two semiological techniques specifically mentioned in them as having been

---

[154] 'Cum enim volumus ut cito consolidetur ... incidimus secundum longum ... Cum vero tardare volumus consolidacionem ... incidimus secundum latum ... ': *Tractatus de con-sideracionibus operis medicine* (ed. Demaitre), p. 234.

[155] 'In massa igitur sanguinis relucet virtus, complexio et operacio membrorum, tam similium quam officialium. Manifestus est igitur quod per sanguinis disposicionem poterimus devenire in cognicionem totius corporis': *De flebotomia*, MS Cues 308, fol. 31vb.

[156] 'Si autem volumus devenire in cognicionem membrorum interiorum nos querimus ea que egrediuntur a corpore, sicut est urina et egestio, etc.; ideo melius et certius possumus devenire in cognicionem nature interiorum per sanguinis disposicionem': ibid.

[157] Representative of this type of literature are the texts studied in two Bonn doctoral theses: D. Blanke, 'Die pseudohippokratische "Epistula de sanguine cognoscendo"' (1973); and H. J. Rommswinkel '"De sanguine humano destillato" Medizinisch-alchemistische Texte des 14. Jahrhunderts über destilliertes Menschenblut' (1974). On diagnosis making use of these means, see G. Keil, 'Makroskopische Hämatoskopie', in *Proceedings of the 23rd International Congress of the History of Medicine* (London, 1974), vol. I, pp. 100–4.

[158] Thus, for example, in Bernard de Gordon's *De flebotomia* five chapters are dedicated to this question.

routine were the examination of patients' urine and that of the blood following phlebotomy.[159]

Observed alterations to the colour of the blood flowing from the wound enabled the physician to confirm the diagnosis at the same time as they indicated to him the necessity of prolonging the evacuation until the blood emerged appearing normal. This last step was interpreted as a sign that the matter causing the illness had been totally eliminated. The advice to continue evacuation until the colour of the blood had changed was already to be found in Hippocratic writings,[160] and it was widely respected by medieval physicians.

For Bernard de Gordon, the quantity of blood that ought to be evacuated was determined by three factors: the disposition of the blood – that is to say, the aspect that its qualities presented to the eye – the need that might be presumed for the patient's individual case, and the state of his or her strength.[161] But the most interesting point is his capacity to correlate these factors with clinical criteria. Thus the polarity between need and state of strength made it possible to establish a priori a scale in the application of phlebotomy, even the frequency with which it was to be carried out being indicated:

If plethora should be intense, the need great and the state of strength precarious, phlebotomy should be carried out frequently and in small quantity; frequently because of the need, but in small quantity because of the state of the strength.[162]

The amount of blood that was to be evacuated also varied according to the type of illness. In cases in which a proportionate increase in the humours existed, that is to say, plethora, bleeding was to take place with greater freedom than if the disorder affected only one of the humours. In the same way, the criterion of the improvement in the patient's health was also used to judge the amount of treatment, as is indicated in Hippocrates' *Aphorisms*.[163] Using all these quantitative and clinical parameters, the physician would estimate the volume that was to be evacuated in the case of each patient.

The state of strength of the patient regulated the employment of the special forms of phlebotomy called *apoforesis* and *secundatio*. The former consisted of interrupting the flow of blood, closing the wound with a finger and opening it intermittently. *Secundatio* or *iteratio*, as its name

[159] McVaugh, 'Bernat de Borriacho ... ', p. 241.
[160] 'Phlebotomo ergo adhibito nullatenus revoces quin tantam minuas quantitatem sanguinis usque dum videlicet illum in splendidum colorem: vel ex splendido in rubeum, aut ex rubeo in nigredinem videas converti': *Regimen acutorum*, in *Articella* (Venice, 1523), fol. 10vb.
[161] 'Quantitas autem evacuaciones [sic] fit secundum disposicionem, necessitatis [sic] et constanciam virtutis': *De flebotomia*, MS Cues 308, fol. 31ra.
[162] 'Si autem plenitudo fuerit multa et necessitas vehemens et virtus debilis, fiat frequenter et in parva quantitate; frequenter propter necessitatem sed parvum propter virtutem': ibid.
[163] See *Aphorisms*, I, 23.

indicates, consisted of repeating the extraction of blood from the same incision and on the same day. With the help of these forms it was possible to practise phlebotomy on individuals who were in a generally weak state, either for natural reasons – children and the elderly – or as a consequence of having suffered an illness.

The physician, once the emission of blood had terminated, had to attend to the patient's recovery. For this purpose, he would dictate a diet or regimen of life, in the wide sense that this had for people in the Middle Ages. This life style, structured around the six non-naturals (*sex res non naturales*) included precise indications on each of these things 'without which it is not possible to be healthy' and which, canonically transmitted by the *Isagoge*, were listed as: surrounding air; exercise and rest; food and drink; sleep and wakefulness; inanition and repletion; and accidents of the soul.

The first non-natural was the surrounding air. In this respect, physicians advised the patient to remain in a place where the temperature was well balanced, neither too hot, nor excessively cold, and they recommended the same as regards the degree of humidity and dryness. The fact that the body of the individual who had undergone phlebotomy was in a state of weakness made them adopt special care regarding these extremes. But the advice to avoid excessive brightness is of greater interest. Physicians suggested that the individual whose blood had been let should stay in a dark place, lying down, with his or her eyes closed,[164] since exposure to excessive light in the three days following blood-letting might be a cause of cataracts, owing to the loss of spirits suffered.[165]

As far as exercise and rest were concerned, the treatises on phlebotomy reminded their readers that after blood-letting the strength was reduced. Therefore, rest was recommended and under no circumstances was the patient to engage in violent exercise. Similarly, bathing should be avoided because it tended to make one weaker, and also because of the risk that the wound might open up on contact with water.

The diet also had to be regulated. Light, easily digestible foodstuffs and beverages were advised, and these were to be taken in small amounts and were to be capable of generating good blood. For this reason, foodstuffs with the same qualities as the life-giving liquid, warm and moist, were recommended because, as they possessed these qualities, they would be more easily converted into blood. Arnau de Vilanova, for instance, advised a diet made up of 'broth made with egg yolks and cooked meat stock and red or white wine'.[166] For Bernard de Gordon, the ideal diet consisted of 'roast meat with plums since, if it is digested, it provides ample, good

---

[164] 'Quiescat super lectum in loco obscuro': *Regimen sanitatis*, c. 37, *Praxis medicinalis*, p. 54.
[165] 'Quamobrem ex negligencia huius regiminis sepissime compertum est plures huiusmodi amittere visum et incurrere catharactas ...': *Tractatus de consideracionibus operis medicine* (ed. Demaitre), p. 255.
[166] '... ut iura ex vitellis ovorum et succo carnium confecta, et vinum subrubeum aut citrinum': ibid., p. 256.

nourishment'.[167] All these foodstuffs were to be administered in frequent meals and in small quantities owing to the weak state in which the stomach found itself after phlebotomy.[168] If the blood-letting was aimed at reducing the amount of blood in existence in the body, the diet should seek the opposite. In such a case it was necessary to avoid those foodstuffs that were easily converted into blood, since the initial situation which required phlebotomy would reappear.

The weakness that set in after blood-letting would seem to make sleep advisable after the process of evacuation. However, physicians warned of the risk that such a position might entail for the body. The reason stemmed from the behaviour of the humours while we sleep. In effect, according to Galenic theory, the humours during sleep tended to congregate in the interior of the body, along with the natural heat, which turned towards the interior to facilitate the digestive process. In contrast, blood-letting provoked the movement of the humoral mass, directing it towards the outside of the body. Sleep and phlebotomy thus had contrary effects on the humours, with the consequence that they were incompatible. On the other hand, sleeping after eating was not prohibited, since in this case sleep was advisable so that the digestive process should be completed.

Of the many things that were regarded as aspects of inanition and repletion, the most striking was that referring to sexual activity after phlebotomy. Physicians reminded their patients of the debilitating effect of intercourse when forbidding sexual relations after the evacuation of blood, at least during the first three days, which were necessary for the body to recover from the loss of blood.

Finally, the accidents of the soul also had to be regulated. The loss of vital spirits evacuated together with the blood made it advisable to avoid those passions that weakened the heart: anger, sadness and desperation had to be eliminated from the life of the patient who had undergone phlebotomy. On the other hand, happiness and joy were recommended since they carried spirits and blood to the heart and thus had a beneficial effect on the internal organs.

This way of life had to be continued for three days, the number necessary for the body to recover from phlebotomy. On this point the medieval texts are also in agreement with the tradition concerning blood-letting in medieval monastic customaries.

---

[167] 'Ut si fuerit fortis cum assatura carnis que fit super prunas quoniam si digeritur multum nutrit et bene': *De flebotomia*, MS Cues 308, fol. 30va.

[168] 'Veruntamem oportet quod fit pauca quantitas quoniam stomachus propter flebotomiam est debilis': ibid.

CONCLUSION

As we have had the opportunity to demonstrate, preventive and therapeutic blood-letting were frequently resorted to as part of the professional practice of medieval physicians, who gave considerable thought to the two methods of revulsion and derivation. Nevertheless, when it came to carrying out blood-letting, were the precise indications concerning the time and place to apply the different methods of derivation and revulsion actually borne in mind? All the evidence leads us to answer in the affirmative when those who practised phlebotomy were those same writers whose recommendations and theories we have been explaining. However, were the barbers and all the physicians and surgeons who were routinely responsible for blood-letting so meticulous? It is difficult to answer this question, for we possess hardly any information on the actual practice of these modest, anonymous practitioners on whose shoulders the weight of medical practice fell. What does seem clear, however, is that the practical use of phlebotomy in the Middle Ages had a considerable and sophisticated theoretical debate behind it.

5

Surgical texts and social contexts: physicians and surgeons in Paris, c. 1270 to 1430

CORNELIUS O'BOYLE

In 1363, the French surgeon, Guy de Chauliac (c. 1290–1367/70), completed a work on surgery which he called an *Inventarium seu collectorium in parte cyrurgicali medicine*.[1] Within a few years, Guy's work – more usually known as the *Chirurgia magna* – was firmly established as a fundamental text on surgery, and remained as such down to the end of the seventeenth century.[2] The popularity of this work is clearly reflected in the relatively large number of manuscript copies and printed editions of the original Latin text which still survive.[3] A brief survey of the fourteenth- and fifteenth-century manuscript copies of Guy's work reveals, moreover, that the complete text was translated into a number of vernacular languages fairly soon after its composition.[4] In addition to the complete versions of the text, there also survives a relatively large number of fragments, summaries and compilations based on Guy's work in both Latin and the

[1] For Guy's biography see Vern L. Bullough, 'Guy de Chauliac', *Dictionary of scientific biography*, ed. Charles C. Gillispie, 16 vols. (New York, 1970–80) (henceforth *DSB*), vol. III, pp. 218–19. See also the modern French edn of the *Chirurgia magna* by Eduard Nicaise, *La Grande chirurgie de Guy de Chauliac* (Paris, 1890), esp. pp. lxxvii–cv.
[2] For a survey of the surviving manuscripts and editions see Jean Enselme, *La longue histoire de la Grande chirurgie de Guy de Chauliac*, Albums du Crocodile (Lyons, 1970).
[3] Twenty-six complete Latin manuscripts survive for the period 1363 to 1424. There are eight editions of the Latin text printed in Venice between 1490 and 1546, and nine editions printed in Lyons between 1499 and 1585: Enselme, *La longue histoire*, pp. 5–15.
[4] There are four complete manuscript copies of the work in French from the fourteenth and fifteenth centuries, and thirty-three editions of the text in French dating from 1478 to 1683; five manuscript copies in Provençal dating from the fourteenth to eighteenth centuries; five fifteenth-century manuscript copies in English, and two sixteenth-century editions in English; one late fourteenth-century/early fifteenth-century manuscript copy in low German; one fifteenth-century manuscript copy in Dutch, and seven editions in Dutch from 1482 to 1650; six editions in Spanish dating from c. 1518 to 1663; one fourteenth-century manuscript copy in Italian, and five editions in Italian dating from 1480 to 1652. There is also one fifteenth-century manuscript copy in Hebrew: Enselme, *La longue histoire*, pp. 15–24, 31–4; Richard J. Durling, *A catalogue of sixteenth century printed books in the National Library of Medicine* (Bethesda, MD, 1967), no. 2246.

vernacular.[5] Guy's work, of course, is not unique in surviving in so many different forms. Indeed, the translations, abridgements and fragments of Guy's *Chirurgia magna* are fairly representative of the various forms in which a number of well-known surgical works from the thirteenth and fourteenth centuries now survive, including the works on surgery by Guglielmo da Saliceto (d. 1277/9),[6] Lanfranco of Milan (*fl.* 1290s),[7] Teodorico Borgognoni of Lucca (*c.* 1210–98)[8] and Henri de Mondeville (*c.* 1260–*c.* 1320).[9] In themselves, these surgical works and their various redactions raise a number of important textual, literary and linguistic questions. Here, however, I wish to investigate the social issues to which these works relate. In particular, I wish to show what these works and their redactions can tell us about the effects that the new university medicine of the thirteenth and fourteenth centuries had upon the role of the surgeon during this period.

MEDICAL PRACTICE IN THE LATE MIDDLE AGES

It has frequently been pointed out that the various forms in which surgical works of the thirteenth and fourteenth centuries survive appear to reflect the categories into which medical practitioners of the late Middle Ages are traditionally divided. In this traditional interpretation of things, the medical needs of people in Western Europe during this period were met by the combined skills of the physician, the surgeon, the apothecary and the

---

[5] There were three widely used summaries of Guy's work: Les fleurs *du Guidon*, which was brought out in at least six versions between 1549 and 1686; Les abrégés *de Verduc* by Laurent Verduc, which was printed twelve times between 1691 and 1790; and De *chirurgica institutione libri quinque* by Tagault, which was printed in Latin thirteen times between 1543 and 1610. There are translations of Tagault in Dutch (1599), French (1549, 1580) and Italian (1550, 1570) as well as a French adaptation (1590) and various English excerpts (1567, 1575, 1586). There are numerous manuscript and printed fragments of Guy's work dating from the fifteenth to seventeenth centuries which concentrate mainly upon the Prologue and the treatises on anatomy, grades of drugs and the treatment of wounds. Enselme, *La longue histoire*, pp. 25–30; Durling, *Catalogue of the National Library of Medicine*, nos. 4296–309 (see also no. 1690).

[6] For Guglielmo's biography see Charles H. Talbot, *Medicine in medieval England* (London, 1967), pp. 99–100. See also Paul Pifteau (ed.), *La Chirurgie de Guillaume de Salicet achevée en 1275* (Toulouse, 1898).

[7] For Lanfranco's biography see Talbot, *Medicine in medieval England*, p. 101. See also Robert von Fleischhacker, *Lanfrank's 'Science of cirurgie'* (Early English Text Society, original series, 102) (London, 1894).

[8] For Teodorico's biography see William A. Wallace, 'Theodoric Borgognoni of Lucca', *DSB*, vol. II, pp. 314–15.

[9] For Henri's biography see Vern L. Bullough, 'Henry of Mondeville', *DSB*, vol. VI, pp. 276–7. See also Eduard Nicaise, *Chirurgie de maître Henri de Mondeville* (Paris, 1893), esp. pp. li–lxii; Julius L. Pagel (ed.), *Die Chirurgie des Heinrich von Mondeville* (Berlin, 1892); and Alphonse Bos, *La Chirurgie de maître Henri de Mondeville*, Société des Anciens Textes Français, 41, 2 vols. (Paris, 1897–8).

empiric.[10] The neat categories of physician, master surgeon and barber surgeon that help to make up this picture of late medieval medical practice appear to explain very nicely the various forms in which surgical works of the thirteenth and fourteenth centuries survive, for it has usually been claimed that complete Latin copies of surgical works were in the possession of learned university-trained physicians who could read Latin; that complete vernacular copies of these works were used by the learned master surgeons of the guilds who could not read Latin; and that the surviving fragments and abridgements were produced for the benefit of barber surgeons who had little theoretical knowledge of their craft.[11]

However, more recent research into the kind of people who were engaged in medical practice in Western Europe during the thirteenth and fourteenth centuries has provided a much richer, more complex picture than the simple physician, surgeon, apothecary model would suggest. In the first place, it is clear that the medical care provided by those who called themselves physicians and surgeons bore little relation to the medical care more usually experienced by the great majority of people in the Latin West. For example, the most recent statistical analysis of medical practitioners in Paris reveals that between 1310 and 1329 there were eighty-four physicians, twenty-six master surgeons and ninety-seven barbers in the city.[12] For a city that had a population of about 200,000 in 1328 these figures would indicate that physicians, master surgeons and barber surgeons represented but a small percentage of the total number of Parisian practitioners, and that they served the needs of probably only a small section of the city's population.[13] By and large, it was also the case that physicians, surgeons and barbers worked mainly in the towns, and therefore their sort of medicine did not necessarily reflect the provision of medical care in the countryside. Furthermore, it appears to have been the case that substantial numbers of physicians and master surgeons were usually to be found only in those relatively few urban centres that supported a university. On the basis of this sort of evidence, then – even when every sort of qualification is placed on such statistical analysis of the surviving evidence – it is hard to avoid the conclusion that the services provided by physicians and master surgeons were unrepresentative of the sort of medical care experienced by ordinary people.

It was not simply the case that these practitioners were unrepresentative.

---

[10] See, for example, Nicaise, *Chirurgie de maître Henri de Mondeville*, pp. vi–xii; *La Grande Chirurgie de Guy de Chauliac*, pp. xlix–lxv; Vern L. Bullough, 'Training of the non-university-educated medical practitioners in the later Middle Ages', *Journal of the History of Medicine*, 14 (1969), 446–58.

[11] Enselme, *La longue histoire*, pp. 5, 15, 25; Bullough, 'Nonuniversity-educated medical practitioners', pp. 449–50, 455.

[12] Danielle Jacquart, *Le milieu médical en France du XIIème au XVème siècle*, Hautes Etudes Médiévales et Modernes, 46 (Geneva, 1981), p. 246.

[13] Jacquart, *Le milieu médical*, pp. 246–7.

A closer examination of the backgrounds of those who called themselves physicians or surgeons shows how very narrow and inaccurate the traditional characterizations of these medical practitioners tend to be.

In general terms, it is noticeable that in the traditional interpretation of things all medical practitioners are assumed to be male. The only exception to this were midwives, for it is often maintained that women's health, at least until the seventeenth century, was treated exclusively as women's business. But more recent research indicates that, despite numerous legal injunctions that attempted to restrict women practising medicine, women practitioners were to be found at all levels of the medical community in the thirteenth and fourteenth centuries, including the physicians and more especially the surgeons.[14]

With regard specifically to the physicians, they are traditionally characterized first and foremost by their university education. No doubt, it was very much in the interest of the universities that all physicians should be graduates of a university faculty of medicine. However, recent studies indicate that in fact not all practitioners of learned medicine were educated at a university. Rather, it appears that it was possible to learn the craft of the physician by apprenticeship. Again, even though their members may have wished it to have been so, the university medical faculties did not have sole discretion in deciding who was to be licensed as a practising physician. Instead, fully trained apprentices in medicine had the right to apply directly to the local authorities for the *licentia practicandi*. This method of licensing appears to have been resorted to even in towns that supported medical faculties, such as Paris and Montpellier.[15]

The traditional characterization of the physician also fails to take account of the fact that there were non-Christians who practised as physicians. It has usually been assumed that the universities did not admit non-Christians, and that therefore all licensed physicians, who are assumed to have been university trained, must therefore have been Christian. It is clear, however, that along the Mediterranean coast there were many Jewish physicians practising within both the Jewish and Christian communities. These Jewish practitioners of learned medicine received their medical education in a variety of ways. There were some cases where universities such as Montpellier did, in fact, allow Jews to graduate as physicians.[16] By and large, however, Jews who wished to practise learned medicine usually received their training within the Jewish community. In some places, Jewish communities maintained their own schools in medicine as well as in Hebrew law. In other places, Jewish communities adopted the method of appren-

---

[14] Monica Green, 'Women's medical practice and health care in medieval Europe', *Signs: Journal of Women in Culture and Society*, 14 (1989), 434–73.

[15] Jacquart, *Le milieu médical*, pp. 84–7.

[16] Harry Friedenwald, 'Jews and the University of Montpellier', in his *The Jews and medicine: essays*, 2 vols. plus suppl. (Baltimore, 1944), vol. I, pp. 241–52.

ticeship for training their physicians.[17] Having learned the art of medicine either at school or by apprenticeship, the Jewish medical student was then able to present himself to the local royal or papal representative as a candidate for the *licentia practicandi*. This licence was usually awarded after the candidate had submitted to an examination in medicine before a panel consisting of both Jewish and Christian learned medical men.[18]

If the category of those who practised as physicians was broader than is usually supposed, then the category of those who practised as master surgeons was broader still. In the past, historians have been impressed by the evidence which suggests that surgery was not undertaken by uni-versity-trained physicians. Some historians have traced this back to the well-documented attempts by the Church throughout the twelfth and thirteenth centuries to prevent, first, the monastic and, later, the secular clergy from practising medicine in general and surgery in particular.[19] In these events historians have seen the beginnings of the separation between the theoretical learned medicine which was studied in the schools by the clerics, and the more practical aspects of medicine such as surgery which were left to be performed by uneducated lay practitioners.[20] Indeed, the actions of university medical faculties would appear to lend further support to the belief that the universities perpetuated a division between theoretical medicine and practical surgery. For example, in 1350, the dean of the medical faculty in Paris, Adam de Francovilla, inserted into the corrected statutes of the faculty a clause obliging all new bachelors of medicine to take an oath promising not to practise manual surgery.[21] Again, in 1408, the Parisian medical faculty accepted as one of its members the surgeon, John of Pisa, on the condition that he swore never to operate manually again.[22] More recent research has revealed, however, that surgery was indeed a subject embraced by physicians as well as surgeons. In the first place, a closer analysis of the Church decrees that have been interpreted as presenting obstacles for clerics who wished to study and practise surgery has revealed that the decrees were not intended to prevent the practice of surgery, and that indeed they did not have the effect of doing so.[23] Moreover, there is evidence to suggest that the universities did embrace the

---

[17] Jacquart, *Le milieu médical*, pp. 84–5.

[18] Harry Friedenwald, 'On the giving of medical degrees during the Middle Ages by other than academic authority', in his *Jews and Medicine*, vol. I, pp. 263–7.

[19] G. C. Coulton, *Medieval panorama: the English scene from Conquest to Reformation* (Cambridge, 1938), pp. 445–7.

[20] Ernest Wickersheimer, *Commentaires de la faculté de médecine de l'Université de Paris (1395–1516)* (Paris, 1915), p. lxxvi.

[21] Joseph F. Malgaigne, *Œuvres complètes d'Ambroise Paré*, 3 vols. (Paris, 1840–1), vol. I, p. cxxix.

[22] *Chartularium Universitatis Parisiensis*, ed. Henri S. Denifle and Aemilio Chatelain, 4 vols. (Paris, 1889–97) (henceforth *CUP*), vol. IV, no. 1853, p. 156.

[23] Darryl W. Amundsen, 'Medieval canon law on medical and surgical practice by the clergy', *Bulletin of the History of Medicine*, 52 (1978), 22–44.

study of surgery. For example, we know that surgery was being taught, at least informally, in Montpellier during the fourteenth century,[24] and that, by the early fifteenth century, the Italian universities had established stipendiary professorships in surgery.[25]

Indeed, the very fact that learned surgical works of the thirteenth and fourteenth centuries appear to be the products of a university setting would seem to indicate that at least some learned medical men were interested in surgery. This is suggested by the fact that the surgical works of Teodorico Borgognoni of Lucca, Guglielmo da Saliceto, Lanfranco of Milan, Henri de Mondeville and Guy de Chauliac were all composed in Latin; they all make frequent citation of the medical authors most extensively studied in the universities, including Galen, Avicenna, Albucasis, Rhazes, Haly Abbas, Hippocrates and Aristotle;[26] and some of these works begin with introductions which correspond more or less closely to the traditional university procedure of introducing texts known as the *accessus*.[27]

The assumption that these works did indeed originate in the university medical faculties is supported by the biographical information we have concerning their authors. All our surgical authors appear to have spent a considerable period of time teaching and practising in and around university towns. For instance, for most of his life Teodorico Borgognoni of Lucca lived in Bologna teaching and practising both medicine and surgery whereby he was reputed to have amassed great wealth. Guglielmo da Saliceto himself tells us that he lectured upon surgery in Bologna and Verona, and that he practised surgery in Cremona, Piacenza, Bergamo and Pavia. Also, Lanfranco, having been expelled from his native Milan by the Visconti, arrived in Paris in about 1295, and at the house of Jean de Passavant, the dean of the medical faculty in Paris, gave a course in surgery that proved to be very popular. Henri de Mondeville is known to have begun his medical studies at Bologna. Guy informs us that, in 1304, Henri was lecturing on anatomy at Montpellier, where he is said to have demon-

---

[24] Vern L. Bullough, 'The teaching of surgery at the University of Montpellier in the thirteenth century', *Journal of the History of Medicine*, 15 (1960), 202–4.

[25] See the Bolognese statutes of 1405 in Carlo Malagola (ed.), *Statuti delle Università e dei Collegi dello Studio Bolognese* (Bologna, 1888), rubric 35, pp. 247–8. See also the 1442 re-establishment statutes of Ferrara (statute 46) translated in Lynn Thorndike, *University records and life in the Middle Ages*, Records of Civilization: Sources and Studies (New York, 1944), pp. 336–7; and Talbot, *Medicine in medieval England*, pp. 98–104.

[26] See, for example, Nicaise, *Chirurgie de maître Henri de Mondeville*, pp. xxx–xxxviii; *La grande chirurgie de Guy de Chauliac*, pp. xviii–xlviii. See also Talbot, *Medicine in medieval England*, p. 102.

[27] Edwin A. Quain, 'The medieval *accessus ad auctores*', *Traditio*, 3 (1945), 215–64; Roger French, 'A note on the anatomical accessus of the Middle Ages', *Medical History*, 23 (1979), 461–8; Per-Gunnar Ottosson, *Scholastic medicine and philosophy: a study of commentaries on Galen's Tegni (ca. 1300–1450)* (Naples, 1984), pp. 65–8. For a summary of the *accessus* to Guy de Chauliac's *Chirurgia*, see below.

strated using thirteen illustrations.[28] Henri himself tells us that he was lecturing in Paris in 1306, and that it was the pressure of students and patients together with his own ill-health that prevented him from finishing his projected book on surgery. Guy's own university connections are still not clear. It would appear from the dedication in his *Chirurgia* that he had studied medicine with masters in Montpellier, Bologna, Paris and Avignon.[29] He may also have studied anatomy at Bologna under Bertrucci, a pupil of Mondino dei Liuzzi. Guy appears to have graduated as a medical doctor since he refers to himself in the preface to his *Chirurgia magna* as a *chirurgicus magister in medicina*. On the basis of the evidence we have that Guy was frequently at Avignon, one historian has concluded that Guy probably received his doctorate at Montpellier which was close by.[30]

The characterization of surgery as a non-university subject, then, would seem to need very careful qualification. A further misconception stemming from the traditional view that the Church forbade clerics to practise surgery was that surgery was an art engaged upon exclusively by the laity.[31] The careers of our surgical authors in the Church suggest that the picture was far more complex. Few of our authors matched the distinction of Teodorico who, early in his career, became a Dominican and was soon appointed as chaplain and confessor to the pope (probably Innocent IV). Thereafter, he secured rapid advancement in his career, being appointed Bishop of Bitonto in about 1262 and then, in 1266, Bishop of Cervia.[32] The ecclesiastical appointments of Guglielmo da Saliceto, Lanfranco and Henri de Mondeville are not so well documented, but they were evidently also in holy orders. The precise details of Guy's career in the Church are more clear. In 1325, he was already a cleric at Langeac. By 1350, he was a residential canon at S. Just in Lyons, and had been appointed eighth physician to Pope Clement VI. Before 1364, he had secured a canonry at Reims and had been appointed second physician to Pope Innocent VI. By the time he wrote his *Chirurgia* he was also Provost of S. Just, a canon of Mende and was first physician and chaplain to Pope Urban V.[33]

Clearly, then, as in the case of the physician, the traditional characterization of the medieval surgeon bears little resemblance to the sort of people who were actually engaged in the art of surgery during the thirteenth and fourteenth centuries.

These more recent findings would appear to raise an interesting problem

---

[28] Loren C. Mackinney, 'The beginnings of western scientific anatomy: new evidence and a revision in interpretation of Mondeville's role', *Medical History*, 6 (1962), 233–9.

[29] 'Et propter hoc mihi ad solatium senectutis et ad solum mentis exercitium vobis dominis meis medicis Montispessulani, Bonoñ, Parisius atque Avinioñ, precipue papalibus quibus me in servitio Romanorum pontificum associavi', Guy de Chauliac, *Chyrurgia* (Lyons, *c.* 1510), fol. 2ra.

[30] Malgaigne, *Œuvres complètes d'Ambroise Paré*, vol. I, pp. lxii–lxiii.

[31] Wickersheimer, *Commentaires*, p. lxxvi.

[32] Wallace, 'Theodoric Borgognoni of Lucca', p. 314.

[33] Bullough, 'Guy de Chauliac', pp. 218–19.

with respect to the learned surgical works we are interested in here. On the one hand, as we have just seen, the neat categories of physician, master surgeon and barber surgeon that help to make up the traditional picture of late medieval medical practice do not accurately reflect the complex social composition of those engaged in medical practice in the thirteenth and fourteenth centuries. Yet the various forms in which learned surgical works now survive do indeed seem to be related very closely to the traditional conceptions of physician, master surgeon and barber surgeon. How, then, are our surgical works, and the traditional categories to which they relate, to be explained? For the purposes of investigating this problem I shall confine myself to the documents relating to medical practice in Paris from about 1270 to about 1430. This analysis is thus concerned specifically with the situation in Paris. Even so, recent detailed studies of late medieval medicine suggest that the Parisian scene bears a strong resemblance to conditions of medical practice elsewhere in Western Europe at this time. For this reason, the conclusions of this chapter may well have a significance beyond the particular circumstance of Paris during this period.[34]

THE MEDICAL MASTERS' PLAN FOR MEDICAL PRACTICE

One of the very earliest descriptions of the traditional medical hierarchy is to be found in the statutes for the medical faculty of the University of Paris dating from 1271. The occasion for these statutes appears to have been the faculty's desire to suppress those who administered dangerous drugs without consulting a physician, as well as those manual operators who continued to practise medicine despite the many ill consequences that the faculty claimed were thereby brought about. The faculty proposed that the prescription of medicines should be a matter reserved exclusively to the industry of the skilled physician. At the same time, it strictly prohibited any male or female surgeons, apothecaries or herbalists from exceeding the limits of their craft secretly or publicly. In future, the surgeon was to engage only in manual practice and the apothecary was to mix only those drugs recommended by the physician. Moreover, both surgeons and apothecaries were strictly forbidden to perform the physician's job of administering or advising upon medicines.[35] By these measures the faculty sought to define the legitimate practices of physicians, surgeons and

---

[34] See, for example, Luis García-Ballester, Michael R. McVaugh and Augustín Rubio-Vela, *Medical licensing and learning in fourteenth-century Valencia*, Transactions of the American Philosophical Society, 79, part 6 (Philadelphia, 1989), pp. 1–55, where the authors show that in fourteenth-century Valencia licit medical practice was increasingly characterized in terms of a definable body of medical *scientia*; that physicians extended their control over medical and surgical practice through new civil legislation and licensing procedures; and that these privileges were increasingly enforced in law by the prosecution of unlicensed practitioners. The authors also discuss the demography of physicians and surgeons in the Crown of Aragon as well as the role of women and non-Christians in medical practice.

[35] *CUP*, vol. I, no. 434, pp. 488–90.

apothecaries in terms of their medical functions, and thereby exclude as illicit charlatans medical practitioners who could not be located within this medical hierarchy.

Of course, these statutes did not provide an accurate description of those who were actually engaged in medical practice in the thirteenth-century Latin West. Rather, they were intended to provide a purely *prescriptive* account of medical practice. Moreover, as a scheme proposed by the Parisian faculty of medicine, it represented the views of a very small number of highly unrepresentative medical practitioners. Yet, as we shall see, by the end of the fourteenth century, the scheme had been adopted as an ideal to be aimed at by all the authorities, including the papal court, the royal court, the local ecclesiastical courts, the local civil courts, the Parlement, and the guilds of master surgeons and barber surgeons. We need to explain, then, how and why this small band of medical men managed to win over to their idealized scheme those groups in society who could assist them in bringing their programme for medical practice into effect. Central to this investigation is an understanding of what these men were seeking to accomplish when they proposed their idealized scheme for medical practice. New light may be shed on this issue by characterizing these learned medical men and their enterprise in terms of the general ecclesiastical and economic circumstances within which they operated.

THE CHANGING SOCIAL CONTEXT OF EDUCATION

As we have seen, one of the earliest expressions of this idealized scheme for medical practice is to be found in the statutes of the Parisian medical faculty dating from 1271. Now most members of the faculty were, of course, practitioners of learned medicine, but the faculty itself was characterized primarily as a fraternity of *teachers* of learned medicine. To this extent, then, the new plans for medical practice should be interpreted as proposals initiated by the masters of medicine.

In part, these medical masters regarded themselves as the direct inheritors of a tradition that was well established in the Latin West of teaching medicine as a learned discipline. This medical scholarship was usually conceived of as part of the broader world of learning in the Latin West that had been fostered by the Church for over eight hundred years. The Church, of course, was engaged in teaching for its own very practical purposes. In monasteries and cathedrals there was an obvious requirement for at least basic levels of literacy among the clergy in order that the divine office could be said, and so that clerics themselves could pursue their own private study of the sacred page. Moreover, the Church was widely regarded as the main provider of educated young men who were required to conduct the administration of secular government. But underlying these practical reasons for the involvement of the clergy in study was the fundamental assumption that all learning was primarily a means of salvation and an aid to restoring man to his original state of perfection. In this scheme of things, all secular studies – in essence, the seven liberal arts of grammar, rhetoric, logic, arithmetic, astronomy, geometry and music – were pursued as part of a preparatory training before one embarked upon a study of sacred scripture, the Church Fathers, the decretals and the liturgy. In this way, the liberal arts, which were acquired by natural reasoning, were seen as leading directly to divine learning, and, in turn, this divine learning was regarded as a process of self-purification that led to salvation.[36]

It was within this context that the study of medicine came to form a distinctive part of the Church's teaching. Of course, the practice of medicine by the clergy sprang initially from the practical needs of providing medical care within isolated religious communities, as well as the obligation to exercise the Christian virtue of charity. But the study of medicine was also included in broader educational plans promoted by those who sought to improve the general education of the clergy. For example, in his *Institutes of divine and secular learning*, Cassiodorus (c. 490–585) recommended to his monks at Vivarium the necessity of studying medicine.[37] Also, in his attempts to instruct the clergy of his diocese, Isidore, the Archbishop of Seville (c. 560–636), devoted one of his twenty books on etymologies to the derivation of medical terms.[38] Again, Rhabanus Maurus (c. 776–856), Abbot of Fulda and Archbishop of Mainz, included in the encyclopaedia he wrote for his clergy, entitled *De universo*, a chapter on biblical references to the nature and parts of man.[39] In the twelfth and thirteenth centuries, learned medicine was also included in the schemes of knowledge drawn up by authors who sought to explain the various disciplines that constituted true Christian knowledge (*philosophia*). For instance, in his *Didascalicon*, Hugh of St Victor (d. 1141) included medicine among the arts that comprised the mechanical branch of *philosophia*.[40] Also,

[36] Cornelius O'Boyle, 'God, medicine and Aristotle in the early universities', *Bulletin of the History of Medicine*, 66 (1992), 185–209.

[37] Magnus Aurelius Cassiodorus, *Institutiones divinarum et humanarum lectionum*, ch. 31, ed. by Jacques P. Migne as *De institutione divinarum litterarum* and *De artibus ac disciplinis liberalium litterarum*, in his *Patrologiae cursus completus* (the *Patrologia latina*, henceforth *PL*), vol. LXX, cols. 1146–7; *An introduction to divine and human readings*, trans. and intro. by L. W. Jones, Records of Civilization: Sources and Studies, 40 (New York, 1946). See James J. O'Donnell, *Cassiodorus* (Berkeley and London, 1979), pp. 202–20.

[38] *Isidori Hispalensis Episcopi etymologiarum sive originum libri XX*, ed. W. M. Lindsay, 2 vols., Scriptorum Classicorum Bibliotheca Oxoniensis (Oxford, 1910; reprinted 1971). See William D. Sharpe, *Isidore of Seville: the medical writings. An English translation with an introduction and commentary*, American Philosophical Society Transactions, new series 54, part 2 (Philadelphia, 1964).

[39] Rhabanus Maurus, *De universo libri XXII*, Book 6, *PL* 111, cols. 137–80. See Everett C. Jessup, 'Rhabanus Maurus: *De sermonum proprietate seu universo*', *Annals of Medical History*, new series 6 (1934), 35–41, and Wilhelm Weber (ed.), *Rabanus Maurus in seiner Zeit, 780–1980* (Mainz am Rhein, 1980).

[40] Charles H. Buttimer (ed.), *Hugonis de Sancto Victore Didascalicon. De studio legendi*, Studies in Medieval and Renaissance Latin, 10 (Washington, DC, 1939), Book 2, chs. 20 and 26,

in his *De divisione philosophiae*, Dominicus Gundissalinus, the mid twelfth-century Archdeacon of Segovia, included medicine among the eight disciplines that comprised *physica*, which, like mathematics and theology, was one of the three branches of *philosophia*. Similarly, in his *De ortu scientiarum*, the English archbishop, Robert Kilwardby (*c.* 1215–79), included medicine among the seven mechanical arts that, together with the moral sciences and trivial arts, made up the practical disciplines of *philosophia*.[41]

In part, then, the medical masters of the thirteenth and fourteenth centuries were the direct inheritors of a tradition in which, for centuries, learned medicine had been studied and practised predominantly by clerics in the monastic and cathedral schools as part of a broader plan of Christian learning.[42] Yet these same medical masters were also the product of the dramatic changes that took place in the twelfth- and thirteenth-century Latin West which, in turn, dramatically reshaped the world of learning and the world of learned medicine. The appearance of market towns populated with new classes of merchants, bankers and artisans; the centralization of secular authority and the expansion of state bureaucracy; and the growth of Church administration reflecting a move towards greater centralization within the papacy and the local ecclesiastical hierarchies; all these changes placed new educational demands upon clerical scholars. In general, these developments necessitated a greatly increased supply of literate and numerate young men as well as scholars trained in the more advanced disciplines of law and theology.[43]

The Church, in particular, had a pressing reason to sponsor a far-reaching programme of educational reform. The reason for the Church's new concern with education was the growing problem of religious dissent that it encountered in the new market towns.[44] Before the twelfth century,

pp. 38–40, 43–4; *The Didascalicon of Hugh of St Victor: a medieval guide to the arts*, trans. and intro. by Jerome Taylor, Records of Civilization: Sources and Studies, 64 (New York, 1961), pp. 74–5, 78–9.

[41] James A. Weisheipl, 'Classification of the sciences in medieval thought', *Mediaeval Studies*, 27 (1965), 54–90, reprinted in Weisheipl, *Nature and motion in the Middle Ages* (Washington DC, 1985), 203–37 at 211–29.

[42] For monastic medical learning see Augusto Beccaria, *I codici di medicina del periodo presalernitano (secoli IX, X e XI)*, Storia e Letteratura, 53 (Rome, 1956); Anne F. Dawtry, 'The *modus vivendi* and the Benedictine Order in Anglo-Norman England', in *The Church and healing*, ed. William J. Sheils (Oxford, 1982), pp. 25–38; David Knowles, *The monastic order in England*, 2nd edn (Cambridge, 1966), pp. 516–18; Frank Barlow, *The English Church, 1066–1154* (London, 1979), pp. 260–4; Brian Lawn, *The Salernitan questions, An Introduction to the history of medieval and Renaissance problem literature* (Oxford, 1963), p. 7. For medical learning in the cathedral schools see Loren C. MacKinney, *Early mediaeval medicine*, Publications of the Institute of the History of Medicine, ser. 3, vol. III (Baltimore, 1937), pp. 26, 49–57.

[43] Richard W. Southern, 'The changing role of universities in medieval Europe', *The Bulletin of the Institute of Historical Research*, 60 (1987), 133–46 at 142–6.

[44] Bernard Hamilton, *The medieval inquisition* (London, 1981), pp. 13–30; Hamilton, *The Albigensian crusade* (London, 1974), pp. 3–16; Rosalind B. Brooke, *The coming of the friars* (London, 1975), pp. 63–88; Malcolm D. Lambert *Medieval heresy: popular movements from Bogomil to Hus* (London, 1977), pp. 3–126.

within the static and stable life of the rural parish community, there was an almost irresistible pressure to conform to the established social customs. By the 1160s, however, urbanization, the growth of trade, the rise of new wealthy, literate, urban classes, and the ever freer movement of people, goods and ideas had all tended to produce a society that was more critical of the Church. But the Church, with its traditional structures and poorly educated clergy, was not well equipped to deal with the growing number of ascetic groups in which this dissent manifested itself.[45] In these circumstances, the papacy soon came to regard the reform of education as an essential element in its strategy to counter these heretical movements. At the most general level, the papacy came to believe that the need to improve the basic level of education among the diocesan clergy – and in particular their skills as preachers (the *ars praedicandi*) – was of primary importance in combating the spread of heresy at its very roots.[46] At another level, the papacy also began to perceive a need for clerics trained in a more systematic view of theology, not only to defend the new exalted claims that the papacy made for itself, but also to provide the Church with a learned body of trusted men who could be called upon to define and defend traditional Church teaching in response to doctrines taught by ascetics that the Church regarded as heretical.

In many senses, the clerical scholars of the cathedral schools were well placed to respond to these new needs in education. In the first place, as we have seen, they were traditionally regarded as the providers of education in the Latin West. To this extent, it was only natural that, in the twelfth century, traders, princes, bishops and popes should have turned to the masters of the cathedral schools in their search for educated young men. Second, the cathedral schools were geographically well placed to respond to the new educational demands. Unlike the rural monastic schools that were separated from the new concentrations of population, the cathedral schools were nearly always located in the centre of one of the new towns. In addition, most royal courts were located in cathedral towns; and, of course, every bishop's court was attached to a cathedral. And third, the traditional disciplines taught by the cathedral school masters were – with generally little adjustment – particularly well suited to the needs of students who wished to take advantage of the new careers that were opening up. By teaching the traditional arts of grammar, rhetoric and logic as well as by introducing new courses in basic writing skills such as the *ars dictaminis*,[47] cathedral school masters were able to provide their students with the requisite skills for a host of new jobs, ranging from scribes and notaries to

---

[45] Clifford H. Lawrence, *Medieval monasticism: forms of religious life in Western Europe in the Middle Ages*, 2nd edn (London, 1989), pp. 239–41.

[46] Brooke, *The coming of the friars*, pp. 77–84, 160–1.

[47] Nancy G. Siraisi, *Arts and sciences at Padua: the studium of Padua before 1350* (Toronto, 1973), pp. 37–9.

envoys, plenipotentiaries and diplomats. Moreover, the masters' specialized knowledge of patristic writings, of the decrees of the Church councils and of scripture made them particularly well suited to teaching students the canon law and sacred doctrine that would fit them for one of the new careers in the Church.[48]

As a result of these new pressures, during the twelfth and early thirteenth centuries a new set of relationships was established governing of the provision of education. On the one hand, cathedral school masters emerged as the main suppliers of educated young men. During this period, ever more masters began to set up their own schools within the shadow of a cathedral, ready to provide students with a training in the basic arts, as well as a training in the more advanced skills of law and theology.[49] To the extent that these masters were indeed providing just such an education, so ever more students, ambitious for social advancement, sought out these masters to secure for themselves a marketable education.[50] On the other hand, in so far as the townsfolk, the state and the Church – who were in need of educated young men – were satisfied with the students being produced by the masters, so they did all they could to protect and foster the work being done in the schools by granting the scholars every sort of privilege.[51]

NEW RESPONSES: LEARNED MEDICAL MEN AND MEDICINE

How did these broader changes in the world of learning during the twelfth and early thirteenth centuries affect the teaching of learned medicine? To some extent, the same new processes that were reshaping the teaching of the basic arts, law and theology were also at work reshaping the teaching and practice of learned medicine. At the broadest level, an increasing population in the new towns inevitably generated a new demand for medical care. More especially, the expanding wealthy upper classes of society generated an increased demand for practitioners of learned medicine.[52] One immediate effect of this was that from among those more ambitious students who wished to make their living by exploiting this end of the medical market there arose a new demand for teachers of learned medicine.

As in the case of arts, law and theology, the clerical masters of the cathedrals schools were once again well placed to respond to these new needs for, as we have seen, there was already a well-established tradition of

---

[48] Southern, 'The changing role of universities', pp. 142–6.

[49] John W. Baldwin, 'Masters at Paris from 1179 to 1215: a social perspective', in *Renaissance and renewal in the twelfth century*, ed. Robert L. Benson and Giles Constable (Oxford, 1982), pp. 138–72.

[50] Baldwin, 'Masters at Paris', pp. 151–8.

[51] For the privileges granted to Parisian scholars see Hastings Rashdall, *The universities of Europe in the Middle Ages*, new edn, ed. by Frederick M. Powicke and Alfred B. Emden, 3 vols. (Oxford, 1936), vol. I, pp. 294–343 and 398–426.

[52] For evidence that physicians catered almost exclusively to the needs of the upper classes see Jacquart, *Le milieu médical*, annexe A, tables 8, 9 and 12, and p. 427.

clerical masters providing instruction in learned medicine. Indeed, the particular case of the schools of Paris provides clear evidence for this increasing interest among scholars in the study of learned medicine during the late twelfth century. If we are to believe the criticisms of contemporary Parisian authors, it would seem that ever more students were rushing through their study of the basic arts with unseemly haste, and were ignoring altogether the more scholarly study of literature and theology in their desire to get a training in a discipline such as law or medicine that would prepare them for a more lucrative career in society.[53] Indeed, such was the demand for medical education that, in the early years of the thirteenth century, some masters such as Gilles de Corbeil, a canon of Notre Dame (d. 1224), and Ricardus Anglicus set up their own schools in Paris devoted exclusively to the teaching of learned medicine.[54] To some extent, then, as with arts, law and theology, the changes in medical teaching in the late twelfth and early thirteenth centuries can also be interpreted as responses to new social needs.

Yet, in one sense, medicine was quite different from philosophy, law and theology. Strictly speaking, philosophy, law and theology could be defined completely in terms of the specific sets of practices that they embodied. Philosophers, lawyers and theologians were, by definition, men who had been trained to engage in discussion with other philosophers, lawyers and theologians in a particular manner over clearly defined philosophical, legal and theological issues. To this extent, the disciplines of philosophy, law and theology could be viewed as direct products of the school environment. Medicine, however, was a rather different matter. There were, in theory at least, no disciplinary boundaries that defined who could and who could not claim to be a medical practitioner. Indeed, there were no disciplinary boundaries that defined a *medical* act *per se*. In the completely open market of medical practice anybody could offer any sort of medical care in the hope of attracting a client. In such a situation non-learned practitioners of medicine were just as keen to exploit the new opportunities that were opening up in the area of medical practice.[55]

In one sense, the physicians were starting from a very weak position

---

[53] See Stephen C. Ferruolo, *The origins of the university: the schools of Paris and their critics, 1100–1215* (Stanford, 1985), pp. 107, 126, 131, 142, 157, 184, 234. For the lucrative nature of medical practice see E. A. Hammond, 'Incomes of medieval English doctors', *Journal of the History of Medicine*, 15 (1960), 154–69; and Carole Rawcliffe, 'The profits of practice: the wealth and status of medical men in later medieval England', *Social History of Medicine*, 1 (1988), 61–78.

[54] Baldwin, 'Masters at Paris', p. 167.

[55] Pearl Kibre, 'The faculty of medicine at Paris, charlatanism and unlicensed medical practices in the later Middle Ages', *Bulletin of the History of Medicine*, 27 (1953), 1–20; Vern L. Bullough, 'The development of the medical guilds at Paris', *Medievalia et Humanistica*, 12 (1958), 33–40 at p. 34; William Eamon and Gundolf Keil, '*Plebs amat empirica*: Nicholas of Poland and his critique of the mediaeval medical establishment', *Sudhoffs Archiv*, 71 (1987), 180–96.

from which to counter this competition. By the thirteenth century, it was usually the case that practitioners of any craft could protect themselves from the rigours of unrestrained competition by gathering together to exert a monopolistic control over the practice of their craft and thus regulate it for their own benefit.[56] But for the learned physicians, because their clients accounted for so small a percentage of the total number of patients and because they themselves accounted for such a small percentage of the total number of medical practitioners, these strategies could not provide them with any effective means of protecting their own livelihoods. In another sense, however, the practitioners of learned medicine were in a very strong position to counter the competition. Their advantage, as we shall see, lay in the fact that they were indeed learned, that is, they had been taught by masters in the schools.

Masters of medicine, of course, were simply doing what they had traditionally done, namely, teaching a system of learned medicine that they no doubt sincerely believed was true and efficacious. Faced, however, with the new competition brought forth by the increased demand for medical care, the medical masters responded in a most natural way. First, instead of competing with one another for students as they had done in the past, they banded together for common protection. The impetus that lay behind this was the same as the impetus that lay behind the formation of the guilds. The only difference was that in the former case the outcome was a fraternity or faculty of teachers, while in the latter case the outcome was a fraternity or guild of practitioners. The results, however, were much the same. In asserting a monopolistic control over the teaching of learned medicine, the Parisian faculty of medicine was able to regulate the teaching, examining and licensing of all practitioners of learned medicine in and around Paris.

The other response of the medical masters was, for a group of academics, even more characteristic. Given that the masters in fact had little control over the market of medical practice, they sought to protect the position of their students in the market place by formulating new arguments in order to defend the status of learned medicine. Now, as learned clerics of the schools, it was entirely consistent that medical masters should turn to Aristotle in search of the sort of defence they were looking for for learned medicine. In Aristotle they found the resources with which to demonstrate, first, that the learned medicine they taught was indeed true medicine and, second, that medical practice was safe and correct only in so far as it was based upon a knowledge of this true medicine. Essentially, they sought to explain the nature of medicine from the point of view of the Aristotelian concepts of *scientia* and *ars*. On the one hand, in discussing whether medicine was an Aristotelian *scientia* or not, masters were attempting to

[56] Richard Mackenney, *Tradesmen and traders: the world of the guilds in Venice and Europe, c. 1250–c. 1650* (London, 1987), pp. xi–xii.

reveal the extent to which medicine could be described as a distinct and demonstrably true body of knowledge that could be derived from first principles drawn from the higher discipline of natural philosophy. On the other hand, in discussing whether medicine was an Aristotelian *ars* or not, they were attempting to reveal the extent to which medicine involved the intellectual skill of applying general theoretical principles in particular practical cases.[57] Rather than examine in detail these discussions about the nature of medicine, I wish to explain how the claims made for learned medicine by the medical masters benefited their students as practitioners of the learned medicine.

Of course, the masters' claims about the nature of learned medicine were directed, in the first instance, towards their medical students who formed the audience for their lectures and commentaries. But, by instructing their students in the nature of learned medicine, masters sought to provide intending physicians with an explanation of learned medicine that would attract the right sort of clientele. Now, by the thirteenth century, the clients of the physicians included many of the wealthiest and socially most exclusive members of society. By this time, a novel situation had also arisen (for the Latin West, at least) in which these members of society were also, by and large, the best educated, for an increasing proportion of them had been trained in the schools. Consequently, because they had been trained in at least the basic arts, it was very likely that they would be receptive to learned medicine in general, and in particular to the new Aristotelian claims that were being made for it. For people trained to accept the validity of certain Aristotelian assumptions and certain Aristotelian ways of thinking, the Aristotelian claims that were made for learned medicine must have had a certain irresistible force to them. Any client who shared these initial assumptions was led to agreeing with the medical masters that the medicine they taught was true. The medical masters' Aristotelian claims for learned medicine, then, were particularly well chosen to appeal to the instincts of precisely those clients whom the physicians wished to attract.

The claims made for learned medicine, however, were of much greater force than simply attracting the right sort of client. By the thirteenth century, it was also the case in the Latin West that among the ranks of the best-educated members of society were not only the wealthiest but also the most powerful members of society. By this time, it was increasingly common to find nobles and courtiers, popes, bishops and other ecclesiastical dignitaries, merchants, bankers, town burghers and others who had been educated in the schools. In so far as a greater proportion of these sorts

---

[57] Nancy Siraisi, *Taddeo Alderotti and his pupils: two generations of Italian medical learning* (Princeton, NJ, 1981), ch. 5; Siraisi, 'Changing concepts of the organization of medical knowledge in the Italian universities: fourteenth to sixteenth centuries', in *La diffusione delle scienze islamiche nel medio evo Europeo* (Rome, 1987), pp. 291–321; Siraisi, 'Pietro d'Abano and Taddeo Alderotti: two models of medical culture', *Medioevo*, 11 (1985), 139–62; Ottosson, *Scholastic medicine and philosophy*, ch. 2.

of people had been educated in the schools then we may conclude that many of the most powerful members of society were similarly very receptive to the new claims being made for learned medicine. Obviously, these were the sorts of people who formed the potential clientele of the physicians, and for this reason alone they would have been the intended audience for the new claims medical masters were making about learned medicine. But they were the intended audience for another equally important reason. In so far as they were able to win the assent of these people for the claims they were making about learned medicine, medical masters were able to secure the support of precisely those groups in society who were able to protect and privilege the physician in the market of medical practice. Here, then, I wish to show how the Parisian masters of medicine deployed their Aristotelian arguments about the nature of medicine in order to persuade the authorities to protect and privilege the practitioners of learned medicine.

Returning to the idealized plan for medical practice proposed by the Parisian medical faculty in 1271, we saw this was a scheme that presented medicine as a practice engaged in by the physician, the surgeon and the apothecary, each of whose roles was clearly established according to function, with the physician placed at the top of the hierarchy. If we look more closely, we can see that this hierarchy was built upon a very specific notion of medical *scientia* and medical *ars*. Thus, the reason given why apothecaries should not make or administer drugs without consulting the physician was because they – unlike the physician – did not have a grasp of true medical knowledge. Instead, they thought up medicine 'out of their own heads', and made them 'not according to art but rather by chance and fortune', and as a result they brought death to many. Surgeons also, it was claimed, administered medicines while being totally ignorant of their 'cause and reason'. It was on these grounds that the medical faculty argued that apothecaries and surgeons should not presume to exceed the boundaries of their respective crafts. Thus, in so far as the Parisian medical masters were promoting a scheme of medical practice that was built upon the Aristotelian notions of *scientia* and *ars*, we may assume that this was a scheme that, of its very nature, was going to appeal to the authorities.

Let us look in detail at precisely how the Parisian masters managed to secure the support of the authorities for their scheme of medical practice. Most important was the medical faculty's right to petition the ecclesiastical authorities for support. This was partly because, in Paris at least, the faculty was composed of clerical masters who received their authority to teach from the Church. But more important was the fact that the licence to practise that the medical faculty secured for its graduates was a licence granted by the Church in the person of the chancellor of Paris. It was therefore the right of the medical faculty to seek the assistance of the Church authorities in suppressing the many medical practitioners in Paris who, the faculty claimed, were practising as physicians without being duly licensed. Indeed, as masters of the Parisian *studium*, it was quite natural for members of the medical faculty to petition directly to the pope for redress against unlicensed medical practitioners. The Parisian medical faculty also had the right – as did any other craft guild – to petition the secular authorities, and even the king himself, to protect the practice of its trade. As we shall see, each time the Parisian medical faculty approached either the ecclesiastical or secular authorities, its strategy was the same. The faculty claimed that there were medical practitioners in Paris carrying out the functions of a physician even though they had not been instructed in the true art and science of medicine, with the consequence that the lives of many Parisians were being put in grave danger.

As we have seen, the papacy already had its own reasons to be well disposed towards the masters of the schools. It is probably not surprising, therefore, that the papacy was generally receptive to the petitions of the Parisian medical faculty. Moreover, a closer examination reveals that the petitions made to the pope by the faculty, as well as the papal injunctions that were secured, were always expressed in terms of the medical masters' Aristotelian argument that physicians alone were trained in the true science of medicine, and that they alone knew how the general principles of medical science were to be applied safely and correctly in particular cases of medical practice. For example, in 1325, Pope John XXII called upon Stephen, Bishop of Paris, to support the medical faculty, which had petitioned him for assistance in stamping out medical practice by people 'wholly ignorant of the art of medicine', who were causing many deaths.[58] In 1330, the pope wrote to the new bishop, Hugh, informing him that the university had again brought it to his notice that medical practitioners 'without the slightest knowledge of the art of medicine' were at large in Paris. He ordered that nobody was to practise medicine other than the masters or those licensed by a council consisting of the dean of the medical faculty and two regent masters 'in the science of medicine'.[59] Again, in 1347, the dean and the faculty of medicine petitioned the pope for aid against men and women in Paris who were audaciously usurping the office of physician and engaging in practice 'without the slightest knowledge of the art and science of medicine'. They asked him to urge the Bishop of Senlis, as Conservator of Apostolic Privileges, to forbid anybody to practise 'the said art and science' unless he was a master of medicine or had been licensed at another university.[60]

The situation was much the same in those cases where the Parisian medical faculty petitioned the French crown for assistance. As we have seen, like the papacy, the French crown had its own interests in attending to

[58] *CUP*, vol. II, no. 844, pp. 285–6.
[59] *CUP*, vol. II, no. 900, pp. 336–7.
[60] *CUP*, vol. II, no. 1138, pp. 602–3.

the needs of Parisian scholars, and so likewise the French crown was always well disposed to the petitions of the medical faculty. Moreover, when we examine the actions taken by the king to protect the physicians we see that they are always justified on the grounds of the Aristotelian arguments put forward by the medical faculty. For instance, in 1352, King Jean was presented with a report that many unauthorized persons – wise women, monks, the uneducated (*rustici*) apothecaries, herbalists, bachelors of medicine and foreigners – were dispensing medicines freely in Paris. But these practitioners, claimed the medical faculty, were ignorant of the 'science of medicine', the complexions and constitutions of men, and the virtues of medicines, and by dispensing dangerous drugs they were imperilling the lives of Parisians. They were also performing operations without the aid of the physicians which, in consequence, were resulting in homicides and abortions. The king ordered, therefore, that nobody was to administer laxatives or opiates except on the advice of a physician who was a master or licentiate in the 'science of medicine'.[61]

The Parisian medical faculty, then, sought to protect the position of the practitioner of learned medicine by securing certain privileges from the secular and ecclesiastical authorities. It also sought to protect the physicians by taking legal action against any non-learned practitioner who infringed upon these newly won privileges. In theory at least, unlike the Church and state, the law courts had no vested interest in favouring the learned over the non-learned medical practitioner. There were, however, a number of reasons why, in fact, advocates and judges tended to be more receptive to the arguments of the medical faculty. Of central importance was the fact that, by the fourteenth century, nearly all advocates and judges were themselves trained in the schools. Indeed, as learned men, lawyers were just the sort of people who we could expect would have turned to the physicians when they were ill. Moreover, despite the tensions that frequently existed between faculties of law and faculties of medicine, lawyers undoubtedly looked upon university-trained physicians to some extent as learned colleagues. Furthermore, lawyers trained in the schools were more likely to be receptive to the sorts of rational arguments put forward by the Parisian medical faculty. Important also was the simple fact that rational arguments, of their very nature, probably carried greater weight in the logical procedures of a fourteenth-century ecclesiastical court. It is not surprising, then, that when we examine the legal proceedings initiated by the Parisian medical faculty we find that its arguments were based upon the same Aristotelian claim that the physician alone had a proper understanding of the true art and science of medicine. The proceedings of the trial of Jacqueline Felice de Almania in 1322 provide an especially well-documented example of this. In the course of the proceedings, the faculty of

[61] *CUP*, vol. III, no. 1211, pp. 16–17.

medicine reminded the court that for nearly sixty years penalties of fines and excommunication had been in operation against ignorant and illicit empirics practising in Paris and its environs. These penalties had been applied with the full force of the Official of the Bishop of Paris and the illustrious Kings of France. But, claimed the faculty, Jacqueline had persisted in acting as a physician although she was totally ignorant of the art of medicine. She was not lettered, and she had not been approved competent in those things which she presumed to treat. Not understanding the causes of illness or the art of medicine, claimed the prosecution, meant that she stood in grave danger of killing her patients. Although a spirited defence was put up on her behalf, the court clearly preferred the arguments of the faculty. Finding her guilty, the court forbade Jacqueline to practise medicine and to exercise the functions of a physician under threat of a fine and excommunication.[62]

From the surviving evidence, then, it would appear that the deployment of arguments about the art and science of medicine formed a central part in the campaign by the Parisian masters of medicine to enrol the support of the most powerful groups in society in privileging and protecting practitioners of learned medicine. But probably even more important was the fact that the deployment of such arguments helped to fix in the minds of the secular and ecclesiastical authorities the notion of a medical hierarchy as something to be aimed at.

NEW RESPONSES: LEARNED MEDICAL MEN AND SURGERY

But how did surgery fit into the plans of the Parisian medical masters and their claims about the nature of medicine? On the one hand, there were some masters such as Turisanus, Pietro d'Abano and Bartholomew of Bruges who concentrated upon establishing the fact that it was the physician alone who possessed demonstrably true medical knowledge. For them, discussions about the more practical aspects of medicine such as surgery were not relevant to their central objective of demonstrating that the medicine they taught was indeed *scientia*. There were other masters, however, such as Lanfranco of Milan, Henri de Mondeville and Guy de Chauliac, who were concerned to demonstrate that it was the physician alone who possessed the skill of taking the general principles of true medical knowledge that had been learned in the classroom and applying them in particular instances of medical practice. Inevitably, then, in seeking to demonstrate that medicine was indeed an *ars*, these medical masters were led to discuss the operations of medical practice.

In reading their works on surgery we must always bear in mind that these texts were written by masters of medicine for students who intended to be practising physicians. We should also remember that these medical masters treated surgery as one specialized example of how the practitioner of learned medicine applied his knowledge of the general principles of true medicine to the particular problems of medical practice. Indeed, these medical masters were at pains to point out that, in order to be a good surgeon, first one needed to be trained as a good physician. Guy de Chauliac's introduction to his *Chirurgia magna* provides an excellent account of the nature of surgery as viewed from this perspective.[63]

As was customary for university masters of the fourteenth century, Guy began his treatise on surgery with a long and elaborate praise of God, calling for divine assistance in completing his work. Guy then adopted the traditional university procedure of introducing his treatise with an *accessus*. First, Guy discussed the use of such a work. He believed that there was a need for a single, general, comprehensive guide to the art of surgery because it was too daunting a prospect for the beginner in surgery to be faced with numerous detailed works on the subject. It was within this context that Guy then explained the title of the work. He was acutely aware that the art was too diffusely taught in several surgical works, and that there was therefore a need for somebody to draw together in a single work an inventory or collection of useful passages on surgery. He then outlined the mode of exposition he was going to adopt. He explained that he would proceed according to the Aristotelian principle that we should begin with a sure understanding of the most general things, and with this knowledge we should then proceed to an understanding of more particular things.

In characteristically scholastic fashion Guy then proceeded to define the subject matter of the work. In his definition of the nature of surgery we should note, first, that Guy regarded surgery simply as one specialized part of medical practice, and second, that – like medicine – surgery should be conceived of as a body of demonstrably true knowledge that could be derived from principles drawn from the higher discipline of medicine, and that – like that of the physician – the skill of the surgeon lay in his ability to apply the general surgical knowledge he had been taught in particular surgical cases.

Guy began this section of his introduction with the most general definition, that surgery was that part of healing conducted by means of incision, cauterization and articulation of the bones. Following Galen, he believed that surgery could be defined either more strictly as the third instrument of medicine after diet and medicines, or more broadly as knowledge which revealed the correct way of operating in order to bring about a cure. Guy elaborated upon this last definition by explaining that surgery could be looked at as either instructive knowledge (*scientia docens*)

---

[63] The following summary is based upon the Vincent de Portonariis edition, Lyons *c.* 1510, fols. 2ra–4va.

or a useful skill (*ars utens*). Surgery could also be described as an art which presumed to provide the correct cure for each illness except where an illness was incurable, or where the illness cured itself, or where one illness foretold another worse one. Guy also defined surgery etymologically as working by hand. Such manual operations had as their subject the human body, and it was the object and intent of surgery to restore the ill human body to health. There again, surgery could be defined with respect to its parts. Surgery, explained Guy, comprised two genera: operations in the soft parts of the human body, and operations in the firm parts. There were also different species of surgery. There was instructive knowledge about wounds, instructive knowledge about healing them, and instructive knowledge about operations concerning phlebotomy and cutting. After describing the instruments of surgery – namely, the surgeon's potions, unguents, emplasters and poultices, and his implements for cutting, for cauterizing, for removing foreign bodies, and for probing – Guy concluded the first part of his introduction by claiming that it was only after acquiring true surgical knowledge that the surgeon was in a position to decide, first, which was the appropriate operation to be carried out in any particular circumstance; second, on what grounds it was to be undertaken; third, whether it was necessary and likely to succeed; and fourth, how one was to proceed.

In the second part of his introduction, after his famous history of surgery, Guy gave an account of the personal qualities of a good surgeon. Here it becomes clear that Guy believed the best sort of surgeon was a learned physician who specialized in the art and science of surgery. First of all, Guy believed that the surgeon should be well read not only in the principles of surgery but also in the theoretical and practical aspects of *physica*. For *theorica* he should have a thorough knowledge of the naturals, non-naturals and contra-naturals, and for *practica* he should have an understanding of the other two branches of medicine, namely, diet and medicines. In addition to all this, he should know the principles of medicine as well as geometry, astronomy and dialectics. Once in possession of this wisdom, the surgeon should then gain experience by witnessing operations, for only in this way, claimed Guy, would the surgeon become truly expert. The surgeon should also be gifted: he should be gifted with good judgement, memory, dexterity, good vision and a sound intellect. He ought to be of graceful appearance, with sensitive fingers, firm hands and clear eyes. Moreover, the surgeon should always be endeavouring to please, fearless in the face of danger, gracious to the infirm, benevolent to his friends, and cautious in prognosticating. He ought to be virtuous, sober, pious, merciful and unlustful. Last but not least, rather than charge extortionate fees he should accept only a moderate salary. When such a surgeon was available, when the sick person was patient and obedient, when the assistants were peaceful, helpful, truthful and discreet, and when the surroundings were conducive to recovery, then, claimed Guy, good surgery was possible.

Like medicine, then, Guy claimed, surgery could be described as a body of true knowledge from which good surgical practice was derived. Indeed, Guy's whole work was an elaboration of precisely this point. He began his work with a treatise on the anatomy of the human body, establishing it as the theoretical framework for the practice of surgery. The following treatises were then given over to descriptions of the growths, wounds, ulcers, fractures and dislocations that could occur in these anatomical parts. By structuring his book in this way, Guy wanted to show how all these practical surgical problems should be understood in the light of a theoretical understanding of human anatomy. Indeed, Guy structured the whole of his book so that it moved from theory to practice, from the general to the particular, and from the unobservable to the observable. Essentially, he was aiming to structure his work on the rational model of cause and effect.

Lanfranco of Milan was another medical master who, like Guy, recognized that there were some physicians who disregarded the more practical aspects of medicine such as surgery. Lanfranco himself, however, stated quite explicitly his belief that to be a good surgeon one first had to be a good physician:

'Why, oh why', he exclaimed, 'is there in our day so great a difference between the physician and the surgeon. The physicians have abandoned all operations to the laity, despising (as some of them put it) to operate with their hands, or rather (as I believe) because they are ignorant as to how to do the operations. This shortcoming has come to the point where the people consider it as impossible that the same man can know both surgery and medicine. But you should know this, that he that has no knowledge of surgery is not a good physician, and conversely, a man cannot be a good surgeon unless he knows *physica*.'[64]

Henri de Mondeville also poured scorn on those of his physician colleagues who despised manual operations, and who therefore chose to treat the most obvious surgical problems with useless medicines. Henri was, however, just as critical of the proud and pompous unlearned surgeons who, to him, appeared to lack any intelligence. They were wicked and cruel men, he claimed, who demanded excessive fees: and what little they did know they knew from physicians such as himself. His fundamental criticism was that they were not given to study. Indeed, only a very few of them were even literate. The real problem, he believed, was that they were all deficient in their understanding of the art and science of medicine, and especially surgery.[65] Clearly, the division foremost in the minds of Lanfranco and Henri was not actually between surgeons and physicians, but between learned medical men who understood the true principles of medicine and the illiterate, ignorant practitioners who did not.

[64] Quoted by Malgaigne, *Œuvres complètes d'Ambroise Paré*, vol. I, p. xlvi (my translation).
[65] Marie-Christine Pouchelle, *Corps et chirurgie à l'apogée du moyen-âge* (Paris, 1983), pp. 25–31.

But, of course, learned physicians such as Guy, Lanfranco and Henri who specialized in surgery accounted for only a very small proportion indeed of the total number of people who made their living at performing medical operations. Most surgeons received no formal training in surgery. Their expertise in certain manual operations was possibly the product of some sort of apprenticeship, but was more probably simply the result of acquired experience. What interest had these sorts of people in the kind of surgery being proposed by the medical masters? In order to understand the responses of the non-learned surgeons in Paris to the new claims being made for surgery we need to investigate the nature and extent of the changes that occurred within the organization of Parisian surgeons during the thirteenth and fourteenth centuries.[66]

NEW RESPONSES: THE PRACTITIONERS OF SURGERY

During this period, the surgeons in the towns, like many other craftsmen, began to organize themselves into fraternities and guilds.[67] As we have seen, these moves sprang from the common interests members felt they shared in protecting their livelihoods. In Paris the earliest signs of these moves among the surgeons appear in the mid 1250s when the Provost of Paris, Etienne Boileau, chose six good and loyal Parisian surgeons to examine all practitioners of surgery in order to prevent inadequately trained people from imperilling the lives of Parisians.[68] The provost enforced this act in 1301 when he named twenty-nine barber surgeons who, under pain of death, were forbidden to practise the art of surgery until they had been examined by masters of surgery known to the provost.[69] Royal force was given to these municipal measures in 1311, when Philip the Fair issued an ordinance against murderers, thieves, foreigners, counterfeiters, spies, robbers, cheats and usurers who practised in Paris as if they were examined surgeons. The ordinance required that all male and female surgeons practising within the city and its environs should be carefully examined and approved by master surgeons appointed by the royal surgeon, Jean Pitart, or his successor, who was to be sworn-in at the Châtelet. These master surgeons were empowered to grant a licence to

---

[66] The standard account is to be found in Malgaigne, *Œuvres complètes d'Ambroise Paré*, vol. I, pp. cxx–clv; Wickersheimer, *Commentaires*, pp. lxxvi–lxxxiv; and Bullough, 'Medical guilds at Paris'.

[67] Mackenney, *Tradesmen and traders*, ch. 1; Antony Black, *Guilds and civil society in European political thought from the twelfth century to the present* (London, 1984), chs. 1–7; Susan Reynolds, *Kingdoms and communities in Western Europe, 900–1300* (Oxford, 1984), ch. 3.

[68] Georges-Bernard Depping (ed.), *Réglemens sur les arts et métiers de Paris rédigés au XIIIe siècle, et connus sous le nom du livre des métiers d'Etienne Boileau* (Collection de Documents Inédits sur l'Histoire de France: Première Série, Histoire Politique) (Paris, 1837), pp. 419–20.

[69] Malgaigne, *Œuvres complètes d'Ambroise Paré*, vol. I, p. cxxiv; Depping, *Réglemens*, note to p. 419.

practise to all those duly examined by them.[70] By the beginning of the fourteenth century, then, surgeons in Paris were already clearly categorized into three distinct groupings, namely, the master surgeons, surgeons who had been duly licensed to practise their art, and those unlicensed surgeons who practised illicitly.

The surviving evidence suggests that these early moves were as much an initiative on the part of the secular authorities as they were on the part of the surgeons themselves. This was probably because the secular authorities were eager to establish some measure of control over the burgeoning but unregulated practice of surgery in Paris. By the mid fourteenth century, however, it is clear that the master surgeons, at least, were taking the initiative by working together to protect their common interests. It appears that in about 1352 the two royal surgeons sworn-in at the Châtelet, Pierre Fromond and Robert Langres, attempted to monopolize the right to examine and license new practitioners, thus denying the rights of the Parisian master surgeons to be a party to the affair.[71] After much negotiation, in 1356, an act of the Parlement confirmed the procedure whereby the representative of the master surgeons – called the provost of the surgeons – shared with the royal surgeons the authority to convoke the master surgeons of Paris for the purposes of examining and licensing.[72] This event suggests that the master surgeons of Paris had, by the 1350s, formed themselves into some sort of organization which was independent of direct royal and civil control, and which elected a representative to protect the master surgeons' right to examine and license practitioners of surgery in Paris.

The first sign that this loose organization had taken on the more concrete form of a confraternity came in a royal statute of 1364 banning illicit surgical practice in Paris. In its preamble the ordinance repeated the ruling that no male or female surgeon should presume to practise the art of surgery either publicly or privately without first being examined and approved. It then proceeded to give formal recognition to the Confraternity of St Cosmas and St Damian, confirming its right to join with the royal surgeons and provost of Paris in examining and licensing surgeons.[73] The confraternity was again addressed by Charles V in 1370 when he ordered that the provost of the master surgeons should report to the provost of Paris all serious wounds that the members of the confraternity were called upon to treat. In the same edict the king granted the master

---

[70] *Ordonnances des roys de France de la troisième race*, 21 vols. plus 2 suppls. (Paris, 1723–1847), vol. I, pp. 491–2. The complete text of this statute is given in the confirmation granted by Jean I in 1352. See *Ordonnances*, vol. II, pp. 496–7.

[71] The 1352 confirmation of the royal edict of 1311 names Pierre Fromond and Robert Langres as the two royal surgeons sworn in at the Châtelet, and describes in detail their powers of licensing. See *Ordonnances*, vol. II, pp. 496–7.

[72] *CUP*, vol. III, no. 1231, pp. 42–3.

[73] *Ordonnances*, vol. IV, pp. 499–501; *CUP*, vol. III, no. 1296, pp. 113–14.

surgeons a special exemption from sentinel and guard duty on the condition that they visited and treated the poor who could not afford to enter a hospital.[74]

Our knowledge of the internal arrangements of the Confraternity of St Cosmas and St Damian comes from its statutes of 1372. These statutes – numbering in all about twenty – describe how a young man wishing to learn the art should apprentice himself in the household of a master surgeon of at least four years' standing. The statutes also outline the stages of bachelorhood and licentiateship. To graduate as a bachelor or as a licentiate the apprentice was required to be examined at a ceremony during which first the masters, then the provost of the surgeons and finally the royal surgeons interrogated the candidate. The ceremony ended with the candidate being obliged to take an oath to uphold the statutes of the confraternity. An entrance fee was also demanded of the candidate before he could take up his new position within the society. For the new licentiate the day ended with an exchange of gifts and an elaborate dinner at the licentiate's expense. The licentiate was then expected to continue practising surgery for four years before proceeding to the ceremony of capping the new master, after which he was then permitted to take on his own apprentices.[75]

More or less contemporary with the development of the Confraternity of St Cosmas and St Damian in Paris was the founding of the Corporation of Barbers. We have already seen how, in 1301 and 1311, all surgeons in Paris were obliged to present themselves before the master surgeons for examination in order to obtain a licence to practise. These barber surgeons were again recognized as a distinct group when, in 1365, Charles V exempted them from sentinel duty.[76] The first evidence, however, of an independent organization of Parisian barbers comes in 1371, when Charles V confirmed the statutes of the Parisian Corporation of Barbers.[77] A statute of the following year provides us with our first description of the sort of surgery performed by members of the Parisian Corporation of Barbers. The preamble to this statute suggests that the barbers had been seeking redress against the master surgeons, who were attempting to prevent them from treating sores, swellings and wounds. After a detailed investigation into the issue, the royal court announced that the barbers were to be permitted to administer 'plasters, ointments and other appropriate medications for swellings, ulcerations and all open wounds ... without being molested, troubled or hindered on their part by the said surgeons and sworn healers'.[78] Thus, by 1372, the independent Corporation of Barbers in Paris had secured for its members the right to carry out a range of basic

---

[74] *Ordonnances*, vol. v, p. 322; *CUP*, vol. III, no. 1360, pp. 191–2.
[75] Malgaigne, *Œuvres complètes d'Ambroise Paré* vol. I, pp. cxxxi–cxxxii.
[76] *Ordonnances*, vol. IV, pp. 609–11.
[77] Ibid., vol. v, pp. 440–2.
[78] Ibid., vol. v, pp. 530–1.

surgical operations without reference to any other group of surgical practitioners.

The economic and social changes of the thirteenth and fourteenth centuries, then, had produced a new and complex picture of surgical practice in Paris. First, there was the small elite band of learned physician-surgeons, who were trained and licensed by the medical faculty, and who acted as advisers, if not actually operators, in those few important cases where a physician's client required a specialized surgical operation. Then there was a small body of master surgeons whose confraternity trained new members by apprenticeship, and licensed them to practise specialized as well as more general surgical operations for the more wealthy inhabitants of Paris. Then there was a relatively large number of barber surgeons to whom the great majority of townsfolk turned for more general, superficial surgical operations. Finally, there were the many illicit practitioners, who made their living at carrying out all manner of surgical operations among the poorer classes of Parisian society.

From this brief sketch we can see that the master surgeons, although in many ways different from the learned physicians, shared with their university-trained colleagues a very similar social and economic position. On the one hand, they shared with the physicians the economic disadvantage of being small in number[79] and serving the needs of relatively few clients. Unable to monopolize the practice of surgery, master surgeons were constantly exposed to competition from illicit practitioners as well as from barber surgeons. Of course, in principle, the livelihood of master surgeons was not threatened by barber surgeons, who practised surgery in geographical areas and among social classes where the master surgeons themselves did not move. But what did reasonably concern them was the fact that the barbers were forming themselves into guilds and securing privileges to protect their rights to practise certain surgical operations. On the other hand, master surgeons shared with the physicians the advantage of counting among their clients the wealthiest, best-educated and most powerful members of society.[80] In these circumstances, it appears that the master surgeons came to regard the plan for medical practice promoted by the physicians as being a plan particularly well suited to their own needs. They perceived that the assumption underlying the plan, that all good practice derived from true knowledge, could be applied in the case of surgery as a means of forwarding their own interests. The physicians had argued that because they alone knew true medical knowledge then they alone could direct good medical practice. In the same way, master surgeons

[79] In 1356 there were nine master surgeons in the Parisian Confraternity of St Cosmas and St Damian. See *CUP*, vol. III, no. 1231, pp. 42–3. In 1396, there were ten members, while in 1424 and again in 1436 there were eleven members. See Malgaigne, *Œuvres complètes d'Ambroise Paré*, vol. I, p. cxlii and note to p. cxliv.

[80] For an analysis of the clients of French master surgeons see Jacquart, *Le milieu médical*, annexe A, tables 8, 9 and 12, and p. 427.

could argue that in so far as they were learned in true surgical knowledge, then they alone could direct good surgical practice. It thus became a matter of great importance for master surgeons to demonstrate that surgery was indeed a learned discipline.

This is revealed in one sense by the fact that the Confraternity of St Cosmas and St Damian increasingly took on the appearance of a university faculty. For example, in 1370, the Parisian master surgeons adopted the titles of bachelor, licentiate and master, titles which had hitherto been restricted to the university faculties.[81] Another indication of this imitation appears in the new statutes of 1396, when the Parisian Confraternity of St Cosmas and St Damian ordered that henceforth all new apprentices should be able to speak and write good Latin.[82] The master surgeons also went out of their way to underline their status as learned scholars. For instance, in 1390, when petitioning the University of Paris for assistance in prosecuting illicit practitioners of surgery, the surgeons of the Confraternity of St Cosmas and St Damian described themselves as 'we your humble scholars and pupils'.[83] Indeed, it appears that, by 1436, the master surgeons had for some time been attending lectures in surgery at the *studium*, for the university statute of this date, which extended to them the privileges attached to the status of being a scholar, was given on the condition that the surgeons continued to attend the lessons of the regent masters of medicine 'as was customary'.[84]

Like the masters of medicine, the master surgeons also defended their privileges on the grounds that they alone possessed the true art and science of surgery. The first evidence we have for this in Paris comes in a royal ordinance of 1372 which permitted barbers to practise minor surgery. The preamble to this ordinance summarized the petitions that had been received by the crown from interested parties. Apparently, the master surgeons and sworn healers of Paris had made a submission in which they had argued that, under royal ordinance, nobody else was permitted to meddle or interfere in the art of surgery because only the master surgeons possessed the true art and science of surgery which should be used to treat all manner of wounds and maladies of the human body.[85] The master surgeons argued along the same lines in their petition to the University of Paris in 1390 for assistance in stamping out illicit surgical practice. They claimed that recently there had appeared in Paris many empirics and unapproved surgeons who dishonoured the science of surgery. According to their royal privileges, they argued, nobody was allowed to practise in Paris or proceed in the science and art of surgery or enter the office or profession of surgeon

---

[81] *Ordonnances*, vol. v, p. 322; *CUP*, vol. III, no. 1360, p. 191.
[82] Malgaigne, *Œuvres complètes d'Ambroise Paré*, vol. I, p. cxli.
[83] Ibid., vol. I, p. cxl.
[84] *CUP*, vol. IV, no. 2496, pp. 594–5.
[85] *Ordonnances*, vol. v, pp. 530–1.

without being examined and approved by the king's surgeon and the provost of Parisian surgeons.[86] Again, in 1436, the University of Paris listened to the petitions of the masters in Paris approved in the science and art of surgery. The University looked favourably upon the argument put forward by the master surgeons that there had recently arisen many quacks and false practitioners not approved in surgery, who were disturbing and cheapening the venerable science of surgery, and who were bringing grave scandal upon the art. All this was occurring, the University was told, even though the crown had granted privileges to the masters of the science of surgery ordaining that only those duly examined were permitted to practise the art.[87]

Again, like the physicians, the master surgeons also used the argument about the relationship between art and science to prosecute those whom they held to be illicit practitioners. For example, in 1411, the master surgeons urged the provost of Paris to arrest Perretta Pettone, a woman who was practising surgery in the rue S. Denis, but who had not been examined or approved by them. They demanded that she should be imprisoned at the Châtelet until they could investigate her knowledge of the art and science of surgery further.[88]

The need to present surgery as a learned discipline also provided the context in which master surgeons used the learned surgical works written by the clerical scholars. In the first place, these works provided them with arguments clearly demonstrating how good surgical practice derived from true surgical knowledge. These texts also provided the master surgeons with the educational tools with which they could instruct their apprentices in learned surgery. Moreover, they provided an examinable body of surgical knowledge which every licentiate could be expected to know. The possession of learned surgical works now became a visible hallmark of what it was to be a good surgeon. It became the habit of a good surgeon to refer to authoritative sources for guidance in carrying out surgical operations. Henceforth, the proficiency of every surgeon – from the most learned to the semi-literate – was to be assessed in terms of his or her understanding of learned surgery. It therefore became essential for all surgical practitioners – even the barbers – to display their knowledge of the theory of surgery. It was thus the case that henceforth every surgeon had to have his surgical text.

CONCLUSION

It is clear that the new works on learned surgery that were written during the thirteenth and fourteenth centuries were products of the changes that

---

[86] *CUP*, vol. III, no. 1586, pp. 534–5; Malgaigne, *Œuvres complètes d'Ambroise Paré*, vol. I, pp. cxl–cxli.
[87] *CUP*, vol. IV, no. 2496, pp. 594–5.
[88] Ibid., vol. IV, no. 1912, pp. 198–9.

were taking place in surgery in response to new social and economic pressures of the period. More particularly, surgery was changing as a result of the rise of the new university medicine. The new university medicine was itself partly a creation of a group of learned medical men who sought to protect and privilege the place of the physician in the competitive market place of medical practice. One of the ways in which these men pursued their objective was by promoting an idealized plan for medical practice which centred upon the notion of a medical hierarchy consisting of physicians, surgeons and apothecaries. In essence, the new works on learned surgery that were written by these learned medical men were attempts to characterize more fully the new notion of the learned surgeon that was embodied in their idealized plan for medical practice.

The new ideal of the learned surgeon received social recognition for two reasons. First, the learned medical men themselves succeeded in enrolling the support of the most powerful and influential groups in society in backing their idealized plan for medical practice; secondly, and more importantly, behind it lay the fundamental principle that all good medical practice rested upon a knowledge of true medical theory. With this authoritative support, the new ideal of the learned surgeon acquired the social legitimacy it required. The learned surgeon became a social reality, however, only when practitioners of surgery realized that it was in their own practical interests to appropriate for themselves the characterization of the learned surgeon. But, of course, this characterization was not credible, nor was it complete, without the necessary symbols of learning, not least of which was the learned surgical text itself.

6

Medical practice in Paris in the first half of the fourteenth century

DANIELLE JACQUART

There are some fields in the history of medieval medicine which still demand to be opened up, whereas others, by contrast, have been explored so many times, at least superficially, that it seems that nothing new can be extracted from them. This last case applies to Parisian medicine during the first half of the fourteenth century. The weight of a priori statements and of frequent polemical intentions has overloaded historiography in this field since the eighteenth century. The rivalries between physicians and surgeons, the competition between the universities of Paris and Montpellier, as well as historians' tendency to combine the intellectual features of the faculties of arts and theology with those of the faculty of medicine – the result of all these factors is that Parisian medicine has rarely been analysed in itself. Despite Eduard Seidler's efforts,[1] it for the most part eludes a clear characterization. The tripartition into *via intellectualis, via scolaris* and *via pragmatica* that the German scholar put forward, as well as his overdone resort to the term 'eclectic', sufficiently suggests, that the dominant characteristics remain in the dark. It seems thus necessary to return to the available sources and to report what they state, in an effort to extricate them from the framework of extrapolating interpretations within which they are usually quoted.

SURGERY AS A CRAFT

In the first half of the fourteenth century, the three professions of physician, surgeon and barber were in place. During the last years of the thirteenth century, the surgeons were given a regulation, emanating from the provost of Paris.[2] Two main concerns emerge from this document. The first one is

---

[1] E. Siedler, *Die Heilkunde des ausgehenden Mittelalters in Paris* (Wiesbaden, 1967) *Sudhoffs Archiv*, 8, and *La médecine à Paris au XIVᵉ siècle* (Paris, 1967) Conférence donnée au Palais de la Découverte le 3 décembre 1966.

[2] There is some doubt whether this document was a part of the compilation called *Livre des métiers d'Etienne Boileau*, dating from 1258; it is more likely that this regulation was issued in the 1280s. Edition: R. de Lespinasse and F. Bonnardot, *Les métiers et corporations de Paris au XIIIᵉ siècle: le livre des métiers d'Etienne Boileau* (Paris, 1879), Histoire générale de Paris,

the fight against criminality: the provost states the fact that many murderers escape from his control, because the injured are secretly nursed by surgeons. According to this regulation, surgeons are obliged to inform the office of the provost, as soon as they are fetched to look after an injured person. The other concern is related to professional competence. Again the regulation starts from an observation: 'comme en Paris soient aucun et aucunes qui s'entremetent de cyrurgie qui n'en sunt pas digne, et perilz de mort d'omes et mehains de membres en aviennent et porroient avenir'. In order to prevent these deaths and maimings due to the practitioners' incompetence, the provost institutes a jury of six surgeons entitled to examine the persons who practise surgery and to determine whether they are skilled in this art or not. The following procedure is established: the sworn surgeons will write two lists, one enumerating the names of practitioners 'dignes d'ouvrer', the other those who are forbidden to practise. Among the six jurors designated in the edict of the provost, only Henri Du Perche and his son are known through other sources as practising in Paris during the years 1282–5.[3]

The regulation of 1301 is in line with the previous measures: it applies to those barbers who labelled themselves surgeons.[4] To be allowed to use this title, they will have to submit themselves to an examination by the master surgeons. In line with the previous regulation, a list of the barbers who were practising surgery without any evidence of their competence is annexed to the regulation of 1301. A second item maintains nevertheless that, in case of emergency, any barber can practise surgery if it is necessary to stop blood flowing or to close up a wound. In the same way as surgeons, barbers will be obliged in such cases to inform the provost of Paris at once.

Probably under the influence of his surgeon Jean Pitart,[5] King Philip the Fair published a decisive edict in 1311.[6] No one is allowed to practise surgery in the town and viscounty of Paris, unless he has been examined and admitted by the sworn surgeons, themselves summoned by, and placed under the authority of Jean Pitart, called by the king *chirurgicum nostrum juratum Casteleti nostri Parisius*. To Jean Pitart and his successors is devolved the power of granting the *licentia operandi*, after the approval of the

pp. 208–9. Reproduction of this edition in E. Nicaise, *Chirurgie de maître Henri de Mondeville* (Paris, 1893).
[3] On Henri Du Perche and his son Vincent, see E. Wickersheimer, *Dictionnaire biographique des médecins en France au moyen âge* (Geneva, 1979, repr. of the edn of 1936), pp. 278 and 774. The other jurors quoted in the regulation are: Robert le Convers and his brother Nicholas, Pierre des Hales and Pierre Joce.
[4] Printed in de Lespinasse and Bonnardot, *Les métiers et corporations*, vol. III (Paris, 1897), p. 628.
[5] On Jean Pitart, see E. Wickersheimer, *Dictionnaire*, p. 465, and D. Jacquart, *Supplément* (Geneva, 1979), p. 175.
[6] Printed in *Ordonnances des roys de France*, vol. I (Paris, 1723), pp. 491–2. Trans. into French in E. Nicaise, *Chirurgie*.

majority of the surgeons who have been summoned. The practitioners who, after the promulgation of this edict, continue to hang out their professional banners, will have them burnt in front of their door and will themselves be taken to the Châtelet, i.e. the criminal jurisdiction of Paris. That is the entirety of the content of this edict, which has been extrapolated by historians of surgery or summed up in a vague way. It repeats for the most part the measures of the regulation issued by the provost of Paris at the end of the thirteenth century. The only novelties are the solemnity conferred by the royal authority and the institution of a kind of 'president of the jury', whose title is not, as it is often said, 'prime surgeon', but only 'royal sworn surgeon of the Châtelet'. Two remarks can be made. On the one hand, as in the previous regulation, mention is made of male and female surgeons, whether legally or not. In the same way, the statutes of the faculty of medicine from 1271 enjoined *cirurgicus seu cirurgica, apothecarius seu apothecaria, herbarius seu herbaria*[7] not to go beyond the limits of their respective competences. Nevertheless, where the edict of 1311 alludes to the sworn master surgeons, we find only the masculine gender.[8] The other remark is that, in this edict, as in the previous regulations, reference is made only to traumatic surgery; the activities which concern dysfunctions arising from pathological origins are not alluded to. The public authority is only interested in what may disturb public order; the division of competences between physicians and surgeons does not fall within its responsibility. Moreover, there are no major conflicts on this point during the first half of the fourteenth century; confrontations really appeared only during the fifteenth century. When in 1331 the faculty of medicine itself obtained a royal edict,[9] the point was not to defend itself against surgeons, but to assert its independence from the chancellor of the university with respect to granting of licences. What is topical in this first half of the fourteenth century is not rivalry in power but rather the affirmation by each profession of its uniqueness and its right to choose its representatives, along with the desire to distinguish itself from empirics.

SURGERY AS A SCIENCE

The end of the thirteenth century and the beginning of the fourteenth was unquestionably an important period for Parisian surgery. In the eighteenth

[7] Printed in H. Denifle and E. Chatelain, *Chartularium Universitatis Parisiensis*, vol. 1 (Paris, 1889), p. 488.
[8] The first sentence is explicit enough: 'Edicto presenti statuimus, ut in villa et vicecomitatu Parisiensi, nullus chirurgicus, nulla chirurgica artem chirurgiae, seu opus quomodolibet exercere praesumat, seu se immiscere eidem publice, vel occulte, in quacumque iurisdictione, seu terra, nisi, per magistros chirurgicos juratos ... et prius examinati fuerint diligenter, et approbati in ipsa arte ...' (*Ordonnances*, vol. 1, p. 491). On the general problem of women's medical practice, see Monica Green's chapter in this volume.
[9] Printed in *Ordonnances des roys de France*, vol. 11 (Paris, 1729), pp. 70–1.

century, François Quesnay[10] endeavoured to give a holy founder to the profession by attributing to King Saint Louis the foundation of the so-called 'College of Saint Cosmas'. It seems, in fact, that it was rather Philip the Fair who played a determining role. We know the names of nine surgeons who were in his service:[11] Ambroise, Arnoul de Mappis, Henri de Mondeville, Jacques de Senis, Jean Le Mire, Jean de Padua, Jean Pitart, a certain P. and Quarreure Nebularius. Philip the Fair's successors, and especially Philip VI,[12] resorted to surgeons to a lesser extent; but Philip V and Charles IV had approximately the same number as that recorded in Philip the Fair's reign, with six surgeons in their service.[13] Philip the Fair had probably understood the value of surgeons in the army; moreover, he saw in their profession a possible help in the maintenance of public order, by the information its members could provide in criminal proceedings. Besides his help in the organization of the profession, Philip the Fair gave his patronage to the most learned among surgeons. Lanfranco of Milan, exiled from Italy, dedicated to him in 1296 his *Chirurgia magna*[14] and Henri de Mondeville, who went into royal service from 1298,[15] did the same later for his *Chirurgia*.

Both these figures embodied the attempt to introduce into Paris a learned surgery, following the Italian model.[16] Besides its purely didactic purpose, Henri de Mondeville's work has a polemical aim and, without claiming it explicitly, presents a kind of project for a new organization of surgical training. The very year (1306) when Henri de Mondeville began his *Chirurgia*, the political writer Pierre Dubois dedicated to the King of England his *De recuperatione Terre Sancte* (On the recovery of the Holy Land)[17], which proposed, in a somewhat Utopian manner, an educative program. A few lines are devoted to medical training in this work.

[10] F. Quesnay, *Recherches critiques et historiques sur l'origine, sur les divers états et sur le progrès de la chirurgie en France* (Paris, 1744).

[11] On these surgeons, see Wickersheimer, *Dictionnaire*; Jacquart, *Supplément* and *Addenda* in Jacquart, *Le milieu médical en France du XIIᵉ au XVᵉ siècle* (Geneva, 1981), pp. 429–80.

[12] We know only three names: Pierre de Genevre, Robert Le Forestier, Thomas Ogier; see ibid.

[13] Surgeons in Philip V's service: Guy (de Condé?), Jacques de Senis, Jean Pitart, Raymond de Thot, Thibaut Benoist, Thomas de Rothomago. Surgeons in Charles IV's service: Enguerrand Desloges, Jacques de Senis, Jean de Busseville, Jean de Cruce, Jean Pitart, Thomas de Rothomago. See ibid. It should be noted that these surgeons were not necessarily in the royal service at the same time; this is the case also with Philip the Fair's nine surgeons.

[14] The best account of Lanfranco of Milan's surgery is to be found in E. Gurlt, *Geschichte der Chirurgie und ihrer Ausübung* (Berlin, 1898), vol. I, pp. 765ff. See also M. Tabanelli, *La chirurgia italiana nell'alto medioevo*, 2 vols. (Florence 1965), vol. 2, pp. 801–1053.

[15] See Jacquart, *Supplément*, p. 117.

[16] On the foundation of a surgery as a learned discipline, see the accounts given in this volume by Jole Agrimi and Chiara Crisciani, Michael McVaugh and Nancy Siraisi.

[17] Printed in C. V. Langlois, '*De recuperatione Terre Sancte*', *Traité de politique générale par Pierre Dubois* (Paris, 1891). On Pierre Dubois see *Lexikon des Mittelalters* vol. III (Munich and Zurich, 1986), cols. 1433–4.

According to Pierre Dubois's views, medicine has to be learned after logic and natural philosophy: up to this point, these views fit perfectly with the university model of the time. What seems more original is the place allotted to surgery:

Those who are less accomplished [*rudiores*] in their studies, after having acquired a little knowledge of logic, and more, if possible, of natural science, will learn surgery, of men and horses; those who are more capable, will add, if possible, the learning of medicine, in order to assimilate the art of surgery with greater advantage [*profectius*].[18]

It is likely that Pierre Dubois and Henri de Mondeville knew each other: both of Norman origin, both having studied in Paris, they were in Philip the Fair's entourage during the same years. Pierre Dubois's program presented surgery in an ambiguous way: considered, in one respect, as a learned discipline, it was, in another respect, made over to the less capable students. Moreover, it suggested the existence of two kinds of practitioners: those who were merely surgeons, whom we can call *chirurgici*, and those who were both physicians and surgeons, or *medici chirurgici*. It would be hazardous to consider Henri de Mondeville's *Chirurgia* as a direct echo of or reply to Pierre Dubois's program, but it is undeniable that it expresses a reaction against the contemporaneous status of surgery. Whereas Pierre Dubois showed this art as being inferior to medicine, Henri de Mondeville undertook to prove its superiority: this claim recurs like a leitmotiv in his book. It has nevertheless to be noted that Pierre Dubois and Henri de Mondeville both provided surgery with a central position in the framework of medical practice: this was probably a major concern in the royal circle at the beginning of the fourteenth century.

In the prologue of his *Chirurgia*, Henri de Mondeville provides some information about his aim and his own personality. This prologue opens by invoking Christ, the Virgin, Saints Cosmas and Damian, the King of France and his sons.[19] We can deduce from this invocation firstly that Henri was probably a member of the Parisian confraternity of Saints Cosmas and Damian,[20] and secondly that he needed the support of his royal patron to promote his ideas. After these invocations, Henri de Mondeville presents himself as surgeon of the king, 'studens et commorans in preclarissima civitate Parisiensi et precellentissimo studio'. This sentence is not

---

18 Langlois, *De recuperatione*, p. 62.
19 Printed in J. L. Pagel, *Die Chirurgie des Heinrich von Mondeville (Hermondaville) nach Berliner, Erfurter und Pariser Codices zum ersten Mal herausgegeben* (Berlin, 1892), p. 10. It seems that the dedication of the work to Guglielmo da Brescia which follows this invocation was not included in the first version dated 1306; it was probably a further addition. Cf. Nicaise, *Chirurgie*, p. 2. We should remember that the *Chirurgia* was written, with some interruptions, between 1306 and 1319–20.
20 The existence of a confraternity does not mean that specific teaching was delivered there; the word 'college', which is often used to designate the confraternity of Saints Cosmas and Damian, is inappropriate, because of its ambiguity.

completely clear, but it seems sensible to assume that Henri de Mondeville had some link with the University of Paris, and more precisely with the faculty of medicine. The verb *studere* can be understood as 'to devote oneself to knowledge', including teaching and research;[21] then, to what kind of school could the expression *precellentissimum studium* apply, except to the university? The existence of a surgical school at this time is very doubtful; Lanfranco of Milan himself seems to have taught in the framework of university teaching and the term *studium* was quite often used to designate the university. It has to be added that we find no text, at this time, which would have forbidden university physicians from practising surgery. According to the eighteenth-century scholar Chomel, the faculty of medicine would have forbidden its bachelors, in 1350, from practising surgery,[22] but we note that, from 1271, it forbade them also from prescribing drugs.[23] In fact, it was from any kind of practice that bachelors were prohibited.

A few lines further on in the prologue, Henri de Mondeville reveals the sources of the knowledge that he intends to present in his *Chirurgia*. After having mentioned the reading of books, mainly Avicenna's *Canon*, Teodorico's and Lanfranco's *Surgeries*, he refers to his own training.[24] He acquired his knowledge by practising (*operando*) and studying (*audiendo*) in Paris and Montpellier; in both places, he taught (*legendo*) surgery several years and, in Montpellier's *studium* alone, he taught medicine. In this latter case also, there is no reason not to understand *studium* as university: in what other place than a university could medicine be taught at that time? The other side of Henri's training was formed by listening to famous masters and by seeing them practising. Among them, the most important was 'master Jean Pitart', surgeon of the king. Jean Pitart is not known to have had any link with the university; he was, on the contrary, a famous representative of surgery as a craft or guild. From his own words, we are allowed to assume

[21] See O. Weijers, *Terminologie des universités au XIIe siècle* (Rome, 1987), p. 287.

[22] J. B. L. Chomel, *Essai historique sue la médecine en France* (Paris, 1762), p. 150. Chomel referred here to the statutes of 1350, which have now been lost. See E. Wickersheimer, *Commentaries de la faculté de médecine de l'Université de Paris (1395–1516)* (Paris, 1915), pp. xli–xlii.

[23] See below.

[24] Printed in Pagel, *Die* Chirurgie, p. 11: 'Retractans ergo praedictorum Magistrorum nostrorum et aliorum cyrurgicorum famosorum diligenter editiones peroptimas jam completas et ea omnia nullo abscondito quae potui perpendere Parisius et in Montepessulano operando, audiendo et per plures annos legendo cyrurgiam publice utrobique et in solo Montispessulanensis studio medicinam praedictis omnibus superaddam cum omnibus similiter quae per experientiam et doctrinam a meis Magistris omnibus et ubique et praecipue a Magistro meo peritissimo in dicta arte, scilicet Magistro Johanne Pitard, illustrissimi praedicti Domini nostri regis similiter cyrurgico, ipsos audiendo docentes et videndo practicantes potui congregare, unde discipuli volentes addiscere cyrurgiam gaudeant et laetentur intelligentes, praecipue literati, qui medicinae saltem principia communia cognoverunt et qui intelligunt verba artis, quoniam pro ipsis opus hujusmodi est principaliter ordinatum. Utrum autem illiteratis proficiat aut non proficiat penitus non excludo'.

that Henri de Mondeville had a double training: by way of university teaching (the erudition of his book reinforces this assumption) and by way of apprenticeship, under several masters in different places (*ubique*), but mainly under Jean Pitart whom he called 'his master'. The first aim of his book is to demonstrate that this kind of double training is necessary. He claims that his work has been arranged in order to teach surgery to literate students, who know the common principles of medicine and are able to understand its technical vocabulary. If illiterate practitioners take any benefit from this teaching, it is good, but the book is not written primarily for them.

In the *Notabilia introductoria* of the second treatise, Henri de Mondeville defines more precisely what surgical training should be.[25] Again, a close reading of this passage is necessary. It starts with a quotation from Holy Scripture: 'Qui intrat in ovile non per ostium, fur est et latro'. Anyone who wants to enter the science and art of surgery without following the right paths is a thief and a traitor, in the same manner as the man who goes into a sheepfold by passing through any way other than the door. Henri de Mondeville, referring to Galen's *De ingenio sanitatis*, states then that any kind of treatment requires firstly knowing with what means it is possible to treat, secondly knowing how to treat with those means. So, the house of surgery has two doors: theory and practice. Two paths lead to the first door: to learn (*audire*) theory with the utmost attention; to teach it (*legere*) and to converse with colleagues (*socii*) about it.[26] Following his Italian predecessors, and particularly Lanfranco of Milan, Henri de Mondeville considers surgery as a science, including both a theoretical and practical side. He repeats many times that it forms the third part of medical therapeutics.[27] Since it is impossible to know one part without knowing the whole, surgeons have to acquire the general principles of medicine ('principia et notabilia medicine communia').[28] Thus, to reach the first door, it is necessary to learn and to teach theoretical medicine. The second door, that of practice, has to be reached also by two paths: by observing surgeons; by practising a long time with other surgeons, and afterwards alone.[29]

---

[25] Ibid., pp. 64–6.

[26] 'Ad unumquodque autem istorum hostiorum dirigit nos necessario duplex via: Ad primum ergo, quod attinet theoricae cyrurgiae, prima via est audire ejus theoriam et ad ipsam attendere cum summa diligentia et adfectu ... Secunda via est legere ipsam et de ipsa conferre cum sociis aliquando ...', ibid., p. 64.

[27] On surgery as the third part of medical art, see the account of Nancy Siraisi in this volume. Johannitius' *Isagoge* was among the most widespread sources which stated this division of medicine into three parts: 'Omnis medicina aut eorum sex quae ante diximus temperata exhibitio, aut potio, aut cirurgia', ed. G. Maurach, in *Sudhoffs Archiv*, 62 (1978), p. 173.

[28] Tr. II, *Notabilia introductoria*: 'Cum ergo sit impossibile aliquam partem perfecte cognosci nisi cognoscatur saltem grosso modo suum totum, impossibile est, cyrurgicum esse sufficientem, qui non cognoscit principia et notabilia medicinae communia', ed. Pagel, *Die Chirurgie* p. 78.

[29] 'Ad secundum ostium, quod attinet practicae, prima via est videre cyrurgicos operari ... secunda via est, quod oportet cyrurgicum operari diu cum aliis et postea totus solus', ibid., p. 64.

If we do not read this passage in an abstract manner, but instead transpose it into the concrete framework of the Parisian medical milieu at the beginning of the fourteenth century, we cannot avoid concluding that, in Henri de Mondeville's view, surgical training should be provided in two places. The first one is the faculty of medicine, where it is necessary both to learn and to teach, that is, to obtain a grade; in the same way that medical learning should be a part of surgical training, surgery should be part of medical teaching, since he who claims to learn the whole of a science, should learn also each part.[30] The second place is the practice of a master surgeon. We know that this bold plan failed. When, a few years after having proposed it, Henri de Mondeville returns to the writing of his book and undertakes to complete it, he expresses his disappointment. He complains, in the prologue of the third treatise, about the king who sent him away from Paris for a while and who issued a bad edict; he is alluding here probably to the regulation of 1316 which fixed the organization of medical and surgical service within the royal household.[31] Presumably there were some restrictive measures in it. He complains also about the surgeons of those days, who were less and less literate, but more and more eager for money. He mainly deplores the fact that surgery was not passed on enough. Henri de Mondeville wrote these lines around 1316, that is, after the royal edict of 1311 which regulated the surgical craft. Historians of surgery used to state that he had a hand in its publication, but it can rather be asked whether he was not disappointed by it. This edict only stated that entry into the surgical art was subject to examination by sworn master surgeons. It protected the guild of surgeons against mere quacks, but did not allude to any particular theoretical training.

Henri de Mondeville's project was probably unenforceable, because it needed to reconcile two opposite rationales: the university's, which was founded on the diffusion of knowledge, through books; the guild's, which was founded on oral transmission from one master to one or a few companions. Henri de Mondeville insists many times on the necessity for surgeons to write books. He states that he was used to teaching *publice*. He caricatures the habit of secrets;[32] he also criticizes the hereditary transmission of the art, which consists in fact in a transmission of ignorance.[33]

---

[30] 'Similiter ex altera parte, cum impossibile sit totum aliquid perfecte cognosci nisi cognoscantur singulae ejus partes, in quantum hujusmodi, impossibile est medicum esse sufficientem, qui artem cyrurgiae penitus ignoravit', ibid., p. 78.

[31] On this regulation, see A. Chéreau 'Les médecins de six rois de France', in *Union Médicale*, 151 (1864), pp. 575–6.

[32] On surgical *practicae* described as revelation of secrets from a father to a son, see J. Agrimi and C. Crisciani, *Edocere medicos. Medicina scolastica nei secoli XIII–XV* (Milan and Naples, 1988), pp. 232–3.

[33] *Chirurgia*, Prologue: 'Sunt enim eorum aliqui quamquam ydiotae et simpliciter ignorantes superbi mirabiliter et elati dicentes, se manualem hujusmodi operationem malis gratibus cyrurgicorum clericorum a tempore, cujus non est memoria, a suis primevis parentibus

The surgical craft in Paris, like elsewhere, was often a family business: among the six surgeons named in the regulation of the end of the thirteenth century, Vincent was Henri Du Perche's son and Nicholas was Robert le Convers's brother. These kinds of practitioners were certainly not prepared to subject their heirs to a long university training and to allow the faculty of medicine to inspect their practice. On the other hand, the university would not have been ready to accept the teaching of medical theory outside its own institution.

Apart from these corporatist rivalries, and the usual reasons that historians put forward, namely the conciliar decisions which forbade clerics to shed blood,[34] and the physicians' contempt for manual operations, is it not possible to discern a stronger and deeper obstacle to the appearance of a scientific surgery? As Henri de Mondeville put it himself, the criterion of efficiency is more imperative in surgery, the effects of which are immediately visible.[35] Could a surgery founded on medieval physiological theory be efficacious? Is it not possible to imagine that the unconscious fear of patent failures also motivated the physicians' reluctance? Surgery in Paris had to find its own way, mainly through practice and empirical knowledge.

PRACTICAL CONCERNS AT THE FACULTY OF MEDICINE

If historians have relatively numerous sources at their disposal concerning the external life of the faculty of medicine (its pursuit of empirics,[36] its control over Parisian practitioners, its argument with the university chancellor),[37] they lack information about the real content of its teaching during the first half of the fourteenth century. For the very first years, Pietro d'Abano's *Conciliator* might provide a remarkable source, but, in the present state of research, it is difficult to determine to what extent this book

similiter illiteratis successivam connaturalem et hereditariam habuisse', ed. Pagel, pp. 11–12.

[34] The weight of this prohibition is excessively emphasized by M. C. Pouchelle in *Corps et chirurgie à l'apogée du moyen âge* (Paris, 1983).

[35] In Henri de Mondeville's view this is one of the reasons which show the superiority of surgery: 'Et in hoc primo maxime apparet praeeminentia cyrurgiae ad medicinam quia curat morbos difficiliores, in quorum curis deficit medicina. Secundo curat morbos, qui nec per se nec per naturam nec per medicinam ullatenus curarentur; medicina enim nullum morbum curat ita manifeste, quin possit dici, quod absque ejus adjutorio curaretur. Tertio quia opera cyrurgiae sunt visui manifesta, et medicinae opera sunt occulta, et in hoc medici plurimi sublevantur, quia, si super patientem erraverunt, eorum error non erit manifestus, et si ipsum interficiant, non fiet in aperto, sed error cyrurgici operantis, ut incisio manus et brachii apparet nothorice cuilibet intuenti nec potest ipsum naturae vel virtuti imponere nec se super hoc excusare nec alium accusare' (Tr. II. *Notabilia introductoria*, ed. Pagel, p. 78.

[36] See P. Kibre, 'The faculty of medicine at Paris, charlatanism and unlicensed medical practice in the later Middle Ages', *Bulletin of the History of Medicine*, 27 (1953), pp. 1–20.

[37] The best account of the faculty of medicine remains the introduction by E. Wickersheimer in *Commentaires*, pp. ix–xcvii.

reflects the teaching of the faculty of medicine.[38] No Parisian master of this period left a work comparable to Jean de St Amand's at the end of the thirteenth century. Although the membership of this author in the faculty of medicine is not attested to by any document, it is likely that he was one of its active members: his whole work has a scholastic and pedagogical character which could hardly be found outside the university framework. The list of the works which are attributed to him reflects both tradition and renewal.[39] It shows commentaries on the texts which were part of the Parisian curriculum in 1270–4:[40] *Antidotarium Nicolai*, Hippocrates' *Prognostics* and *Regimen on acute diseases*, Isaac Israeli's *De dietis*, Johannitius' *Isagoge*, Philaretus' *De pulsibus*, Theophilus' *De urinis*. But it attests also to the introduction of important new texts, through the commentary on a part of Avicenna's *Canon* (lib. 4, fen 1) and, above all, through the *Revocativum memorie*, the main aim of which was to make the Galenic translations of the twelfth century accessible.[41] While one part of this didactic set consists of mere summaries of some Galenic treatises, the *Concordancie*, in their presentation of topics in alphabetical order, rely mainly on the same Galenic treatises. Another feature of Jean de St Amand's entire work is the emphasis which is laid on practical issues, mostly on therapeutics. The part of the *Revocativum memorie* which is called *Areole* deals entirely with drugs; besides the *Antidotarium Nicolai*, Jean de St Amand seems also to have commented on pseudo-Mesue's work and on *Tacuinum sanitatis*, both being therapeutical guides.

The two main aims of Jean de St Amand's works, namely to provide students with an *aide-mémoire* by gathering the essential points of Galenic doctrine together, and to concentrate on issues related to therapeutical method, marked a tradition which remained active at the faculty of medicine. In the second half of the fourteenth century, Pierre de St Flour[42] undertook to complete the *Concordancie*, thus indicating that this work was still used in his time. Concerning therapeutical issues, the question of 'specific form', which had an important part in Jean de St Amand's work,[43] seems

---

38 Pietro d'Abano is known to have spent some years at Paris studying or teaching; he started on his *Conciliator* there, but returning to Padua around 1306–7, he finished it after 1310. See N. G. Siraisi, *Arts and sciences at Padua: the studium of Padua before 1350* (Toronto, 1973), p. 121, and E. Paschetto, *Pietro d'Abano medico e filosofo* (Florence, 1984), pp. 28–9.

39 List of Jean de St Amand's works in Wickersheimer, *Dictionnaire*, pp. 476–8, and Jacquart, *Supplément*, p. 179.

40 On this curriculum (ed. in *Chartularium* I, p. 517), see D. Jacquart and F. Micheau, *La médecine arabe et l'occident médiéval* (Paris, 1990), ch. 5.

41 See L. García-Ballester, 'Arnau de Vilanova (*c.* 1240–1311) y la reforma de los estudios médicos en Montpellier (1309): el Hipócrates latino y la introducción del nuevo Galeno', in *Dynamis*, 2 (1982), pp. 105–6, 153–4; L. García-Ballester and E. Sanchez Salor (eds.), *Commentum supra tractatum Galieni de malicia complexionis diverse* (Barcelona, 1985), *Arnaldi de Villanova opera medica omnia* (AVOMO), vol. XV, pp. 15, 23–31, 92, 122–3.

42 Pierre Gas or de St Flour became master of the faculty of medicine in 1349: see Wickersheimer, *Dictionnaire*, pp. 634–5.

43 See the detailed account of this question in M. R. McVaugh (ed.), *Aphorismi de gradibus* (Granada and Barcelona, 1975), AVOMO, vol. II, pp. 31–51 (pp. 48–51 edition of the *questio famosa* contained in Jean de St Amand's commentary on *Antidotarium Nicolai*:

to have continued to be topical in the Parisian discussions. Jean de St Amand set out this question in different places: in his commentary on *Antidotarium Nicolai* as well as in the *Areole* and in the *Concordancie*. In this last work, three expressions are put forward to designate the specific virtue of a simple or compound medicine which, according to Avicenna, cannot be deduced from the elementary qualities of its components but is known only through experience: *tota substantia, forma specifica, tota species.*[44] The third expression seems to have been the most commonly used in the framework of Parisian discussions. In the *Questiones attrebatenses* that Thomas Le Myésier addressed to Ramon Lull in 1299,[45] there were five questions which concerned medicine. One of these five questions is about the action of rhubarb which 'attracts bile *a tota specie*', asking 'what is this *tota species*[?]'.[46] Another indirect testimony of the continuing topicality of this question is given a few years later by Henri de Mondeville. In the *Notabilia introductoria* of the second treatise, written between 1306 and 1308, he violently condemns superstitious attributions of diseases to the influence of the saints. He relates that some rural surgeons take refuge in these beliefs in order to hide their incapacity to treat. He then compares these practitioners to 'physicians who, when they are unable to explain something, say that it happens *tota specie*'.[47]

Besides indirect testimonies of this kind and the possible echo that Pietro d'Abano's *Conciliator* provides of some features of Parisian teaching, we know almost nothing about the functioning of the faculty of medicine during the first twenty years of the fourteenth century and, in particular, about its masters. The occasion of the first trial against an empiric in 1312 gives us the name of a dean.[48] It is only for the years from 1322 that some

'utrum medicina composita ut tyriaca operetur per formam medicinarum simplicium quas recipit, aut per formam totius resultantem, ex mutua actione et passione per quod fit earum excellentiarum confractio').

[44] Printed in J. L. Pagel, *Die Concordanciae des Johannes de Santo Amando* (Berlin, 1894), pp. 350–1: 'Ad videndum quid sit toat substantia'.

[45] The date on which Thomas Le Myésier became master in medicine is not known; in 1299, he lived in Arras. See Jacquart, *Supplément*, pp. 274–5. Analysis of his works: J. N. Hillgarth, *Ramon Lull and Lullism in fourteenth century France* (Oxford, 1971).

[46] Q. xxix 'Item nos dicimus quod reubarbarum attrahit coleram a tota specie. Queritur quid est tota illa species', The other questions concerning medicine are the following: q. xxv 'Dixit Avicenna quod calor radicalis nostri corporis non cessat depascere suum humidum radicale donec veniat unicuique mors quod destinata est sibi per naturam, utrum sit verum hoc dictum'; q. xxvii 'Utrum vita hominis possit prolongari per naturam et artem'; q. xxxv 'Utrum humidum spermaticum viri cadat in substantiam fetus'; q. xxxvi 'Utrum in generatione sit necessarium mulierem spermatizare'. See the Lyons edition of 1491.

[47] Ed. Pagel, p. 320.

[48] We should bear in mind that the available registers of the faculty of medicine provide information only from 1395; for the first half of the fourteenth century, the main source is constituted by the *Chartularium universitatis Parisiensis*, vol. II (Paris, 1891). In 1312 the dean was 'Iohannes de Miciclis' (ibid., p. 150) about whom nothing else is known. The names of the deans are given at the end of this chapter, Appendix 1; this list is based on Ernest Wickersheimer's *Commentaires*, pp. xcv–xcvi.

names of professors occur regularly,[49] and from 1325 that we find the names of the deans for almost every year. It should be noted also that none of the deans nor of the *magistri regentes* made his mark in the history of medicine, that is, apart from one possibility, which has more often than not been dismissed, recently again by Nancy Siraisi.[50] Among the few professors of Italian origin, most of whom had temporarily left their country for political reasons, there appears between 1325 and 1330 a certain Petrus de Florentia, who died before 1335. The assertion of Filippo Villani (writing in 1381–2) that Turisanus or Pietro Torrigiano had written his *Plusquam commentum* on Galen's *Tegni* at the end of his life and during the same years as Dino del Garbo was teaching in Bologna (that is between 1305 and 1319), seems to exclude the possibility of identifying him with Petrus de Florentia. There are nevertheless some disturbing similarities between these two masters, who were both from Florence: Turisanus is supposed to have been an ecclesiastic, while the faculty proposed Petrus de Florentia for a chaplaincy in 1325;[51] moreover, to both of them is attributed an interest in theology. Anyway, if we reject this identification on the basis of Villani's assertions, we have to trust his assertion that Turisanus taught in Paris during the period we are studying here. This fact cannot be without significance for the history of Parisian medicine.

Apart from this question of the Parisian part of Turisanus' activity, the lists of *magistri regentes* do not reveal any famous author. For the period which ends in 1348 with that original initiative – the collective consultation on the plague – only two medical works are known to have been written by masters *actu regentes*: a *Regimen sanitatis* by the Milanese Maynus de Mayneriis, professor from 1326 to 1331, and a commentary on the third book of Galen's *De crisi*, composed in 1339 by Pierre Chauchat.[52] This last author is a perfect representative of Parisian medicine: he studied arts and medicine in Paris, was *magister regens* of the faculty of medicine from 1330 and acted as dean three times (in 1329–30, 1333–4, 1342–3). Like most of his colleagues, he acquired several ecclesiastical benefices. In his practice, he was in some seigneurs' service, but entered the royal court only in 1352, under Jean II. His commentary on *De crisi*, which is preserved in manuscript 1014 of the Bibliothèque municipale in Reims,[53] consists, on the one hand, in a literal explanation of the Galenic text, and, on the other hand, in a kind of introduction summarizing the ways of recognizing crisis, according to the time and the nature of symptoms. This commentary does not include any *dubia*. It looks rather like a guide to applying Galenic principles. In the

[49] See the examples of a few years in Appendix 2: the lists are drawn up from the information found in Wickersheimer, *Dictionnaire*, and Jacquart, *Supplément*.
[50] N. G. Siraisi, *Taddeo Alderotti and his pupils* (Princeton, NJ, 1981), pp. 64–6.
[51] See *Chartularium*, vol. II, p. 287.
[52] On both authors, see Wickersheimer, *Dictionnaire*, p. 533–4, 625–6, and Jacquart, *Supplément*, pp. 202–3.
[53] Fols. 65r–75v, 89rv (another work by another author is interpolated fols. 77r–88v).

course of his commentary, Pierre Chauchat takes the opportunity to specify what seems to him to be most useful for the training of young physicians. Without entering into a long discussion of this topic, he contents himself with quoting the introductory definition of medicine which is given in Averroes' *Colliget* ('the art of medicine is an operative art drawn from true principles'), and with recalling that, according to Galen's *De ingenio sanitatis*, it is better for a disciple to learn the 'way and method of operating' (*viam et modum operationis*) rather than to discourse on the principles which rule them. Pierre Chauchat's conclusion is this: 'in order to succeed in the art of medicine, it is better and more useful to verify principles through operations than to question oneself about these principles through a *propter quid* demonstration'.[54] Since Pierre Chauchat did not linger much over the definition of medicine nor over the method proper to this art, it would be risky to extrapolate and, for instance, to draw a parallel between his commentary and Turisanus' *Plusquam commentum*, which, in a more detailed and thorough philosophical context, also attributes to *propter quid* demonstration (i.e. absolute demonstration from the reasoned cause) a limited part in medicine.[55] Pierre Chauchat's statement, which emphasizes the formative character of 'the verification of principles through operations', seems more obviously to fit in with the actual orientation of Parisian medicine. Indeed, this statement was particularly topical, since in 1335, that is, four years before the writing of the commentary on *De crisi*, the faculty of medicine had made practical training obligatory. There is still room for doubt concerning the level of studies at which this experience had to be acquired. In 1335, it was stipulated that, 'nobody will be promoted to master's degree, unless he has practised during two summers outside Paris, or continuously during two years in Paris under the supervision of another matter'.[56] According to this document, it seems that practical training had to take place after the licence,

---

[54] 'G[alenus] ostendit [in *De ingenio sanitatis*] quod sufficit quod sciat [discipulus] viam et modum istius operationis preterquam inquit de principiis eius … Patet probatio intenti quod erat probari quod modus proficiendi in hac arte medicine melior et utilior discipulo est verificatio principiorum per operationes et non inquisitio de eis per demonstrationem propter quid' (fol. 73r).

[55] 'Adhuc autem, cum medicina sit applicabilis ad opus, opus autem omne circa singularia et sensibilia, oportet quod ab his, quae sensibus subiacent, certificentur, quae a sensibus sunt remota, haec autem accidentia et posterior natura, quare etiam naturalior est medicinae demonstratio quia, vel doctrina compositiva quam demonstratio propter quid vel doctrina resolutiva. Adhuc autem magis proprium videtur esse medici ostendere aegritudinem inesse corpori per signa et accidentia comitantia aegritudinem quam e converso per aegritudinem et causam estendere effectus, qui sequuntur…': *Plusquam commentum* (Venice edition 1557), fol. 6A, quoted by P.-G. Ottosson, *Scholastic medicine and philosophy* (Naples, 1984), p. 119. For a detailed account of Turisanus' statement about demonstration *propter quid*, see Siraisi, *Taddeo Alderotti*, pp. 128–37.

[56] 'Die mercurii post Pascha ordinavit facultas per cedulam vocata, ut moris est, quod nullus deinceps ad magisterium valeret promoveri nisi per duas estates practicaverit extra Parisius, vel continuaverit per duos annos practicam Parisius in comitatu alterius magistri, Iohanne de Villanova decano' (*Chartularium*, vol. II, p. 454).

just before the granting of the master's degree. Yet when, in 1450, the faculty repeats this statute, reference is clearly being made to bachelors.[57] It is impossible to decide whether it was always the rule or whether a change happened between 1335 and 1450. We notice nevertheless that practical training in the town of Paris had to be done under a master's supervision.

THE CONTROL OF THE MEDICAL PROFESSION

The emphasis on practical issues, which seems to characterize the teaching of the faculty of medicine during the first half of the fourteenth century, bears some probable relationship with the specific conditions of medical practice in Paris. Complaining about the existence of quacks had no doubt been a *topos* of medical literature since antiquity, but the picture of Parisian medicine that Henri de Mondeville paints may be considered realistic to some extent: beside the crowd of barbers, sorcerers, alchemists and midwives, there were those, even in the upper-classes, who acted as medical practitioners on the basis of a presumed divine gift.[58] The proceedings that the faculty of medicine instituted against empirics testify similarly to the existence of a great mass of untrained practitioners. Rather than suggesting a general mistrust of scientific medicine or skilled surgery, the resort that patients made to them suggests an insufficient number of trained practitioners in a town of around 200,000 inhabitants.[59] The efforts of the faculty of medicine echo in some way the program that Henri de Mondeville planned for surgery: firstly, to fight against illiterate practitioners; secondly, to limit access to the profession to literate practitioners able to teach theory.

From the 1271 statutes of the faculty of medicine onwards, every prescription of drugs in the town of Paris was to be subject to the approval of a master. This general rule, which was mainly directed at manual practitioners such as surgeons, apothecaries and herbalists, provided for a special clause concerning students in medicine: they were threatened with the deprival of promotion if it so happened that 'they prescribe for any healthy or sick person some fortifying, altering or laxative drugs, without

---

57 'Quantum ad secundum, ego [Guillermus de Camera, decanus facultatis] narravi super reformatione baccalariorum quod in quodam statuto facultatis cavebatur quomodo quilibet baccalarius tenebatur ante licentiam per duas estates practicare Parisius cum aliquo magistrorum, vel per duos annos extra sine magistro, quod tamen minime faciebant ... Quoad secundum articulum, conclusit facultas quod in fine dicte congregationis et in presentia facultatis, decanus exortaretur baccalarios de juramentis per eos prestitis et signanter super statuto quo cavebatur quod debent practicare Parisius, cum magistris ante licentiam per duas estates, vel extra per duos annos ...' (Wickersheimer, *Commentaires*, p. 189). Compared with the previous regulation (as it is preserved in the *Chartularium*), this text shows another difference: the period of two years is assigned to practice *extra Parisius*, and the period of two summers to practice *Parisius*.

58 Henri de Mondeville, *Chirurgia*, Tr.II, *Notabilia introductoria*, ed. Pagel, p. 65.

59 This number is nowadays generally agreed on: see J. Dupâquier, editor in chief, *Histoire de la population française*, vol. I, *Des origines à la Renaissance* (Paris, 1988), pp. 305–7.

the presence of a master in medicine'. Students were also forbidden 'to visit a sick person more than once, without being accompanied by a master who advises them and shows them the way to act'.[60] This clause calls to mind what we read in the regulations established for surgeons and barbers; the former were allowed to examine a wounded person only once, before informing the provost; the latter were allowed to stop the bleeding of a wound, even if they had not been approved as surgeons. The exception of the first visit, which is made concerning the practice by students in medicine, corresponds probably to the same demand: in case of emergency, it is permitted to take initiatives before having the master's degree. It can be added that the restriction to a single visit precluded the possibility of having a regular practice in town, and so of competing with the masters. Thus, when, in 1335, the masters of the faculty of medicine instituted a practical training period, they were no doubt induced to do so by their stand on the definition of medicine and their views on medical education. Meanwhile they did not lose sight of the control they intended to exert over Parisian practice. While they did not mind if inexperienced students treated patients in other towns, they did not tolerate the practice in Paris, either for fear of competition or through a real concern for public health in the town placed under their control.

We can consider here the profound difference that existed between medical practice in university towns and medical practise elsewhere. The master's degree seems to have been necessary in order to practice in Paris. The report of the conflict[61] which opposed the faculty of medicine to the university chancellor in 1330–2 raises the question of the status of the licence. We find here the only evidence for the existence of a *licentia ad practicam* which could be granted without the *licentia ad theoricam*. The origin of the conflict lay in the fact that, contrary to the advice of the faculty, the chancellor had granted Alphonse Dionysii, who was patronized by the King of Portugal, the *licentia ad theoricam et practicam*, and a certain Guido de Novara, the *licentia ad practicam* alone.[62] Since this last restriction did not seem to have raised any problem, we may suppose that it was not exceptional. Nevertheless, we do not know for what kind of students it was meant, what kind of studies it sanctioned, or what kind of

---

[60] 'Et quoniam nonnulli sunt qui simul querunt scientiam et modum sciendi, quod est inconveniens maximum, cum eorum error etiam in principio non modicus maximus sit in fine, idcirco sub penis prefatis et specialiter sub privatione cujuscumque promotionis in facultate medicine habite et habende universis scolaribus et etiam singulis inhibemus firmiter ne aliquis eorum sano seu etiam infirmo aliquod medicamentum confortativum alterativum seu etiam laxativum sine alicujus magistri in medicina presencia subministret, nec etiam, excepta prima vice, visitet, nisi secum affuit magister aliquis qui ipsum dirigat et modum operis ostendat' (*Chartularium*, vol. I, p. 488).

[61] This conflict is related at length in *Chartularium*, vol. II, pp. 352–99 ('Lis facultatis medicine contra cancellarium Parisiensis').

[62] Ibid., p. 398.

practice it allowed. I have pointed out in a previous study[63] that the proportion of licentiates who had not passed the master's degree seems to have been higher in Paris than in Montpellier. May we suppose that a proportion of these licentiates had only been granted the *licentia ad practicam*? If this kind of licence did really exist, it is likely that it did not allow one to practise within the town of Paris.

MEDICINE, ASTROLOGY AND ROYAL SERVICE

Within the framework of this Parisian teaching which during the 1330s stressed practical training, is it possible to detect the role of astrology? It is obvious that an astrological tradition existed at the faculty of medicine and that it continued through the Middle Ages, but its true impact eludes easy evaluation. In 1267 and 1270, the dean was Pierre de Limoges, who, despite Ernest Wickersheimer's reservation, it is sensible to identify with the theologian and astronomer of the same name.[64] This author's commentary on Richard of Fournival's *Nativitas* provides several examples of comments which concern medical astrology, for instance, on how to establish diagnosis, to prescribe drugs and bleedings, or to determine critical days.[65] At the end of the Middle Ages, in 1452, the faculty officially recognized its interest in astrology when it graduated bachelor a student who had not studied for enough months. In order to compensate this failing, the candidate promised to offer to the faculty every year both 'the large and the small almanacs'.[66] But, it is necessary to add that, in the same period, Jacques Despars, master of the faculty of medicine, was not favourable to the use of astrology.[67]

One indication of the place of astrology within Parisian medical teaching at the end of the thirteenth century may be drawn from Jean de St Amand's *Concordancie*, which remained a basic source for years. A few topics lead the author to tackle this problem, for instance, the entries *luna, stella, monstra, natura, sol* and, of course, *phlebotomia*. Except for the engendering of monsters, the astrological explanation of which relies on the pseudo-Galenic *De spermate*, the other entries consist mainly of quotations from Galen's *De diebus decretoriis*. Predictably, the term *phlebotomia* gives rise to several questions (*multa dubitabilia*), one of which deals with the appropriate time for bleeding. It opens with the usual distinction, set forth in Avicen-

---

[63] Jacquart, *Le milieu médical*, pp. 59–63.

[64] See Wickersheimer, *Dictionnaire*, p. 645; Jacquart, *Supplément*, p. 237.

[65] A. Birkenmajer, 'Pierre de Limoges commentateur de Richard de Fournival', in *Isis*, 40 (1949), pp. 18–31; repr. in *Studia Copernicana*, vol. I (Cracow, 1970), pp. 22–35.

[66] 'Et fuit sibi facta ista gratia sub ista conditione quod de cetero singulis annis, circa festum Nativitatis Domini, ipse dabit facultati unum almanach magnum et unum parvum' (Wickersheimer, *Commentaires*, p. 193).

[67] See D. Jacquart, 'Theory, everyday practice, and three fifteenth-century physicians', *Osiris*, 6 (1990), 140–60.

na's *Canon*,[68] between a bleeding of choice, of a prophylactic nature, and a bleeding of necessity, of a therapeutical nature. Astrology is involved only in the first case, and in a rather incidental manner. The emphasis is more on climatic considerations. A few lines are nevertheless devoted to astrology for the benefit of those who want to use it:[69]

> If you want to know in what quarter of the moon it has to be done, I say that the first quarter is similar to Spring, the second to Summer, the third to Autumn, the fourth to Winter; just as bleeding has to be done in Spring, it has to be done in the first quarter of the moon.

This correlation of the seasons with the phases of the moon, which medieval authors deduced from Ptolemy's *Quadripartitum*,[70] is the only astrological information provided about bleeding. The reader who wants to use astrology can nevertheless apply to the phases of the moon all that is said about seasons. The entry *luna* provides him also with some basic rules drawn from Galen's *De diebus decretoriis*.[71] In conclusion, the resort to astrology does appear in Jean de St Amand's *Concordancie*, but only discreetly.

Apart from the time for bleeding, the question of crisis generally offers authors another occasion to resort to astrology, in the context of the prediction of critical days. In his commentary on Galen's *De crisi*, Pierre Chauchat could hardly avoid this problem and, in fact, he included a long astrological digression,[72] dealing with the influence of the moon on epileptics, on the menses, on the movement of humours, and dealing above all, with the computation of the medical month. The resort to astrology is less discreet than in Jean de St Amand, but it remains within the limits fixed by Galen's *De diebus decretoriis*. Even if knowledge of astrology – probably acquired at the faculty of arts – is obvious, no explicit quotation is made from purely astrological writings. For a time Pierre Chauchat's colleague at the faculty of medicine, Maynus de Mayneriis, master regent from 1326 to 1331, was undoubtedly as much astrologer as physician, at least when he was in Bernabo Visconti's service from 1346.[73] In his *Regimen sanitatis*, written during his stay in France and dedicated to Andrea Ghini de Malpighi, Bishop of Arras between 1331 and 1333, astrology is not predominant, but appears on expected topics: bleeding, cupping-glasses

---

[68] Avicenna, *Canon*, lib. I, fen 4, c. 20; see Pedro Gil-Sotres' paper in this volume.

[69] *Concordancie*, ed. Pagel, p. 123.

[70] See P. Gil-Sotres and L. Demaitre, *Tractatus de consideracionibus operis medicine sive de flebotomia* (Barcelona, 1988), AVOMO, vol. IV, p. 87.

[71] *Concordancie*, ed. Pagel, p. 170.

[72] MS Reims, Bibl. mun., 1014, fols. 70r–72v.

[73] Petrarch mentioned him as the chief of a group of astrologers at the Visconti court; he wrote in 1358 a *Theorica corporum celestium*, and on the occasion of the 1360 epidemic a treatise on the plague combining astrology with medicine: see L. Thorndike, *A history of magic and experimental science*, vol. III (New York and London, 1934), pp. 520–1.

and purges.[74] Concerning the prescription of this last treatment, emphasis is laid on the importance of astrological consideration: 'It should be seriously considered that the moon is not in Leo ... It should be seriously considered that the moon is not in conjunction with Jupiter ... nor with Saturn etc.'[75] In the chapter on bleeding, Maynus de Mayneriis certainly resorts to astrology to a greater extent than Jean de St Amand: not only the phase of the moon ('etas lune') but its position in the Zodiac ('locus eius similiter autem et coniunctio et aspectus') has to be taken into account, in order to determine, besides the appropriate time for bleeding, the part of the body which has to be incised or spared.[76]

Just as Maynus de Mayneriis developed his astrological practice mostly when he was at the court of Bernabo Visconti, so in Paris astrology seems to have been more a concern for royal physicians than for masters of the faculty of medicine. Despite their title of 'physicians of the king',[77] some practitioners were mainly astrologers. Arnoul de Quinquempoix, who was in the service of four successive kings (from Philip the Fair to Charles IV) endeavoured to translate into French some of Albumasar and Abraham ibn Ezra's works. Similarly, Robert Le Febvre and Geoffroy de Meaux are known for their astrological knowledge.[78] The *Astronomie iudicialis compendium* of the last-named deals, to a large extent, with astrological medicine. Composed of scholars, more often than not of clerics provided with benefices, sometimes of exceptional figures, such as Guido da Vigevano,[79] whose *Anatomia* written in 1345 reflects Mondino de' Liuzzi's teaching, the circle of the physicians at court during this period does not seem to have had close links with the faculty of medicine. For instance, we do not notice

---

[74] *Regimen sanitatis Magnini Mediolanensis* (Louvain, 1482), pars v, cc. 1, 2, 5.

[75] 'Multum considerandum est quod Luna non sit in Leone et quod Leo non sit ascendens et universaliter quod Luna non sit signo fixo. Sit igitur Luna in signo mobili et frigido et humido. Unde inter omnia signa mihi videtur quod Cancer est convenientius signum ad farmaciam et deinde Piscis, hec enim signa non sunt fixa et sunt aquatica, frigida et humida. Scorpio est signum conveniens quia aquaticum frigidum et humidum, sed est signum fixum. Multum etiam considerandum est quod Luna non sit coniuncta Iovi nec corporaliter nec per aspectum et quod etiam non sit coniuncta Saturno. Nam coniunctio cum Iove debilitat virtutem medicine et fortificat virtutem naturalem corporis. Medicina autem laxativa non evacuat virtutem nisi superando virtutes naturales corporis. Amplius coniunctio cum Saturno immobilitat humores et sic impedit operationem farmacie' (ibid., pars v, c. 5).

[76] Ibid., pars v, c. 1.

[77] A list of these royal physicians is given in Appendix 3 below. It is based on the information drawn from Wickersheimer, *Dictionnaire*, and Jacquart, *Supplément* and *Addenda*.

[78] Robert Le Febvre is known as the author of a nativity (*Supplément*, p. 260); apart from the *Astronomie iudicialis compendium*, Geoffroy de Meaux wrote several astrological works, as well as a treatise on the conjunction of 1345 which preceded the plague (*Dictionnaire*, p. 180; *Supplément*, p. 83).

[79] Like several other physicians in the reign of Philip VI (see Appendix 3 below), Guido da Vigevano seems rather to have been in the service of the queen (*Dictionnaire*, pp. 216–17; *Supplément*, pp. 96–7). On Guido da Vigevano and crusade plans, see C. Samaran, *Projets français de croisades de Philippe le Bel à Philippe de Valois*, in *Histoire Littéraire de la France*, vol. XLI (Paris, 1981), pp. 72–4.

any *magister regens*. A certain rivalry can even be discerned through the conflict which opposed Jean Hellequin, physician of the kings till 1322, when he proposed a candidate for the licence to the university's chancellor.[80] A radical change took place in the reign of Jean II, during which several *magistri regentes* entered the court: Dominique de Martiniaco de Clavaxio, who was also an astrologer, Gérard de St Dizier, Gervais Chrestien, Jean de Coucy, Jean de Guiscry, Pierre Chauchat and Guibert de Celsoy. The first signs of change can be perceived in the reign of Philip VI. Just as surgeons at the beginning of the century had had the support of Philip the Fair, so the university physicians appealed to Philip VI during their conflict with the chancellor. They thus obtained in 1331 a royal edict which confirmed their exclusive authority in the examination of candidates for the licence.[81] But the decisive act was the consultation on the plague, the *Compendium de epidemia* that the college of physicians addressed to the king, probably around October 1348.[82] In the rhetoric of their presentation, the authors speak of their intention of working for the people's sake. They skilfully introduce themselves to a monarch by divine right, himself thaumaturge, as representatives of a divine creation, that is, the medical art.[83] From the second half of the fourteenth century, it became quite usual for the *magistri regentes* to go into the king's service. Did the epidemics play a part in this? As Katharine Park has shown, in Florence the plague brought university physicians to the realization that the authority of theoretical knowledge was not sufficient and that they had to increase their political influence.[84]

The *Compendium de epidemia* is often put forward by historians to prove the interest of the masters of the faculty of medicine in astrology. This is not actually very clear. Indeed, at the beginning of their treatise, the Parisian physicians put forward the astronomers' statement, according to which the primary and remote cause of the epidemics was 'aliqua constellatio celestis',[85] namely, the 1345 conjunction between Saturn and Jupiter. After this statement, the text deals exclusively with the specific and

---

[80] *Chartularium*, vol. II, pp. 349–50.
[81] See above.
[82] See A. Coville, *Ecrits contemporains sur la peste de 1348 à 1350*, in *Histoire Littéraire de la France*, vol. XXXVII (Paris, 1937), p. 339.
[83] 'Amplius pretermittere nolumus, quod quando epidimia a voluntate divina procedit, in quo casu non est aliud consilium nisi quod ad ipsum humiliter recurratur, consilium tamen medici non desperando. Altissimus enim de terra creavit medicinam; unde sanat solus langores Deus qui de fragilitatis solo producit in largitate sua medicinam. Benedictus Deus, gloriosus et excelsus qui, auxiliari non desinens, certam curandi doctrinam timentibus explicavit', printed in E. Rebouis, *Etude historique et critique sur la peste* (Paris, 1888), p. 92. On medicine as *donum Dei*, see J. Agrimi and C. Crisciani, *Medicina del corpo e medicina dell'anima* (Milan, 1978).
[84] K. Park, *Doctors and medicine in early Renaissance Florence* (Princeton, 1985), p. 239.
[85] 'Dicamus igitur quod remota causa et primeria istius pestilentie fuit et est aliqua constellatio celestis ...' (ed. Rebouis, p. 76).

immediate cause, that is the corruption of the air.[86] We find no other allusion to astrology, either in the account of individual predispositions or in the advice concerning one's dwelling, where mention is made only of geographical factors and exposure to the winds. We again have to conclude in favour of a discreet resort to astrology. As far as it was practised in connection with medicine, this art seems to have been, in the first half of the fourteenth century, mostly the prerogative of royal physicians, whose predictions had probably both a medical and political aim.

SOME NUMERICAL ASSUMPTIONS

The half century preceding the Black Death was marked by an intense activity on the part of the representatives of physicians' and surgeons' groups to reinforce their professional autonomy and to extend their social influence. At first surgeons, then physicians, saw in royal power a valuable support for their ambitions. As is well known, the barbers, making use of their probable numerical superiority, tried to find a place between these two groups.

Quantitative estimates from the available sources remain fragmentary and highly hypothetical.[87] One of the most reliable indications is the number of barbers (156) who practised during the second half of the thirteenth century, since it is almost entirely based on the statement of the 'taille' of 1292, which did not omit many taxpayers. The slight fall noted for the first half of the fourteenth century can be explained in part by the fact that the main source – that is the statement of the 'taille' of 1313 – concerned fewer taxpayers.[88] In the meanwhile, also the regulation of 1301 was passed, which instituted an examination for barbers who wished to practise surgery. It is possible that some of the barbers who passed this examination preferred to be called surgeons. The number noted for the second half of the fourteenth century is only a reflection of the poor state of our sources. As for physicians, whose appearance in the sources is more regular, the estimate for every period of twenty years gives a consistent

---

[86] 'Credimus autem presentem epidimiam sive pestem ab aere corrupto in sui substantia, et non solum in qualitatibus alterato, immediate provenire' (ibid., p. 80).

[87] I refer here to the numbers proposed in Jacquart, *Le milieu médical*, pp. 242–7, 414:

	1250–99	1300–49	1350–99
Physicians	69	160	176
Surgeons	19	33 (+54?)	45 (+54?)
Barbers	156	112	27

[88] See R. Cazelles, *Paris de la fin du règne de Philippe Auguste à la mort de Charles V, 1223–1380* (Paris, 1972), *Nouvelle Histoire de Paris*, pp. 131–3.

enough result,[89] with a maximum (ninety-nine) during the years 1330–49 and a fall (sixty) in the years immediately following the Black Death.

The major query concerns surgeons, whose names are not recorded in the statements of the 'taille', nor in the university documents. The only reliable numbers – and they are very small – of thirty-three and forty-five for the first and the second half of the fourteenth century respectively are not, perhaps, so derisory as first appears, if we consider the difficult situation of surgeons, who were forbidden to practise medicine and who had left the practice of bleeding to barbers. Katharine Park notes that in Florence too there were fewer surgeons than physicians.[90] There still remain the fifty-four names that François Quesnay listed for the fourteenth century, with no more precise date, and that no other available source mentions. The polemical nature of Quesnay's work prevents us from taking these names into consideration.[91] Nevertheless, even if the eighteenth-century physiocrat was writing a fanciful history of surgery, this introduction of names, invented or not, shows quite well the importance of the fourteenth century, and particularly of its first years, for the founding of the surgical profession. After Jean de St Amand, the most significant author linked to the Parisian medical milieu was Henri de Mondeville, who chose to practise and to teach surgery: this was not completely by chance and attests to the growth of this art in the Parisian framework. Eduard Seidler saw in Henri de Mondeville a representative of what he called (following Pierre Dubois) *via pragmatica*.[92] In fact, this tendency also seems to characterize the faculty of medicine during the 1330s. Two principal reasons can be advanced for the emphasis on practical concerns: above all, the necessity of training practitioners in a town with a numerous population; and the taking into account of an empiricist approach at a time when Ockhamism was making a disturbing entry into the faculty of arts and Jean Buridan became rector of the university. These reasons could have played a part but, in the present state of research, they remain mere assumptions.

---

[89] See Jacquart, *Le milieu médical*, p. 244:

1290–1309	42
1301–1329	84
1330–1349	99
1350–1369	60
1370–1389	86
1390–1409	79

[90] Park, *Doctors*, p. 75. In Florence the proportion of physicians mostly increased from the fifteenth century. City tax rolls indicate: in 1359, 9 physicians, 8 surgeons; in 1399, 16 physicians, 8 surgeons; in 1427, 19 physicians, 7 surgeons; in 1451, 14 physicians, 2 surgeons.

[91] It has to be remembered that Quesnay's book (*Recherches critiques*) was written in order to obtain from the king a new regulation for the College of Parisian surgeons.

[92] E. Seidler, *Die Heilkunde*, p. 109.

Appendix 1 Deans of the faculty of medicine

The names are quoted in the form in which they appear in Ernest Wickersheimer, *Dictionnaire*. The same rule applies to Appendix 2 and Appendix 3.

1311–1325	Jean de Miciclis
1325–1325	François Du Castel
1326–1327	?
1327–1328	Jean Pipe
1328–1329	François Du Castel
1329–1330	Pierre Chauchat
1330–1331	Philippe de Curia
1331–1332	Regnault de Cornemare (*locum tenens decani*)
1332–1333	Regnault de Cornemare
1333–1334	Pierre Chauchat
1334–1335	François Du Castel
1335–1336	Jean de Villanova
1336–1337	Jean de Coucy
1337–1338	Pierre Lemonnier
1338–1339	Hugues Sapientis
1339–1340	François Du Castel
1340–1341	Barthélemy de Alkeriis de Brixia?
1341–1342	Jean de Boisseyo
1342–1343	Pierre Chauchat
1343–1344	Jean de Clermont
1344–1345	Jean de Coucy
1345–1346	?
1346–1347	Pierre Bonefidei
1347–1348	Gérard de Saint Dizier
1348–1349	André de Rippecourt?
1349–1350	Gérard de Saint Dizier
1350–1351	Adam Bercheril de Francovilla

Appendix 2 Some *Magistri regentes* of the faculty of medicine

1274 Jean de Roseto (dean) – F. Brito – Hugues de Parma – J. de Cathalano – Jean de Nigella – J. Normanni – J. Parvi – Pierre d'Auvergne – P. de Novo Castello – R. Meldensis – V. Bouret

1322 (Dean ?) – Gilles de Raveriis – Herman Lombardus – Jean Bostol – Jean de Monasterio – Rémy de Mariniaco – Etienne Spetiarii

1326 François Du Castel (dean) – Etienne Spetiarii – Geoffroi de Gonsalac – Gilles de Raveriis – Herman Lombardus – Ivain de Janua – Jean de Basoles – Jean Bourgot – Jean Fayni de Dia – Jean Pipe – Jean de Pontneuf – Maynus de Mayneriis – Manfred de Coppis – Pierre de Damouzy – Pierre de Florentia – Pierre Pigouche – Regnault de Cornemare – Rémy de Mariniaco

1331 Regnault de Cornemare (*locum tenens decani*) – Aimon Seant de Filigeriis – Denis Saffray – Etienne Spetiarii – Gilles de Grimberge – Gilles de Raveriis – Jacques de Cantarana – Jean Bourgot – Jean de Coucy – Jean Fayni de Dia – Jean de Hallines – Jean de Jotro – Jean Pipe – Jean de Pontneuf – Jean de Portuepiscopi – Maynus de Mayneriis – Manfred de Coppis – Philippe de Curia – Pierre Chauchat – Pierre Pigouche – Rémy de Mariniaco – Sello de Puteo – Thomas de Saint-Georges

1349 Gérard de Saint Dizier (dean) – Adam Bercherii de Francovila – Barthélemy Boneti – Jean de Coucy – Jean de Guiscry – Laurent de Boescure – Thibaud Rotarii de Lanis – Thomas Le Ghisnoys – Nicolas de Goudriaan – Pierre Bonefidei – Pierre Lupi de Montibus

Appendix 3 Physicians in royal service 1300–1350

King	Name	Provided with ecclesiastic benefices	Astrologer	Physician of the queen
Philip the Fair (1285–1314)				
	Arnoul de Quinquempoix		X	
	Etienne de Neufchastieu	X		
	Gilet			
	Guillaume de Baufet			
	Henry Du Puy			
	Jean			
	Jean Hellequin			
	Jean de Lyons			
	Jean Lombart de Roya			
	Jean de Padua			
	Jean de Paris			
	Maurice			
	Robert Le Febvre		X	
Louis X (1314–1316)				
	Arnoul de Quinquempoix		X	
	Guillaume Aymart	X		
	Jean Hellequin	X		
	Jean de Lyons	X		
	Jean de Pavilly			
Philip V (1316–1322)				
	Arnoul de Quinquempoix		X	
	Geoffroi de Corvo	X		
	Geoffroi de Meaux		X	

King	Name	Provided with ecclesiastic benefices	Astrologer	Physician of the queen
	Guillaume Aymart	X		
	Jean de Chalon	X		
	Jean de Lyons	X		
	Jean de Mariniaco	X		X
	Jean de Pavilly	X		
	Pierre Borelli	X		X
	Thomas Le Myésier	X		X
Charles IV (1322–1328)				
	Arnoul de Quinquempoix		X	
	Geoffroi de Corvo	X		
	Geoffroi de Meaux		X	
	Gilbert Hamelin	X		
	Guillaume Aymart	X		
	Herman de Pontramble	X		
	Jacques Gaufridi	X		X
	Jacques de Priceno	X		X
	Jean de Lyons	X		
	Raoul de Bellay	X		
	Regnault de Creciaco			
	Thomas de Pont de l'Arche			
Philip VI (1328–1350)				
	Bartholomew of Bruges	X		
	Etienne de Chaumont	X		
	Etienne Dufresne	X		
	Gilbert Hamelin	X		
	Guido da Vigevano			X
	Jean de Besançon	X		
	Jean de Lyons	X		
	Jean de Prulliaco	X		X
	Pierre			X
	Pierre de Alesto	X		X
	Raoul de Bellay	X		X
	Robert			X
	Robert de Annevilla	X		
	Simon de Lantages			X

7

Royal surgeons and the value of medical learning: the Crown of Aragon, 1300–1350

MICHAEL R. McVAUGH

I

What did it mean to call oneself a surgeon rather than a physician at the beginning of the fourteenth century? A natural starting point would seem to be the distinction drawn in contemporary texts between their respective spheres of activity: the former, says Henri de Mondeville, treats external complaints – wounds, ulcers, abscesses, haemorrhoids, and skin diseases, as well as dislocations and fractures – while the latter cares for ailments within the body.[1] Yet immediately we have to ask whether this distinction was really observed in practice, and whatever the answer, it still will not carry us very far: we would like to know, too, about the surgeon's place in society, the status of his occupation and the value assigned to his services, and his own perception of the possibilities for advancing both. Can we say anything about such comparatively subjective matters?

We have one unusually full description of the surgeon's situation at that very moment. Henri de Mondeville's *Surgery* appears to offer, in the *notabilia* preceding its second book, a uniquely reflective analysis of the relations between the two health occupations around 1300. It paints a picture of generally ruthless competition, where both physicians and surgeons try routinely to secure patients who would nominally be attended by the other.[2] Whatever this may imply about ethics in this pre-professional age, it certainly suggests that the separation of medicine and surgery

---

[1] Henri de Mondeville, *Chirurgia*, III, proemium; Pagel, 41 (1891), 937; Nicaise, p. 495. I use this work in exemplification because Mondeville will subsequently be an important witness on other matters. The *Chirurgia* has been edited by Julius Leopold Pagel, and was published as *Die Chirurgie des Henri de Mondeville* (Berlin, 1892), but this edition is difficult to obtain. Exactly the same text was published by Pagel in instalments as 'Die Chirurgie des Heinrich von Mondeville (Hermondaville)', *Arch. f. klin. Chirurgie*, 40 (1890), 253–311, 653–752, 869–904; 41 (1891), 122–73, 467–504, 705–46, 917–68; 42 (1891), 172–228, 426–90, 645–708, 895–924, and because this version is much easier to obtain I have referred all my citations to the *Chirurgia* to it. I have also provided references to the French translation of E. Nicaise, *Chirurgie de maître Henri de Mondeville* (Paris, 1893).

[2] Pagel, 40 (1890), 662–3; Nicaise, pp. 99–101.

was not strictly observed. Indeed, in practice it was hard at times to draw the line between them, even for a scrupulous practitioner. Mondeville imagines a patient with an incipient abscess: once the abscess matures it will be the undoubted province of the surgeon to open it, but, before that stage, should the patient consult a surgeon or a physician? If he decides on a surgeon, an unprincipled one will try to bring the abscess to a head immediately so that he can operate upon it, even though it would be better for the patient to bring about its resorption by medical means; a conscientious surgeon, however, either will advise the patient to begin by consulting a physician or will himself adopt the physician's role and try to resorb the abscess with diets, purges and dressings.[3] Evidently the frontier between the two worlds could be given only a rough demarcation: part of the practice of a thirteenth- (or fourteenth-) century surgeon was bound to be 'medical' in character.[4]

To be sure, Mondeville can scarcely be considered representative of his craft. For a number of years he had practised, studied and taught medicine at Montpellier and surgery at Montpellier and Paris. He had been formed in an academic medical environment, as most surgeons were not. It is reasonable to imagine that this thorough exposure to a professionalizing medical education might have coloured his views, might have created the defensiveness apparent in his contention that surgery is more certain, more desirable, nobler, more perfect, surer, more necessary, more lucrative, and indeed in every respect better than medicine.[5] How far, therefore, can this obviously self-conscious text be taken as typical of the attitude of other surgeons? How did they feel about their craft vis-à-vis the newly emerging learned medicine? Did they share Mondeville's belief in its superiority – and its greater profitability? Appealing to a different sort of evidence may take them unaware, so to speak, and permit us to judge them by their actions, their career decisions. Let us see what the archival record tells us about Mondeville's contemporaries, their income and their practice.

We will do so by focusing on a region near that where Mondeville trained and taught, the Crown of Aragon in northeastern Spain.[6] This political entity came into being in 1150, when Ramon Berenguer IV, Count of Barcelona, married the Aragonese heiress Petronilla. Petronilla's Aragon, stretching from Pyrenean Jaca south to cities newly recovered from Islam like Zaragoza (1118), Calatayud and Daroca, was largely organized into military tenancies that could consolidate the reconquest; except for the fertile Ebro valley, it was relatively poor and thinly popu-

---

[3] Pagel, 40 (1890), 667–8; Nicaise, pp. 107–8.

[4] See Christian Probst, 'Der Weg des ärtzlichen Erkennens bei Heinrich von Mondeville', in Gundolf Keil et al. (eds.), Fachliteratur des Mittelalters (Stuttgart, 1968), pp. 334–6.

[5] Pagel, 40 (1890), 675–6; Nicaise, pp. 118–20.

[6] The conclusions that follow are based on a decade's systematic examination of archival materials in the Crown of Aragon from the first half of the fourteenth century; I am preparing a broader survey of medicine and society in those realms during that period.

lated. Ramon Berenguer's Barcelona had established itself as pre-eminent among the old Carolingian counties of the northeastern coast (extending from the Roussillon region to Tortosa, and known generally as Catalonia) by virtue of its increasing commercial importance; Catalonia had passed only partially and briefly under Muslim control, and had strong cultural and historical ties with Languedoc and Provence. Aragon and Catalonia, then, were quite distinct societies – the former speaking Aragonese, the latter Catalan – and were really unified only in the person of their common ruler, the count-king. The Crown of Aragon was enlarged in 1238 by the conquest from Islam of Valencia, the enormously fertile coastal strip stretching south from Catalonia to the river Segura, south of Alicante. Valencia remained a separate kingdom within the wider Crown, shaped primarily by Catalan (rather than Aragonese) institutions and language. The fourteenth-century Crown of Aragon was thus a composite political creation in which the wealthier and more populous regions of the Mediterranean seaboard enjoyed the most influence, a fact that does much to explain the expansion of the Crown eastward – to the Balearics, Sardinia, and even Greece – as the century wore on.[7]

II

It is by virtue of its tradition of service to the count-kings of Aragon that we can say so much about one particular surgical dynasty there, the ça Riera family of Gerona in Catalonia.[8] However, the first ça Riera of whom there is any record, Guillem, is poorly known. He received a grant of 300 *sous* yearly from King Pere III in June 1284, an income reconfirmed by Alfons III in May 1285 and paid on Geronan revenues from at least 1287.[9] There are archival records of further grants to him, one for clothing while in attendance on the infante Alfons in Zaragoza in November 1284,[10] but no concrete information about his practice; he may have served the army in 1290.[11] By September 1294 he was dead,[12] and now a new generation of surgical ça Rieras came into the king's employ: Guillem's son Jaume and his nephew Berenguer. The cousins were closely associated in practice for a decade and more, but I will limit myself to discussing Berenguer's career, which is the more revealing – partly because of the

---

[7] For a recent concise account of the Crown, see T. N. Bisson, *The Medieval Crown of Aragon* (Oxford, 1986).

[8] A brief account of this family has been given by A. Cardoner Planas, 'Los cirujanos ça Riera del siglo XIV', *Medicina Clínica*, 2 (1944), 160–2.

[9] Archivo de la Corona de Aragón, Cancillería (hereafter ACA) 62, fol. 71v (15 kls. June 1285); ACA 64, fol. 154v (13 kls. Mar. 1286/7). Here and subsequently I refer to the monarchs of the Crown of Aragon by their Aragonese (rather than Catalan) regnal numbers, as perhaps better known.

[10] ACA 71, fol. 157 (7 id. Nov. 1284).

[11] ACA 82, fol. 168v (2 non. Oct. 1290).

[12] ACA 89, fol. 8 (16 kls. Oct. 1294).

nature of his practice, partly because his role seems to have evolved from giving health care to being entrusted with a wide range of royal commissions. Eventually he became much more than a surgeon.

Berenguer first appears in the Aragonese archives in May 1298, during the planning for King Jaume II's expedition against Sicily, and he was present in the army at Syracuse in that autumn.[13] In 1299 he was promised an annuity of 600 *sous* (twice what his uncle's annual fee had been) from the revenues of Gerona.[14] Such an annuity was apparently distinct from the formal medical contracts one sometimes finds in the later Middle Ages, which specified continuing attendance on the donor as demanded. The annuities granted by the Aragonese monarchs to their medical personnel, like those granted to other favoured subjects, seem to have been retainers with no contractual element, and once granted could apparently be binding on the ruler even though the recipient might have left the kingdom.[15] They must certainly have been made, however, with some exception of undefined but willing reciprocation. In Berenguer's case, he attended the king closely for the next five years. He accompanied the host to Murcia in 1300[16] and went on another military engagement in 1302,[17] and he appears regularly in household accounts through 1303.

During these years Jaume II had not formally set up a medical staff; he seems to have kept the ça Riera cousins on hand and to have consulted other practitioners locally as he travelled through the kingdom. Then, in 1304, the king adopted a different posture towards medical care, appar-

---

[13] ACA 264, fol. 315 (non. May 1298); ACA 264, fol. 338 (14 kls. June 1298); ACA 265, fol. 102 (6 id. Oct. 1298).

[14] ACA 197, fol. 18v (id. Nov. 1299). The document explains that the annual grant is made because of past and future services 'et que cotidie facere non cessaris'. Such a grant was occasionally loosely referred to as a *violarium*, a term which normally denoted an annuity purchased for a certain sum rather than, as here, received in expectation of medical attention; see C. E. Dufourcq and J. Gautier-Dalché, *Historia económica y social de la España cristiana en la edad media* (Barcelona, 1983), pp. 243–4.

[15] An exceptional case suggests the strength of the obligation incurred. Guillem de Béziers came from Montpellier in 1301 to teach medicine in Jaume II's new university at Lerida. Once there, he was called on repeatedly to act as physician to the royal family, and in June 1303 he was promised 1,500 *sous* annually 'dum vita fuerit vobis' by the king (ACA 201, fol. 7v). Over the next few years Guillem was harassed by the competing demands of Lerida and the king, his annuity was often in arrears (ACA 270, fols. 41v (10 kls. Nov. 1305) and 180r–v (4 id. Sept. 1306)), and by 1307 he seems to have returned to Languedoc, perhaps to teach at Montpellier; his pension went unpaid. Subsequently he entered the service of the Avignonese papacy, and in the spring of 1321 the pope's nephew wrote to Jaume II expressing surprise that the stipend had been discontinued. The king's reply has a defensive tone – 'quia dictus magister G. per modicum temporis spacium hic remansit et ad propria remeavit, istud siquidem causa fuit quare dictum violarium non accepit' (ACA 301, fol. 123) – and he reinstated the *annua pensio*. José Martínez Gázquez and I will give a fuller biographical account of Guillem in our forthcoming edition of the brief *Informatio* that he prepared for his students.

[16] ACA 266, fol. 364v (5 id. Nov. 1300); ACA 268, fols. 69v–70r (7 kls. Apr. 1301); ACA 294, fol. 47v (5 id. May 1302).

[17] Eduardo González Hurtebise, *Libros de tesorería de la casa real de Aragón*, vol. 1 (Barcelona, 1911), pp. 23, 479; docs. 80, 479 (8 Apr., 20 Nov. 1302).

ently deliberately choosing to appoint a staff possessed of the academic training that he obviously admired: he hired two physicians, Armengaud Blaise (Montpellier-trained) and Martí de Calça Roja, giving the former seniority. When Armengaud left the court at the end of 1306, Joan Amell (who also had an academic background) replaced him at the court as principal physician. After 1304, therefore, Berenguer's medical role at court diminished sharply, and he begins to appear in very different settings: between 1304 and 1306 as bailiff (*baiulus*) of Gerona,[18] in 1306 as royal ambassador to treat in Montpellier with representatives of the Genoese.[19] He was now acting primarily as royal official and agent, though his medical involvement was not at an end; he travelled with the army to Almería on the crusade-expedition of 1309. His last commission from the king was to arrange the cutting of stones for the tomb of Queen Blanca, who died in October 1310.[20] Two months later Berenguer himself was dead.

What sort of rewards could such a diligent royal servant command?[21] On paper they are impressive, but the actuality seems to have been much less so. Take, to begin with, Berenguer's annual stipend from the king of 600 *sous*, granted in November 1299 on the revenues of Gerona. In May 1300 the grant was shifted to the revenues of Barcelona because the Geronan income was not adequate to pay it.[22] By May 1302 (and perhaps earlier) the grant was again in arrears,[23] and the king had to insist that it be paid – vainly, for he issued the same command in August 1303.[24] Still in arrears, it was shifted back to a Geronan source in June 1304.[25] For June 1305 a financial statement survives: after five and a half years of service, Berenguer was owed 2,216 *sous* 8 *diners* of the 3,300 *sous* due him from his annuity:[26] thus he had averaged only about 200 *sous* a year from the grant. In April 1306 the grant was moved to a new source, the rents of Palafrugell and Cerviá,[27] and two months later he obtained the right to sell the grant for whatever he could get.[28] What Berenguer was able to recover from the annuity thereafter we do not know. By May 1307 he had been paid another 176 *sous* 8 *diners* on the old account, by February 1309 a little more – but

---

[18] Berenguer is cited as *baiulus* on 5 kls. Nov. 1304 (ACA 202, fol. 172v) and is still identified as such on 8 id. Mar. 1305/6 (ACA 236, fol. 137).

[19] ACA 236, fols. 185r–v, 201v (kls. June and 10 kls. Aug. 1306).

[20] ACA 147, fol. 52v (17 kls. Nov. 1310).

[21] This question is treated generally for the thirteenth–fifteenth centuries by L. Comenge, 'Formas de munificencia real para con los archiatros de Aragón', *Boletín de la Real Academia de Buenas Letras de Barcelona*, 2, año 3 (1903), 1–15.

[22] ACA 197, fol. 115v (kls. May 1300).

[23] ACA 269, fol. 50 (5 id. May 1302).

[24] ACA 269, fol. 232v (6 kls. Sept. 1303).

[25] ACA 202, fols. 147v–148 (3 id. June 1304), amplified by ACA 295, fols. 5–6 (letter of 12 kls. July 1305).

[26] ACA 295, fols. 5–6 (12 kls. July 1305); ACA 296, fol. 75 (5 kls. June 1307).

[27] ACA 203, fol. 150v (id. Apr. 1306).

[28] ACA 203, fol. 173 (13 kls. July 1306).

over 400 *sous* were still outstanding on the salary promised him a decade before.[29]

Or consider Berenguer's payment for military service. For the expedition to Murcia, he was owed 1,807 *sous* 'by certain nobles and knights, being one day's fee when they were with us in the kingdom of Murcia'; and similar language in connection with the crusade against Almería is used to account for a debt of 7,196 *sous* 8 *diners*. Evidently he had contracted with several hundred individuals among the host to provide medical care to them as necessary in exchange for one day's worth of their fee from the king for military service; in effect, offering them a system of prepaid medical care.[30] But of course it was then the king's responsibility to pay him, and again payment was belated. The Murcia money was promised in January 1301; 742 *sous* 8 *diners*, two-fifths of the total, were still unpaid in May 1302.[31] Berenguer died before the fee for his Almería service had been paid, and it proved to be even more difficult for his heirs to exert sufficient pressure to collect; his surgeon-nephew Ferrer Moragues was still receiving money on this account in 1316.[32] The 500 *sous* owed to Berenguer for supervising Blanca's tomb, just before his death in 1310, were still unpaid in 1331, despite his son's most intense efforts.[33]

This last debt reveals that apparently petty sums were no easier to collect than large ones. In February 1302, in attendance at court, Berenguer was

[29] ACA 296, fol. 75 (5 kls. June 1307); Arxiu de la Catedral de Barcelona (hereafter ACB), Manual de Bernat de Vilarrúbia for 1307–1309–1312, fol. 71 (9 kls. Mar. 1308/9).

[30] In 1296 a knight was paid 4 *sous* per day by the king for himself and the support of his horse; by the time of the Sardinian campaign of 1323 the stipend had increased to 4 *sous* for the man and a further 4 *sous* for his horse: Charles Emmanuel Dufourcq, 'Prix et niveaux de vie dans les pays catalans et maghribins à la fin du XIIIe et au début du XIVe siècle', *Le Moyen Age*, 71 (1965), 507. When the surgeon Bernat Pertegaç accompanied the army to Sardinia in 1323, he made similar contracts with no fewer than five different groups of 'barones et milites exercitii': for 4,944 *sous*, 1,472 *sous*, 1,347 *sous* 10 *diners*, 481 *sous* 10 *diners*, and 640 *sous*: ACA 421, fol. 16r–v (3 kls. May 1325). To get an idea of the value of money: Dufourcq ('Prix et niveaux', pp. 512–17) suggests that one could live reasonably well on 2–3 *sous* per day. Berenguer's royal grant would thus by itself have not supported him, even if it had been promptly paid.

[31] ACA 294, fol. 47v (5 id. May 1302).

[32] ACA 277, fols. 113, 264 (3 kls., 2 non. Sept. 1316). The later document shows Ferrer transferring the king's debt in order to settle his own indebtedness to a third party; he was thus able to collect on the obligation in spite of the king's pennilessness.

Ferrer Moragues' family was Valencian; he was still a minor in 1290 (Archivo del Reino de Valencia (hereafter ARV), Justícia de Valencia 20, s.f. (c. non. June 1317)). Jaume II commended him as a surgeon to his brother Frederick of Sicily/Trinacria in 1294 (ACA 99, fol. 308v); he was back in the Crown of Aragon nine years later, when Jaume II granted him property in newly conquered Murcia (ACA 201, fols. 42, 117v). He went with his uncle on the expedition to Almería in 1309 (ACA, Real Patrimonio 272, fol. 50r), and attended the king briefly in 1312 (ACA, Real Patrimonio 275, fol. 60v) and for a longer period in 1320–1 (ACA, Real Patrimonio 285, fol. 74v; 287, fol. 54v). In 1323 he joined in the conquest of Sardinia (ACA 177, fol. 153r–v) and thereafter is lost from sight. None of the material on Ferrer's career sheds any light on the character of his formation or orientation as a surgeon.

[33] ACA 560, fols. 231v–232r (10 kls. July 1330); ACA 498, fols. 184r–185r (3 kls. Oct. 1331); ACB, perg. C–15 2427 (17 kls. Dec. 1331).

promised 300 *sous* for clothing; only 50 of that had been paid by November. In December 1306 Berenguer was due to receive 500 *sous* from the king in settlement of a nobleman's estate – but the king asked him to wait until Easter to collect.[34] In fact, what could be collected depended partly on chance. If an order for payment was presented to the treasurer at the moment when some receipts happened to come in, a part of what was owing might be paid over; otherwise debts would continue to accumulate – sometimes very rapidly, as the 8,000 *sous* given to Berenguer on account in the autumn of 1301 suggest.[35] On the other hand, because cash was so short, the treasury might refuse to turn over receipts that had been specifically assigned to the person requesting payment. A letter survives from Berenguer to the king reminding him that a part of the overdue account was to have been settled with money from fines imposed on Jews who had trafficked illegally with Muslim Alexandria, and complaining that the treasurer would not release the funds; eventually Berenguer managed to obtain nearly 1,000 *sous* on account from this source in February 1309.[36]

In such conditions, where the king was so short of cash, other kinds of reward would seem more valuable: rights, for example. In September 1301, Berenguer and his cousin Jaume jointly bought from the king the rights to Palau and Quart for 5,000 *sous* of Barcelona, but paid him in cash only 214 *sous* 3 *diners*: the remainder simply cancelled sums already owing to them.[37] We may well imagine that Berenguer's appointment as bailiff of Gerona was potentially more remunerative than any cash he might expect from the king. The difficulty was that offices and rights, too, were limited: they could not be indefinitely created. In June 1304 Berenguer obtained from the king a royal mill in Gerona, but only by supplying the 3,500 *sous* necessary to recover it from the estate of the man to whom it had been granted by Jaume's late brother, Alfons.[38] The king himself had nothing to give – and gave nothing.

III

We have very little concrete information about the medical care that the ça Riera cousins provided to the court. The only specific case of which there is a record is Berenguer's treatment (*c.* 1308) of Arnau Amaneu, the papal nuncio to England, for an ailment in the knee and a dislocation

---

34 ACA 140, fol. 12 (6 kls. Jan. 1306/7).
35 ACA 294, fol. 52.
36 On 9 kls. Mar. 1308/9 he was paid 957 *sous* 9 *diners*; ACB, Manual de Bernat de Vilarrúbia 1307–12, fol. 71r.
37 The original *albaranum* is in ACA, Cartas Reales Diplomáticas (hereafter CRD), Jaume II, extra-series 1696, dorso; see also the copy in ACA 198, fols. 375–6 (5 kls. Oct. 1301 – a note says final payment was made up 8 id. May 1302).
38 ACA 202, fol. 140r–v (kls. June 1304).

(*deslogament*) of the hip. We have Berenguer's own assurance to the king that Arnau obtained in Catalonia 'what he had not found from the physicians of the king of England, nor in the kingdom of France, nor at Montpellier, nor anywhere': the hip returned to its place and the knee improved significantly. But we have no details of the cure.[39]

Nevertheless, some further cautious inferences as to his approach to surgery are certainly possible. Eighty years ago Rubió y Lluch called attention to a curious transaction linking Berenguer ça Riera to medical learning. In September 1301 Jaume told his bailiff for Catalonia that he badly needed the copy of Avicenna (probably the *Canon*) that Berenguer had recently pawned for 500 *sous*, and that the book should be reclaimed and the pledge paid out of the revenues of Catalonia.[40] The king repeated the command in March and again in May 1302,[41] and finally in November the royal treasurer gave Berenguer the 500 *sous* necessary to reclaim the volume.[42] The book had originally been given to Berenguer as a pledge for a debt of 500 *sous* owed to him by the king; as we have seen, the annuity promised in 1299 had fallen immediately into arrears. The renewed need for the volume does not seem to indicate a medical emergency, because Jaume's requests for the volume were spaced out over a year or so, and in any case we know of no problems with the health of the royal household in 1301–2. We may tentatively imagine that it was Berenguer who found the *Canon* useful, who wanted it on hand, and that it was at his urging that he personally was finally enabled to reclaim the volume. The suggestion that *he* was the Avicennan at court receives some support from the fact that in September 1303, as Berenguer was ending his period of close attendance on the king, Jaume granted him 250 *sous* to buy a copy of Avicenna for himself ('ad opus sui').[43]

The discrepancy between this sum and the pledged value of the king's own copy, 500 *sous*, could be explained in many ways. One would be that Berenguer was concerned to possess only a portion of the *Canon*, most likely Book IV, which covers diseases and devotes three fen to specifically surgical problems – tumours and apostemes, wounds and ulcers, dislo-

---

[39] Antoni Rubió y Lluch, *Documents per l'història de la cultura catalana mig-eval*, vol. II (Barcelona, 1921), pp. 53–5, doc. 56; Berenguer seems to have been directed to this patient by the king. Cardoner, 'Cirujanos', notes 'debemos decir, en honor a la verdad, que hasta el siglo XIX se dió el nombre de "deslogament", en catalán, o de "luxación espontánea del fémur" a cualquier artritis de la cadera, porque durante el curso de éstas a veces sobreviene una subluxación' (p. 161). The document is undated, but because it includes a complaint that he has not yet been paid the money assigned him from fines assessed on Geronan Jews who had illegally trafficked with Alexandria, it presumably predates February 1309, when he was paid from this source (document cited above, n. 35).

[40] Rubió y Lluch, *Documents*, vol. II, p. 13 (doc. 15); ACA 268, fol. 217v.

[41] ACA 269, fol. 26v, and ACA 294, fol. 45; Rubió y Lluch did not find the first of these. Nowhere in the documentation is the volume actually identified as the *Canon*, but the high monetary value placed upon it strongly suggests that this is what it was.

[42] González Hurtebise, *Libros de tesorería*, vol. I, pp. 120–1; doc. 480.

[43] Rubió y Lluch, *Documents*, vol. II, p. 15 (doc. 19); ACA 294, fol. 131v (3 kls. Aug. 1303).

cations and fractures. Equally well, however, Berenguer may have wanted the *Canon* complete, and Jaume may have been willing or able to furnish only a part of the purchase price. For Berenguer certainly had a broad mastery of a more generally medical (as distinct from surgical) learning. Arnau de Vilanova – medical master, physician and confidant to the royal family – had by 1307 completed a Latin *Regimen sanitatis* designed for Jaume II, and Jaume's queen, Blanca, sponsored its translation into Catalan. The work is typically Arnaldian and, though by no means technical in language, clearly reflects Arnau's academic background and knowledge of Galenic physio-pathological theory. Hence it is noteworthy that the queen asked her surgeon Berenguer to make the translation; after all, the court now had two specifically medical men permanently in its service, Joan Amell and Martí de Calça Roja, and the former, the king's principal physician, was that rare thing in the early fourteenth century, an academic master. Evidently Berenguer must have been well acquainted with medical learning, not merely empirical surgical techniques, or the queen would have turned to her physician for the desired translation. Indeed, Berenguer's preface to the translation – the only scrap of medical writing we have from him – shows his familiarity with Galenic medical thought in its explanation that 'health is equivalent to a balanced complexion, and a balanced complexion is equivalent to a tempering of the humours'.[44]

It is virtually certain that Berenguer was personally acquainted with Arnau de Vilanova, for the latter visited the court to oversee the queen's pregnancy while Berenguer was in attendance there in 1302,[45] and it is not inconceivable that Arnau could have seen and approved Berenguer's version of the *Regimen*, which is a close and accurate one. It *is* certain that Berenguer knew well Arnau's nephew Armengaud Blaise, another Montpellier academic, who was in royal service intermittently until 1306. They must have encountered one another in Gerona, where Armengaud had arrived to practise by 1296.[46] In 1297 Berenguer told the king that

[44] 'Sanitat no es sinó per egualtat de compleccion, e egualtat de complecion no és sinó per temprament de les humors' (p. 99): the translation has been edited by Miquel Batllori, in Arnau de Vilanova, *Obres catalanes*, vol. II (Barcelona, 1947), pp. 99–200; he discusses the translation at pp. 74–9, without however identifying the translator with the surgeon who figures in Rubió Lluch's *Documents* (p. 75). The Latin *Regimen* will be edited by Ana Trías Teixidor in the *Opera Medici Arnaldi*; a discussion of its contents may be found in Arnau de Vilanova, *El maravilloso regimiento y orden de vivir*, (ed. Juan A. Paniagua Arellano, Zaragoza, 1980), pp. 63–77.

[45] Michael McVaugh, 'The births of the children of Jaime II', *Medievalia*, 6 (1986), 11–12.

[46] For a general outline of Armengaud's career, see 'Armengaud Blaise', in Ernest Wickersheimer, *Dictionnaire biographique des médecins en France au Moyen Age, Supplément* (ed. Danielle Jacquart; Geneva, 1979), pp. 25–6. 'Magister Ermengaudus Blasini phisicus Gerunde' acknowledged receipt of 1,000 *sous* of Barcelona from the abbot of Amer on 8 id. Sept. 1296 – 500 *sous* repaying a loan, 400 *sous* for a mule, the rest for a *vixellam argenti*: Arxiu Diocesà de Giorona (hereafter ADG), serie G: Notularum, 1, fol. 37v. Armengaud was made physician to Queen Blanca by 1301 (ACA 294, fol. 19v (11 kls. Nov. 1301)), went back to Montpellier early the next year (ACA 120, fol. 190v. (4 non. Jan. 1301/2)), and was called back to serve the royal family in 1304 at a salary of 2,000 *sous* from the king

Armengaud owned a useful book on the treatment of haemorrhoids, a chronic complaint of the young monarch (Arnau devoted a special chapter to it in his *Regimen* ten years later), and Jaume then ordered Armengaud to send him the book and to pass on to Berenguer any further advice that he might have to contribute about how to cure the ailment.[47] The picture of Berenguer that thus begins to emerge from these fragments of documentation is of a surgeon, no doubt, but a surgeon who is well acquainted with the world of more purely medical learning.

Before the cousins became attached to the court, they had been practising for several decades in Gerona. It is not particularly surprising that we have no documents that refer to this, what we might call their 'private' (as distinct from royal or military) practice, for thirteenth-century records of any sort are comparatively scarce. Yet the surviving account of a Geronan inquest from the first decade of the fourteenth century does shed some light on their medical role within the city at the same time that it confirms what we have just inferred about their approach to surgery.[48]

On Good Friday in an undetermined year, while some young clerics were standing on the great stairway leading up to the Geronan cathedral and ('as the custom was') were pelting the Jews and their houses below with stones,[49] the sling of one slipped and the stone hit a boy behind him, Nicolau, in the head. Women passing by heard the boy call out 'Ladies, help me', and a bystander (a canon of the cathedral) took Nicolau to his home, where he inspected the wound. It did not appear to be serious – there was little swelling and almost nothing of a cut – and the canon himself bandaged it. Nicolau returned to work in the shop of the silversmith he served, and paid no attention to his wound, despite medical advice; he soon discarded the bandage and continued to go out through the streets of Gerona following the Easter processions (*coreas*), careless of the wind, vigorously battering Jewish houses with sticks and stones. But within two weeks he had worsened dramatically, and at this point Jaume and Berenguer ça Riera, 'by general consent among the best surgeons in all Catalonia', were called in. Neither they nor other surgeons could do anything for the boy, however, and he died in the third week of the injury.

At the inquest, the surgeons were asked to assign the cause of death in order to determine where responsibility for the death lay: was the young

---

[47] Rubió y Lluch, *Documents*, vol. II, p. 12 (doc. 14); ACA 106, fol. 132v (6 id. Dec. 1297).

[48] The following account is based on ADG, serie C (procesos), 20 (old 69, fasc. 5). The date of the inquest is largely illegible: all that can be read is 'anno domini m°.ccc.° ***'.

[49] The Jews of Gerona were still complaining about this practice in 1345 (ACA 632, fol. 54r–v). By 1436 municipal ordinances had been introduced to prevent it; see Luis Batlle y Prats, 'Ordenaciones relativas a los judíos Gerundenses', *Homenaje a Millás Vallicrosa* (Barcelona, 1954), vol. I, pp. 83–4.

and 4,000 *sous* from the queen (ACA 294, fol. 195v, and 202, fol. 167r–v (16 kls. June and kls. Oct. 1304)). He is last found alive in the archives on 5 id. Oct. 1306 (ACA 203, fol. 195), evidently making plans to leave the kingdom. There is considerable additional material in the ACA on Armengaud's career which I hope eventually to publish.

cleric whose sling had slipped responsible? Had it been an inevitably fatal injury? Berenguer ça Riera, called to testify, said that he had seen such stone-throwing for twenty years in Gerona, Barcelona, Valencia and elsewhere in Catalonia. As soon as he had observed Nicolau, he had known that the boy was sure to die of his head wound, either because he had received bad medical treatment or because of his own imprudent behaviour (*regimen*). His cousin Jaume concurred; *he* had had *thirty* years' experience, and he agreed with his cousin that the art of surgery led them to conclude that the boy would not have died if he had had a good doctor (*medicum*) and had taken proper care of himself, 'as could be seen from the nature of the blow and of his symptoms'.[50] It was Nicolau himself who was to blame for his own death, for not having obeyed advice to follow a sensible and healthy routine.

What should Nicolau have done? Presumably he should have rested and kept the wound bandaged – but there is more, as we learn from the testimony of yet another surgeon, Ramon de Cornellà.[51] The boy, he testified, was 'incorrigible, because he ate beef with cabbage, and raw lettuce with vinegar, and drank a lot of water – all of which is bad for the wounded, according to surgery as practised in these lands'. Ramon himself had told the boy that he shouldn't have drunk water, but Nicolau had retorted that 'he didn't have any wine, and he was thirsty'.[52]

The testimony of the ça Rieras and Ramon de Cornellà thus confirms that, in turn-of-the-century Catalonia, surgery was not at all (as perhaps we tend to imagine it today) a primarily invasive activity, but involved, rather, consciously ordered procedures linked to preventive medicine – to rest and diet – in accordance with principles based upon physiological theory. This approach is very much in line with the thirteenth-century emergence, in the north Italian schools, of surgery as a subject with its own written tradition akin to and devolving from medical authority.

The new Italian interpretation of the nature of surgery as a rational procedure sharing common ground with medicine is clearly reflected in Henri de Mondeville's claim to be writing his book especially for 'students wanting to learn surgery ... particularly the educated, those who at least

---

[50] One witness testified that when the cousins first viewed the patient they said 'quod si ante fuisset eis hostensus quod potuissent ei dare consilium'.

[51] In this document Ramon claimed thirty-five years' experience, but he first appears in the archival record as a surgeon appointed (for an annual salary of 100 *sous*) to care for the bishop and cathedral chapter of Gerona, in April 1296 (ADG, Notularum 1, fol. 26), and thereafter he crops up regularly in the Geronan documentation until he drew up his will in March 1313: Josep Maria Marquès i Planagumà, *Pergamins de la Mitra (891–1687): Arxiu Diocesà de Girona* (Gerona, 1984), doc. 648.

[52] '[Erat] incorrigibilis quod comederat carnes vaccinas cum caulibus et lactucas crudas cum aceto, et potuerat satis de aqua: que omnia sunt contraria vulnerato secundum practicam cirurgie que observatur in hac terra ... Et recordatur ipse testis quod cum idem testis inculparet dictum puerum quia potaverat aquam, idem puer dixit quod non habebat vinum, et sitiebat.'

know the general principles of medicine and understand its language', because 'it is impossible for a surgeon to be competent if he has not mastered the basic principles of medicine; likewise ... it is impossible for a physician to be competent if he is thoroughly ignorant of the art of surgery'.[53] Henri went on:

> Let us give a concrete example drawn from surgery. A surgeon seeing an aposteme knows that it is a disease [*morbus*], because it sensibly harms the activity of the organs; he knows that it is a compound *morbus* because it combines all the three kinds of illness, namely bad complexion, malformation, and breaks in continuity ... he recognizes the signs of the complexion of the aposteme, and from these he knows its material cause – for example, that it arises from blood. The surgeon knows all these things from his mastery of theory, though he cannot go further in knowledge or effect a cure without passing on to operative surgery.[54]

Evidently at least some surgeons explicitly admitted the value of medical learning and tried to ground their practice upon it.

The Geronan surgeons' criticism of Nicolau's behaviour ought to be examined, therefore, against the background of contemporary surgical writing on the theoretical principles underlying wound treatment and its associated diet, and it is interesting to find what seems to have been a difference of authoritative opinion on the subject. From the Italian Guglielmo da Saliceto: 'let [someone with a head wound] utterly abstain from wine until he is nearly cured, for there is nothing that harms the head as much as wine, bringing matter to the brain – nothing else that so induces a relapse and weakening of the brain and the flow of humours there as does wine'.[55] From what might be called the western Mediterranean tradition,

---

[53] 'Unde discipuli volentes addiscere cyrurgiam guadeant et laetentur intelligentes, precipue literati, qui medicinae saltem principia communia cognoverunt et qui intelligunt verba artis, quoniam pro ipsis opus hujusmodi est principaliter ordinatum.' 'Impossible est cyrurgicum esse sufficientem, qui non cognoscat principia et notabilia medicinae communia; similiter ... impossibile est medicum esse sufficientem qui artem cyrurgiae penitus ignoravit.' Pagel, 40 (1890), 263, 675; Nicaise, pp. 4, 117. See also Pagel, 40 (1890), 657; Nicaise, p. 91.

[54] 'Verbi gratia ponamus exemplum sensibile familiare cyrurgicum: Cyrurgicus videns apostema cognoscit, quod est morbus, quia infert actioni membrorum sensibile nocumentum, et quod est morbus compositus, quia in eo sunt omnia vel tria genera morborum, scilicet mala compositio cum mala separatione et disjunctione partium membri apostemati facta ex imbibitione materiae apostematis inter ipsas et pectus in forma membri sicut eminentia vel tumor. Deinde cognoscit signa complexionis apostematis, deinde per signa cognoscit causas ut materiales, ut: quod est sanguineum etc. Et haec omnia cognoscit cyrurgicus per theoricam suam, nec per ipsam ulterius potest cognoscere nec accedere ad curam apostematis nisi transeat ad cyrurgiam operativam ... ' Pagel, 40 (1890), 666–7; Nicaise, p. 105.

[55] 'Summo opere a vino abstineat usque quasi ad perfectam curationem, quia nichil est quod ita percutiat capitem et protus **it materiam ad cerebrum quemadmodum vinum nec aliquid quod inducat ita residivacionem et debilitatem cerebri et cursum humorum ad cerebrum ut vinum.' *Cirurgia*, II.I. I follow the text in Oxford, St John's College MS 76, fol. 36r; the word I have been unable to read is rendered 'protrahat et conculcet' in the text printed in *Ars Chirurgica* (Venice, 1546), fol. 326vb.

however, the counsel was rather different. Teodorico Borgognoni of Lucca dedicated his surgery to the bishop of Valencia in the 1260s; it was translated twice into Catalan, and was probably the most widely disseminated surgical text in the Crown of Aragon.[56] Teodorico has no specific diet for head wounds, but he does say of wounds in general (following Ugo da Lucca) that

the drink which master Ugo used to give ... was the best wine which could be found, without the admixture of water. And the wine which he asserted would be most amicable to the human constitution is a white wine, delicately aromatic, pleasant to drink. For he used to say that this was a wine from which blood is generated with no intermediary, as it were, and that nature operates best in wounds with such a wine. And I myself have always followed him in that respect, supported by the authority of Galen, who says in his book on the technique of healing, that wine must under no conditions be denied to the wounded unless a hot abscess should appear.[57]

Henri de Mondeville adhered to Teodorico's position, though he was even more explicit about the scientific reasons for the use of wine:

Good wine is the most appropriate food for generating blood, and consequently for generating flesh. The antecedent is proved by the authority of the Philosopher [misquoting Aristotle, *De generatione animalium* 723a?], who says that good wine passes more or less directly into the blood and is changed into blood. Moreover, of all foods wine is most like blood in substance and colour, and it is easier for similar things to change into one another. Thus wine is the most appropriate food for producing blood. The consequent is proved because flesh can be created only from blood, so that what is appropriate for producing blood is appropriate for producing flesh. Teodorico adds that incompetent surgeons fail to understand this and insist that the wounded maintain a strict diet and abstinence ... They cannot commit a more serious error than to thus thin the blood, which in all wounds has the task of repairing what has been lost, of filling cavities and reuniting the flesh.[58]

Henri goes on thereafter to condemn beef as well as vegetables, water and all moist foods: obviously, Nicolau had indeed followed the worst possible regimen. It would plainly be a mistake, therefore, to understand the 'practica in hac terra' upon which our Geronan surgeons insisted as alluding to a course of treatment based purely upon experience; rather, it was heavily theory-laden, rooted in the Galenic tradition and even in natural philosophy.[59]

---

[56] Antonio Contreras, 'La difusión de la Cyrurgia de Teodorico Borgognoni en los paises de habla catalana', Tesis de Licenciatura en Medicina (University of Cantabria, 1986).

[57] Teodorico, *Cirurgia*, 1.25; *The surgery of Theodoric*, trans. Eldridge Campbell and James Colton, vol. 1 (New York, 1955), p. 93. The Galenic passage in question is probably *De ingenio sanitatis* VIII.3; *Opera Galeni* (1490), II, 194va.

[58] Mondeville, II.i.i.6. Pagel, 40 (1890), 902; Nicaise, p. 284.

[59] It should be remembered that surgeons continued to acknowledge disagreement on this issue: in the mid fourteenth century Guy de Chauliac depicted Teodorico and Henri as standing out alone against Bruno Longoburgo and Lanfranco, Haly Abbas and Galen in defending a 'dietam vinosam et calidissimam' for such patients (*Chirurgia magna*, III.1.i).

We can now see that a sharp distinction between surgeons and physicians was made even more difficult because of the desire of some surgeons to graft their subject onto the stock of medical learning. Berenguer and Henri are just two of many European practitioners who by the turn of the century foresaw that both intellectual substance and social status might be conferred if surgery were acknowledged as founded, like medicine, on scientific principles, and if its proponents were recognized as belonging to the learned tradition. Far more critical to them than the physician/surgeon distinction was a distinction between the literate surgical practitioner, who can build on that tradition, and the illiterate empiric who has only limited and misunderstood experience to guide him and is really no better than a charlatan. Henri quotes Galen to show that the ability to practise rationally is the mark of a true 'medicus' (a term customarily used as denoting both *phisici* and *cirurgici*), and he rails angrily against those who falsely pretend to such ability,

all those illiterates – barbers, sorcerers, landlords, tricksters, counterfeiters, alchemists, bawds, go-betweens, midwives, old women, converted Jews, Saracens – all those who have foolishly squandered what they have and proclaim themselves surgeons so that they can make a living, hiding their wretchedness, poverty and lies under the cloak of surgery.[60]

Henri's intensity of language expresses his frustration that, in spite of their intellectual superiority, learned surgeons are still not properly appreciated and are at an economic disadvantage compared to empiric practitioners of the craft: 'ignorant frauds grow wealthy and gain renown in it, while the learned [*scientes*], honest and knowledgeable, are oppressed and live like paupers or beggars'.[61] He could not have been alone in feeling this frustration. When the ça Riera cousins were finally called to the bedside of the dying Nicolau, they discovered that an empiric had first been given charge of the patient; it is hard not to hear resentment in their protest that 'We could have cured him had we been called in at the outset.'[62]

IV

In a variety of ways, the circumstances of the career of Berenguer's son Arnau are quite different from those of his father's. The most distinctive

---

[60] 'Omnes illiterati, sicut barberii, sortilegi, locatores, insidiatores, falsarii, alchemistae, meretrices, metatrices, obstetrices, vetulae, Judaei conversi, Sarraceni et quasi omnes, qui bona sua fatue consumpserint, qui fingunt se cyrurgicos aliquando, ut habeant, unde vivant, et ut sub pallio cyrurgiae cooperiant miserias suas, paupertates et etiam falsitates.' Pagel, 40 (1890), 661.

[61] 'Deceptores ignorantes lucrantur et in ipsa magnifice exaltantur, et scientes, veridici et experti opprimuntur et vivunt saepe pauperes et mendici.' Ibid.

[62] This interpretation rests on my reading of a defective passage in the Geronan document (above, n. 47) that cannot be fully reconstructed due to severe deterioration of the paper on which it is written. What is legible says, ' . . . qui quidem R. Johannis diligentiam quam habuerat circa curam Nicholay **** sui et quem ut filium dilig ***, et neglig *** empirici

feature of Arnau's career is certainly the nature of his professional formation. His father no doubt gave Arnau practical training in surgery, but he may have hoped that he would go on and profit from the learned tradition as well: Berenguer's will specifies that his books are not to be dispersed but should be passed on as a whole to his heir.[63] Nor did Arnau's acquaintance with scientific medicine end there, for it has recently been discovered that he was university trained. By a happy chance, his academic licence from fourteenth-century Lerida has survived – the only licence from any of the faculties there to have done so. It appears to show that Arnau received at least the training of a bachelor of medicine at Montpellier in the late 1320s, studying with Jean Maseti, and practised there for several years; and that he was subsequently awarded the title of *magister* at Lerida in 1344.[64] Significantly, most public documents referring to Arnau identify him as *physicus et cirurgicus*, and his gravestone insists on his title of *magister in medicina*. The dual role we have inferred his father to have played is thus made explicit in Arnau's career.[65]

Along with certification of professional training seems to have gone full-time attention to medical responsibilities as distinct from broader political or administrative service; at the same time, a higher value was placed on those responsibilities. Arnau's service to the crown apparently began in 1334, when he was summoned urgently from Gerona to attend Alfons IV in Tortosa.[66] He was one of many physicians whose presence was commanded from all over the kingdom – Besalú, Tarragona, Zaragoza – for Alfons was undergoing a serious crisis in an illness caused by 'an overheated liver and blocked spleen' that seems to have begun the previous year. But Arnau's treatment was evidently perceived as particularly successful, for four months later he was singled out for an annuity of 1,000 *sous*, payable on the king's revenues from the Jewish community (the *aljama*) of Barcelona,[67] and he stayed with the king as 'master of medicine

---

medici videlicet **** cirurgici Geru[nde] propter quam ***** ...'. I have concluded that this passage reveals the unsuccessful treatment given Nicolau by an empiric surgeon of Gerona, but of course it is susceptible of other interpretations as well.

63 'Volo quod libri mei non alienentur, immo conserventur et traduntur heredi meo.' ADG, Pia Almoina 7691. Berenguer's heir, his namesake Berenguer, was the only one of his sons who had attained his majority when the surgeon died in 1310. Berenguer *fils* went on to a career as *iurisperitus*, and it is perhaps plausible to think that he was intended to turn the medical books over to his younger brother. In any case, the language of the will certainly makes plain the importance that the father placed upon the written tradition.

64 Michael McVaugh and Luis García-Ballester, 'The medical faculty at early fourteenth-century Lérida', *History of Universities*, 8 (1989), 1–25.

65 I find it significant that the earliest record we have (1330) of a case undertaken by Arnau testifies to his treatment of a woman with a breast tumour (a condition normally dealt with by surgeons) and specifies that the success of his treatment is to be evaluated by 'duorum cirurgicorum vel medicorum'; yet it is careful to refer to Arnau as *fisicus*. Arxiu Històric Provincial de Girona (hereafter AHPG), Notari-Girona 1, reg. 7 (5 kls. May 1330).

66 ACA 536, fol. 42v (4 non. Oct. 1334).

67 ACA 468, fol. 173v (10 kls. Apr. 1334/5).

and surgery', providing medical care,[68] until Alfons died in January 1336 (though Arnau does not appear to have been on hand at the deathbed). Alfons' son and successor, Pere IV, not only continued his father's grant but added a further 3,000 sous to it, praising Arnau as 'expert in the science of medicine', in June 1336;[69] so Alfons' death was evidently not attributed to Arnau's poor care. In August 1336 the grant was shifted from the Barcelonan to the Geronan aljama, to make it easier for Arnau to collect it.[70] From 1336 to 1341 Arnau appears regularly in attendance on the new monarch, and in May 1334 – three months after receiving his degree from Lerida – he was paid 4,800 sous due him by the treasury.[71] He continued to draw his annuity until his death in the 1348 plague.[72]

What explains these much higher rewards for Arnau? Are they only superficially higher – that is, was there an inflation that reduced their real value between 1300 and 1335? Not, certainly, of the order of 650 per cent (comparing Arnau's 4,000 sous with his father's 600).[73] An increased availability of money to the treasury might seem another possible explanation: Pere had enough spare cash in hand, for example, to make Arnau a spontaneous de gratia payment of 300 sous in December 1336.[74] The annuity granted in March 1335 was paid in full by August; 2,000 sous more were paid (on the enlarged annuity) in December 1336.[75] But such behaviour was most unusual, for the royal treasury was still stretched beyond its limits.[76] Pere, like his father and grandfather, was usually in arrears to his physicians, and he sometimes tried to reassure them that their fees would be paid if they came to attend him; indeed, it has been shown that the Aragonese monarchs routinely put off paying their medical personnel through at least the end of the fifteenth century.[77]

In order to assess the meaning of Arnau's new stipend intelligently, it is necessary to step back and consider the reputed wealth of the medieval medical practitioner, a subject that has long excited comment. Chaucer is

---

[68] 'Mestre Arnau de Riera metge de ffisicha e de cirurgia' was paid 95 sous of Barcelona on an order of 1 July 1335 'per algunes coses medicinals que compra per fer anguens et empastres obs de la persona del dit SR'. ACA, Real Patrimonio 307, fol. 52v.

[69] ACA 858, fol. 142v (15 kls. July 1336). Whereas the original annuity from Alfons IV was merely 'for past services', the additional 3,000 sous was identified specifically as for Arnau's provisio and quitacio as part of Pere IV's household (domesticus).

[70] ACA 858, fols. 220v–221 (6 kls. Sept. 1336).

[71] ACA, Real Patrimonio 322, fols. 118v–119.

[72] Arnau's widow Caterina gave the Jews a quittance for the sum on kls. Dec. 1349 (AHPG, Notari-Girona 3, reg. 1). To the documents cited in McVaugh and García-Ballester, 'The medical faculty', as providing a basis for following Arnau's career can now be added ACA 632, fol. 109v; 1295, fol. 76; 1296, fols. 22v–23; 1297, fols. 158 and 179; 1300, fol. 19v; 1301, fol. 127r–v; 1304, fol. 48; 1306, fol. 131; ACA, Real Patrimonio 778, fol. 41.

[73] Dufourcq, 'Lex prix', p. 477, suggests that between 1285 and 1330 the Barcelonan sou lost about one-third of its value against the gold dinar.

[74] ACA, Real Patrimonio 309, fol. 129.

[75] ACA, Real Patrimonio 307, fol. 38v, and 309, fol. 117v.

[76] Dufourcq and Gautier-Dalché, Historia económica y social, pp. 232–35.

[77] Comenge, 'Formas de munificencia', pp. 8–10.

only the most famous contemporary critic of the physician's avarice, and modern historians, acknowledging that Chaucer's physician is not a universally valid type, still tend to stress the rewards of practice.[78] Often the practitioner's wealth is attributed to his grasping habits and his exorbitant fees; Henri de Mondeville is often quoted in this connection, too, for his candour offers critics a cutting weapon:

The surgeon should pretend that he has no living nor capital except his profession, and that everything is as dear as possible, especially drugs and ointment; that the fee is as nothing as compared with his services; and the wages of all other artisans, masons for example, have doubled of late.[79]

We must grant, certainly, that, as their wills show, surgeons like Berenguer ça Riera and Ramon de Cornellà were financially well off, even if the specific sums mentioned tell us little about the surgeons' standing relative to the merchants and lawyers of Gerona.[80] What is harder to believe is that their wealth was founded on haggling over broken legs at fees of 200 *sous* per case, that such methods – even if Mondeville does not overstate them – really represent the way in which the most successful physicians and surgeons acquired their wealth, when much larger sums might be forthcoming in annuities.

What seems to me an important difference between a fee for a particular service and an annuity has never been stressed by historians who discuss practitioners' income – such discussions tend merely to list the different forms that income took. I believe that these two types of reward express fundamentally different perceptions by the client of the value of medical care. A patient who calls on a surgeon for treatment of a particular problem will haggle over price because the operation is in effect a market commodity – he may be able to get it elsewhere more cheaply, no worse performed. He does not expect a recurrent need for this particular surgeon's services; 'his chief object', as Mondeville sourly explained, 'and the one idea which dominates all his actions, is to get cured, and [therefore]

[78] Chaucer's example has helped draw particular historical attention to the English scene: see E. A. Hammond, 'Incomes of medieval English doctors', *Journal of the History of Medicine*, 15 (1960), 154–69; and Carole Rawcliffe, 'The profits of practice: the wealth and status of medical men in later medieval England', *Social History of Medicine*, 1 (1988), 61–78.

[79] Cited by E. A. Hammond, 'Incomes', p. 156.

[80] The Geronan merchant Pere Vilar, who died *c.* 1333, was owed slightly over 10,000 *sous* by his customers at his death; he must still have been placed modestly within the city's merchant community, for his contemporary, Bononat Bordils, was able to invest 2,500 *sous* in cash plus nearly 24,000 *sous* more in credit in a single commercial enterprise in 1326: Christian Guilleré, *Diner, poder i societat a la Girona del segle XIV* (Gerona, 1984), pp. 35–6. These data may be compared with the sums mentioned in Berenguer ça Riera's will: he left the unspecified bulk of his estate to his son and namesake, but left 5,500 *sous* to his daughter Guilelma and 2,500 *sous* each to his two other sons. He made further scattered bequests totalling 2,000 *sous*, but he commanded prudently that these last should be paid 'de peccunia quam dominus rex mihi debet et de assignationibus quas inde mihi fecit' (ADG, Pia Almoina 7691). These minor legatees probably had to wait a long time before they could collect their inheritance.

once he is cured he forgets his own obligations and omits to pay'.[81] An annuity, on the other hand, expresses broad confidence in a particular practitioner's skills; the grantor wants to ensue the recipient's continuing concern and good will. From a surgeon's point of view, an annuity must usually have seemed more desirable: it promised him an income on which it was in his client's interest not to default (for fear of losing his services), and it did not necessarily impose arduous conditions. But it also gave him an incentive to keep his client healthy, lest in a crisis he lose his reputation or, at his patient's death, his salary; Mondeville acknowledges as much in a passage that is not usually given its full weight.[82] Seen in this light, the steadily increasing royal annuities being given to the ça Rieras should probably be understood as in the surgeons' interest, of course, but also as an expression of royal confidence in them and in the approach to surgery that they had come to espouse. When Pere IV granted Arnau 600 sous in April 1347 to buy a 'book on medicine',[83] just as his grandfather had bought an Avicenna for Arnau's father, he was reaffirming their common belief in the value of a fusion of medical learning with surgical technique. In turn, Arnau's decision to acquire formal training in that learned tradition reflects a surgeon's response to the new valuation of academic medicine, his willing acquiescence in it.

v

There is inevitably the danger that we are treating Arnau as representative when he was actually atypical – after all, his Leridan license is unique. On the other hand, there are other indications that the ties between surgery and a more particularly medical learning were strengthening in the first half of the fourteenth century. One is the surprising fact that surgery had been introduced into the Leridan studium by 1330. When the school was founded in 1300, it had one – purely medical – master, Guillem de Béziers; ten years

---

[81] Quoted by Hammond, 'Incomes', p. 159, who misidentifies the source; it is taken from Nicaise, p. 111.

[82] Mondeville distinguishes four types of clients by the fees that can be expected from them, of whom the last 'is a class who pay in full, and in advance, and they should be prevented from getting ill at all, because we are paid a salary to keep them in health'. Quoted from Hammond, 'Incomes', p. 155; not taken from p. 91 of Nicaise, as he says, but p. 110. This passage is often selected to illustrate Mondeville's concern with fees, but it should be remembered that it is actually part of a larger section acknowledging that preventive care is the best form of medicine.

Elsewhere (p. 159) Hammond states that 'Mondeville's experience had led him to the conclusion that it was more satisfactory for a physician to be paid an outright fee for his services than to contract for an annuity.' He does not identify his source for this statement, however, and so far I have not been able to find any such passage in the Surgery. Rawcliffe ('Profits', p. 65) argues the same for England in the late fourteenth and fifteenth centuries. The problems that she suggests were associated with such contractual agreements were not, I believe, shared by the looser annuities granted by the Aragonese monarchs.

[83] ACA 1311, fol. 56 (prid. kls. Apr. 1347); published by J. M. Madurell i Marimon, 'Documents culturals medievals (1307–1485)', Bol. R. Acad. B. Letras, 38 (1979–82), 309.

later there was still a place for only one, medical, master. In 1302 the Valencian surgeon Guillem Correger had had to travel abroad in order to study (*audire*) surgery because there was no school where it was taught in the Crown of Aragon.[84] A quarter of a century later, however, at the end of the 1320s, the Leridan *studium* had a master lecturing on surgery (for 400 *sous* yearly) in addition to its medical masters.[85]

Moreover, Arnau was not the only surgeon's son in the early fourteenth century who tried to broaden the traditional family base – Guillem Correger's son, Pere, is another. Guillem had practised surgery in Valencia for at least fifteen years before deciding to leave the kingdom to pursue his subject in books;[86] six years after his departure, in 1308, he displayed his new commitment to a learned surgery by preparing a Catalan translation of Teodorico's *Surgery*[87] – a work marked precisely by its insistence that the best surgical practice is one firmly embedded in Galenic medical doctrine.[88] The Pere Correger whom we find practising in Valencia from 1313 to 1347, evidently Guillem's son, was identified as *cirurgicus* when he was paid 300 *sous*, in 1323, for caring for the infante Alfons after he fell while hunting boar.[89] Yet a decade later he turns up as *fissich* to an ailing patient, and in the same year his former patient Alfons (now king) alludes to him as 'phisicus et cirurgicus noster'.[90] In that same decade of the 1330s, the city of Valencia established a two-man tribunal to examine the qualifications of anyone wishing to practise medicine or surgery there, making sure that

84 'Fidelibus suis universis officialibus et subtitis ad quos presentes pervenerint etc. Cum G. Corrigiarii civis Valencie presencium exhibitor exeat terram nostram ad partes alias accessurus pro audienda arte cirurgie cum de arte ipsa in terra nostra non legatur ad presens, ideo vobis et cuilibet vestrum dicimus et mandamus quatenus dicto G. Corrigiarii familia equitaturis vel rebus suis nullum in exeundo terram nostram ex dicta causa impedimentum vel contrarium faciatis nec ab aliis fieri permitatis. Datum Gerunde idus Oct. [1302].' ACA 125, fol. 96v.

85 McVaugh and García-Ballester, 'Medical faculty'. The stipend of the medical master was 600 *sous*. The Leridan currency was the Aragonese money of Jaca, which exchanged about 6:11 with the less valuable money of Barcelona.

86 In 1288 Guillem was granted 300 *sous* for expenses and another 300 *sous* as a fee for having travelled from Valencia to Zaragoza to treat Alfons III's brother Pere; ACA 79, fol. 40 (2 non. May 1288).

87 The language of Guillem's introduction to his translation is significant: 'En nom de la senta e non depertable Trinitat ... comens jo G. Correger, de Mayorcha, aprenant en la art de cirurgia, a translatar de latí en romans catalanesch aquesta obra de cirurgia ... Per asso jo veent que alcuna partida de los surgians qui son en la seyoria del noble en Jacme per la gracia de Deu rey dArago no entenen los vocables latins, cor tots los homens daquestes nostres encontrades obren mes per pratica que per teorica ... ': Alfred Morel-Fatio, *Catalogue des manuscrits espagnols et des manuscrits portugais* (of the Bibliothèque Nationale) (Paris, 1892), p. 33, quoting from MS 94.

88 On this characterization of Teodorico, see Chiara Crisciani, 'History, novelty, and progress in scholastic medicine', *Osiris*, 2nd series, 6 (1990), 118–39 at 133.

89 'Pro salario cure quam nobis fecit de casu quem fecimus in venacione porci.' ACA 387, fols. 197, 198 (18 kls. Feb. 1332/3).

90 Pere Correger is owed 40 *sous* for the 'cura de la malaltia del dit defunt de la quel morii': AMV, Justica de 300 sueldos, 4, fol. [34]v. Alfons so describes him in ACA 456, fol. 6v (17 kls. Feb. 1332/3).

applicants had a training equivalent to four years' study in a medical faculty; Pere Correger was named to the panel three times between 1336 and 1342.[91] Here, apparently, we have another case of a surgical family coming to acknowledge the importance of learning and of medicine over and beyond surgery.

Yet another parallel instance seems to be provided by the two Jacmes d'Avinyó, father and son, though they are not always easy to distinguish in the documentary record. The father was practising surgery in Valencia by 1295,[92] and his successes soon came to the attention of the royal family. He was summoned to Teruel to treat Jaume II in 1310 and again to Burriana in 1312,[93] and in 1323 he joined Pere Correger on the case of the infante Alfons.[94] He was still alive in 1324.[95] The son was of age to act as legal witness in 1309,[96] and by 1317 he was identified as *phisicus*. He and his father had not gone separate ways in practice, however, for only a few years later we find them associated in a case: 'en Jacme d'Avinyo cirurgia i en Jacme d'Avinyo fill d'en Jacme d'Avinyo fizich' testified before the court in 1321 that the apothecary Llorenç Limosi had never been paid for 'sugar, syrups, unguents, clysters, electuaries, and other medicinal items' supplied to their patient.[97] It is difficult, therefore, to believe that surgery and medicine were really differentiated by these two practitioners, all the more since in 1333 Jacme d'Avinyó – 'cirurgicus', but by now evidently the son – was recorded as having treated a patient with a wound[98] and then in 1338 and 1341 sat on the municipal tribunal for would-be medical practitioners.[99] The two generations of d'Avinyós seem to have followed the same path as the Corregers towards a broader professional expertise, though perhaps a little less quickly. The facts are susceptible of many explanations, of course, but it may be significant that when in 1323 he and Pere Correger both cared for the infante Alfons after his fall, Jaume d'Avinyó senior – the older practitioner, with many more years of practical surgical experience – received only two-thirds the fee of Pere, the young

[91] In 1336, 1339 and 1342; Luís García-Ballester, Michael R. McVaugh, and Agustín Rubio-Vela, *Medical licensing and learning in fourteenth-century Valencia*, Transactions of the American Philosophical Society, 79 (1989), part 6, Appendix 1.

[92] ARV, protocols 2631, where he appears as witness to a document of 12 kls. Aug. 1295.

[93] ACA 297, fols. 242v–243r; 298, fols. 99–100.

[94] ACA 386, fol. 198; Jacme's fee was 200 *sous* of Barcelona (18 Feb. 1322/3).

[95] Called Jacme d'Avinyó 'major de dies', he is named as a municipal councillor on 3 non. June 1324 (Archivo Municipal de Valencia, Manuals de Consell, A–1, fol. 219).

[96] ARV, Justícia de Valencia, 11, fol. 18. They are identified as 'en Jacme davinyo cirurgia i en Jacme davinyo fill seu' (6 id. Apr. 1309).

[97] ARV, Justícia de Valencia, 37, s. fol., entry of id. Feb. 1320/1; their testimony is given 6 non. May 1321.

[98] ARV, Justícia de 300 sueldos, 4, fol. [21] (8 kls. May 1333).

[99] 'Jaime Aviñón, médico de Montpellier', purchased a house in Valencia in 1352 (Elias Olmos y Canalda, *Pergaminos de la catedral de Valencia* (Valencia, 1961), p. 290, doc. 2478) – it is tempting to anticipate future historical research and imagine that Jacme *fils* was now completing his formation as physician in an academic environment.

heir to a more intellectual approach to their common craft. Learning may here have earned a tangible reward.

The growing importance to surgeons of a specifically medical learning in the generation between Berenguer and Arnau can be further corroborated from the history of a private library. In June 1319 the king (Jaume II) wrote to the infante Jaume to ask him for the 'surgical books and tools' of master Roger, who had died the year before. Roger had treated Queen Blanca, and in 1312 he had been promised 2,000 sous by Jaume for his services to her[100] (they were still unpaid in 1316[101]); by 1315 he had become rector of Vallbona and chaplain (as well as occasional surgeon) to the infante and his household, only to die in 1318.[102] As King Jaume now explained to his son, he wanted to pass on Roger's books and equipment to his own surgeon, Bernat Serra.[103]

In so far as we can reconstruct it, Bernat's professional relationship to the court was not unlike Berenguer's.[104] His surgical career can be traced back to 1309,[105] but he seems first to have attended the king in 1317, when a series of grants from the monarch began that continued until Jaume's death ten years later: the grant of 1,000 sous to buy a home in Valencia;[106] grants of grain and wood and permission to export them;[107] a present of 4,000 sous towards his marriage, in 1324;[108] gifts of items confiscated from the Templars in Tortosa;[109] income from Sasser, in Sardinia;[110] and regular

[100] ACA 298, fol. 112v (8 kls. July 1312).
[101] ACA 277, fol. 140v (4 non. May 1316).
[102] Roger's name suggests that he may have been English, as his nephew and heir Nicholas certainly was: ACA 359, fol. 24 (2 id. Apr. 1319). In that case, he is perhaps to be identified with the *fisicus* Rotxerus Anglicus who in 1299 in Barcelona was hired to treat Rodericus Petri, a soldier of Casseda 'qui loqui non potest' – the complaint might very well have been committed to a surgeon's expertise: Archivo Histórico de Proto-colos de Barcelona, sección histórica (hereafter AHPB); Manual de Pedro Portell, fol. 30v (17 kls. Nov. 1299). The infante sent at least two members of his company to Vallbona for treatment: ACA 353, fol. 82 (4 id. July 1315); ACA 362, fol. 40 (3 non. July 1316). Roger was alive in April 1318 (ACA 357, fol. 62) but dead by July (ACA 357, fol. 172).
[103] J. Ernesto Martínez Ferrando, *Jaime II de Aragón: su vida familiar* (Barcelona, 1948), vol. II, p. 205 (doc. 283; 2 kls. July 1319).
[104] The fullest account to date of Bernat's life is that of Ricard Carreras Valls, 'Introducció a la història de la cirurgia a Catalunya: Bernat Serra i altres cirurgians Catalans Il.lustres del segle XIV', in Societat de Cirurgia de Catalunya, *Tres Treballs Premiats en el Concurs d'Homenatge a Gimbernat* (Perpignan, 1936), pp. 1–63, which nevertheless treats only a portion of the documentation in the ACA concerning Bernard's career.
[105] ACB, Manual de Bernat de Vilarrúbia, 8/1308–4/1309, fol. 161 (4 id. Jan. 1308/9), where Bernat Serra figures as a witness. Bernat was born in Santa Cecília de Voltregá, north of Vic (Vic, Arxiu de la Curia Fumada, manual 74 [7 id. July 1319]).
[106] ACA 259, fol. 42v (5 id. Nov. 1317). Of this sum, 471 *sous* were still unpaid in January 1320 (ACA, Real Patrimonio 284, fol. 36).
[107] ACA 216, fol. 79 (6 kls. Sept. 1318); 218, fols. 45, 100 (2 kls. June, 10 kls. Sept. 1320); 423, fol. 21v (13 kls. July 1320).
[108] ACA 302, fol. 114v (3 id. Jan. 1323/4).
[109] ACA 283, fols. 171–3 (8 id. Mar. 1321/2).
[110] Carreras Valls, 'Introducció', p. 13.

payments for clothing for himself and his wife.[111] Payment on the promises was naturally always in arrears – in early 1327 Bernat agreed to settle one debt of seven years' duration by accepting a Saracen woman instead[112] – and it is hard not to be surprised that Bernat was willing to loan the king 10,000 sous towards the conquest of Sardinia in 1323.[113] Alfons IV, in his turn, continued to show favour to Bernat, in 1328 granting him 600 sous yearly on the income of Molins de Rei once the previous grantee's rights had expired.[114] Bernat's income from the mills should have begun in June 1331 but had not been paid by the following March,[115] and the annuity had eventually to be drawn from another source.[116] King Alfons was still heavily in debt to his surgeon in March 1334,[117] and it was perhaps in compensation that by 1333 he had appointed him bailiff of Camprodon.[118]

Bernat died thirty months after his royal master, in June 1338, and fortuitously the inventory of his estate has survived.[119] It includes a long and detailed list of surgical tools and also enumerates more than thirty technical books found in an iron chest by the executors. Some or all of these books and instruments may once have belonged to master Roger in the teens; it is impossible to tell whether Bernat coveted Roger's library and persuaded the king to get it for him or built the collection up in other ways. The books included a remarkably comprehensive collection of the current technical surgical literature – Teodorico Borgognoni, the 'Four Masters', Rolandino, Roger Frugard, Bruno Longoburgo, Lanfranco, Albucasis, Rhazes – but they include a striking range of more directly medical texts as well: Macer's herbal, Trotula, Galen's *Megategni*, Rhazes' *Almansor*, the *Viaticum*, the *Compendium Salerni*, the *Aggregator*, Hippocrates' *Aphorisms*, Iesu Haly *De oculis*. Some of these have more apparent relevance to surgery than others, but as a whole they provide a solid introduction to medical science, to physiology, pathology and therapeutics. Wherever Bernat got them, the works he owned vividly illustrate the increasing availability of books as well as the increasing authority of medical learning for surgeons in the early fourteenth century.

[111] ACA 303, fol. 43 (id. Dec. 1325); ACA, Real Patrimonio 293, fol. 88 (id. Dec. 1325); Real Patrimonio 294, fol. 58 (Sept. 1326).

[112] ACA 286, fol. 97v (9 kls. Mar. 1326/7).

[113] ACA 302, fol. 88 (11 kls. Oct. 1323); the repayment schedule is discussed in ACA 302, fols. 131v–132r (kls. Apr. 1324).

[114] ACA, CRD, Alfons IV 465; ACA 476, fols. 255r–v, 263v (4 kls. July 1328).

[115] ACA 497, fol. 98r–v (prid. id. June 1331); 498, fols. 281v–282r (7 kls. Mar. 1331/2).

[116] ACA 495, fol. 70r–v (kls. May 1330); 443, fol. 63r–v (4 id. May 1331); 468, fol. 212 (7 kls. Sept. 1335).

[117] Carreras Valls, 'Introducció', p. 13, identifying one debt of 4,000 sous.

[118] ACA 507, fol. 182v (8 kls. May 1333); Bernat exercised the office through a substitute.

[119] Attention was first drawn to the inventory by Carreras Valls, 'Introducció', who transcribed and translated into Catalan those portions of the inventory that described Bernat's books and tools; his transcription is sometimes inaccurate, since a number of the book titles were unfamiliar to him. The inventory itself is in AHPB, Manual de Pere Folqueres for May–Sept. 1338.

VI

What do these admittedly scattered pieces of evidence have to suggest about the answer to my opening question? We have found that a number of Catalan surgeons at the turn of the fourteenth century had come to share the conviction of the Italian surgical writers that their subject should be studied as a learned subject like medicine. Furthermore, in some respects their practice merged into areas nominally the province of physicians. A surgeon like Berenguer ça Riera was in contact with academic medical masters, read texts embodying learned medicine, and knew and applied its theory. As Henri de Mondeville seemed to suggest, there was not necessarily a sharp cleavage, intellectual or social, between physicians and surgeons in 1300.

Our evidence also strongly suggests that some in the next generation of Catalan surgeons – the generation of Arnau ça Riera and Pere Correger – tried to take advantage of this overlap between medicine and surgery in their pedagogical and practical aspects, so as to claim outright the status of a physician as well as that of a surgeon.[120] We are fortunate to be able to establish that surgeons might go so far as to get formal training and certification as academically qualified physicians; others presumably merely asserted their claim to the title on a basis ranging from study and apprenticeship down to the mere possession of medical texts.

We must not think that every surgeon reacted in this way to the increasing prestige of medicine and tried to remake himself professionally: indeed, Arnau ça Riera's younger brother, Bernat, chose instead to continue in the family occupation.[121] Bernat ça Riera appears to us first in February 1336, as surgeon to the new king Pere IV.[122] He served on the king's campaign in Majorca in 1343, and bought ointments and other medicines to use on Pere's reduction of Roussillon the next year.[123] Bernat continued to hold his post into the 1350s, surviving the plague (and hence outliving his brother); he died in 1371. Like Arnau, Bernat was given an annuity on the Gerona *aljama* by Pere IV, but one worth only 2,000 *sous*, half his

---

[120] Other examples might be added to those we have studied above – for example, that of Ramon de Pulchro Die of Alzira, licensed to practise surgery, to whom in 1347 Pere IV allowed a limited medical practice as well, despite his never having been examined in the latter subject (ACA 882, fols. 144v–145). A particularly vivid instance of a continuing quest for status is that of Domènech de Tolosa of Valencia, who called himself *barberius* in 1308 (ACA, Cancillería, pergaminos Jaime II, 2519) but *sirurgicus* in 1326 (ARV, Justícia Civil 19, fol. 37) and by the time of his will of May 1334 had become 'magister Dominicus de Tolosa fisicus' (ARV, protocolos 4313, cover).

[121] Arnau's seniority is implicit in the wording of their father's will (above, note 62). The family relationship between the physician Arnau and the surgeon Bernat is made explicit in ACA 1306, fol. 131.

[122] ACA 1301, fol. 128, a letter of 3 kls. Aug. 1340 embodying bills for service of 12 Feb. and 31 Aug. 1336 and 7 Jan. 1337.

[123] ACA, Real Patrimonio 320, fol. 154v; Real Patrimonio 322, fol. 112v.

brother's stipend.[124] Bernat's professional goals were evidently traditional ones, distinct from and perhaps less ambitious than Arnau's – and they seem to have been financially less rewarding. The stability inherent in a family surgical tradition that is evident in Bernat's career thus throws into still sharper relief the move into medicine that his brother and others decided to make.[125]

Why was there this movement – a movement evidently all in one direction, since my survey has turned up no cases of Catalan physician families moving to add surgery to their repertoire? Sheer intellectual conviction that, as Henri de Mondeville argued, no surgeon can be competent unless he knows medicine, may have played a part. The rising social prestige of *scientia*, of medical learning based on natural philosophy, is a still more plausible motive – but in that case, why did such prestige, within what must have been a relatively restricted circle of patients prepared to appreciate the academic tradition, seem valuable to surgeons? To whom was the additional label of *phisicus* designed to appeal?

Here the evidence is still less conclusive. I would suggest, however, that the interest of the Aragonese royal family may have played a decisive role in influencing certain surgeons – talented, literate, and ambitious – to broaden their assertions of expertise. There is ample evidence that Jaume II and his descendants were ardent proponents of learned or academic medicine: they supported the translation of medical works and commissioned treatises on scholastic medical theory; they appointed academic masters to treat their ills and deliver their wives of their children; they created a national university and supported the claim that academic credentials should be the minimal qualification for medical practice; and they imported the most famous university masters to attend them *in extremis*, rewarding them hugely.[126]

Pere's IV's priorities are particularly clear. In the very year that Arnau ça Riera took his degree at Lerida – 1344 – King Pere drew up *ordinacions*

---

[124] ACA 864, fol. 128 (15 kls. Nov. 1338); Bernat's stipend was unchanged fourteen years later (AHPG, Notari-Girona 6, reg. 46).

[125] Perhaps I should recognize that of the twenty-five archival references to Bernat I have discovered, one (ACA 1306, fol. 208v) does speak of him as 'cirurgicus et fisicus' and another (ACA 1304, fol. 48) refers to him and his brother as 'fisicis nostris magistris Arnaldo de Riaria et Bernardo de Riaria'; with these exceptions, however, he is always identified simply as 'cirurgicus'.

[126] Evidence for all but the last of these statements has already been provided above. Towards the end of Alfons IV's illness, master Jordan of Turre was brought in from Montpellier for consultation and was given, over and beyond his expenses, the very considerable sum of 100 gold florins. Jordan's fee of 100 florins is revealed in ACA 503, fols. 177–8 (7 id. Dec. 1335). His expenses were paid in four instalments and totalled 894 *sous*; they are recorded in ACA, Real Patrimonio 307, fols. 45v, 48v, 57v, 58. On Jordan and his attendance on the Aragonese royal family see further Michael R. McVaugh, 'The two faces of a medical career: Jordanus de Turre of Montpellier', in Edward Grant and John E. Murdoch, eds., *Mathematics and its applications to science and natural philosophy in the Middle Ages* (Cambridge, 1987), pp. 301–24, esp. pp. 302, 312.

describing the duties and privileges of officials at his court. Under the rubric 'on medical practitioners', he laid down that

there shall ordinarily be present in the court two practitioners [*metges*] learned and experienced in medicine or physic who will carefully look after the preservation of our health, and will ensure that we do those things that will keep us healthy while avoiding those that will be harmful; they will inspect our urine every morning so as to be aware of the state of our health, and if they detect any worsening they will immediately prescribe a satisfactory remedy. Moreover, if we come to suffer from any bodily ailment they will treat it diligently.

After explaining that these physicians were to treat members of the royal family and household 'in accordance with their understanding of the art', Pere ordained that,

if only one of our physicians should be *maestre en medicina*, he should be given precedence over the other; if both are, or if they are of equal status in some other respect, the precedence should fall to him who has been longer in our service.[127]

The *ordinacions* went on to consider much more briefly the duties of the royal surgeons ('meges de cirurgia'); while two of them are to be present at court in case of need, they have little or no role to play in the routine maintenance of health. Their expertise is useful primarily in treating accidents or in time of war.[128]

King Pere here made explicit the hierarchy that had evidently been developing at court since his grandfather's reign: it is physicians rather than surgeons whose art is now publicly acknowledged as more valuable to ordinary life, and the academically trained physician is most prized of all. Arnau ça Riera's new degree was thus of particular advantage to him as physician to Pere IV – he might even have chosen to incept at this moment with the forthcoming *ordinacions* in mind. It is not implausible, therefore, that other surgeons who were aware of the king's priorities and who hoped to gain increased favour and patronage from the royal family should have taken advantage of the undefined boundary between their field and medi-

---

[127] 'E donchs ordonam que en la cort nostra ordinariament sien dos metges instruyts e provats en medecina o phisica qui diligentment insisten per la conservacio de la nostra salut e a nos parlen e diguen sens dubte que preceesquam e usem daquelles coses que seran a nostra salut profitoses et encara aquelles que nocives seran esquivem: e cascun dia de mati la urina nostra esguarden per tal que la disposicio de nostre cors regonegen e si hauran vist en nostre cors alcun piyorament decontinent curen de remey salutari proveyr: e encara si per alcuna corporal necessitat o per qualque altre infirmitat lo cors nostre agreviat esser veuran de la nostra curacio ab no enujada e curosa diligencia curar facen ... En apres si dels metges nostres la un tan solament sera maestre en medecina aquell en prerogativa donor al altre sera davant anant: si empero amdos maestros o en altra manera de par condicio seran lavors aquell deura esser en la honor pus poderos qui primerament al nostre servey sera appellat.' 'Ordenacions fetes per lo molt alt senyor en Pere terç rey Darago sobra lo regiment de tots los officials de la sua cort', *Procesos de los antiguos cortes* ...; Próspero de Bofarull y Mascaró (ed.), *Colección de documentos inéditos del archivo general de la corona de Aragón*, vol. v (Barcelona, 1850), pp. 76–7.

[128] Ibid., p. 78.

cine so as to lay claim to a still higher status, and thereby to expect higher fees than their less broadly competent colleagues could hope for or demand – a not inconsiderable advantage in a period when only a fraction of every fee was collectible.

Let us close by giving Henri de Mondeville a chance at the last word, for his gloomy assessment in 1306 of the support for learned surgery might seem to cast doubt on this suggestion:

> It is the habit of all princes, prelates, and ordinary people these days in all the western lands – it may not be so in hotter regions – not to trust any medically learned surgeon [*medico cyrurgico scientifico*] very far, for they say that a surgeon ought not to be a cleric because, while a cleric is in the schools, the layman is learning the technique of manual operation.[129]

'All princes' and 'all the western lands'? Henri's pessimistic generalizations, if they were well founded, would force us to wonder whether surgery in the Crown of Aragon could be an exception. On the other hand, it is not altogether easy to take this complaint seriously from someone who boasts (at the beginning of Book III of the *Surgery*) that he is surgeon to King Philip IV of France and subsequently reveals that the king's brother (Charles of Valois) has been his patron and has endorsed his approach to wound treatment without suppuration.[130] Perhaps Henri's career is better testimony than his treatise; perhaps in France, as in Catalonia, the fusion of medical learning with surgery was lending a formerly empirical craft a new social prestige.

---

[129] 'Nunc est consuetudo omnium principum, praelatorum et vulgarium in omnibus regionibus occidentis, et forte in calidis regionibus non sit ita, quod de nullo medico cyrurgico scientifico confidunt nisi parum, dicentes quod cyrurgicus non debet esse clericus, quia interim quod clericus intrat scolas, laicus addiscit modum manualiter operandi.' Pagel, 40 (1890), 664; Nicaise, p. 102. I have slightly altered Pagel's punctuation.

[130] Pagel, 41 (1891), 935; 40 (1890), 721; Nicaise, pp. 492, 188.

8

Facing the Black Death: perceptions and reactions of university medical practitioners

JON ARRIZABALAGA

INTRODUCTION

Between late 1347 and early 1348 a great disaster, which is nowadays known as the Black Death, began to spread all over Europe. By 1351 this terrifying plague, which plunged people into panic and distress, had killed 25–50 per cent of Europe's inhabitants.

Much historical work has been done which stresses the importance of the effects of the Black Death of 1348 in many areas – demographic, economic, political and cultural – and its central role in the so-called 'European crisis of the fourteenth century'.[1] This global crisis has been seen as the first major step in the transition from feudalism to capitalism. Of course, historians have often exaggerated the impact of the Black Death on Europe through the late Middle Ages, even going so far as considering this disease as the turning point between the medieval and the modern world.[2] Despite such exaggerations, it continues to be unquestionable that, while it was not unique, the Black Death was nevertheless a first-order historical event in late medieval Europe.[3]

Historians have paid much more attention to the attitudes of European

---

[1] For an overall view of and bibliography on this topic, see P. Ziegler, *The Black Death*, (London, 1969; repr. 1982); R. S. Gottfried, *The Black Death. Natural and human disaster in medieval Europe* (London, 1983). Very useful is the long bibliographical chapter provided by J.-N. Biraben, *Les hommes et la peste en France et dans les pays européens et méditerranées*, 2 vols. (Paris and The Hague, 1975–6), vol. II, pp. 186–413.

[2] A good example of this historiographical trend is shown by Gottfried, *Black Death*.

[3] If we just take present-day historians' views on the demographic impact of the disease as an impressionistic example of the overall consequences of this disaster, we can see that the plague pandemic of 1347–50 is currently assumed to have been one of the significant causes (along with subsequent epidemic crises, famines, wars, natural catastrophes and periods of shortage) for the demographical losses throughout Europe during the fourteenth and fifteenth centuries. For the case of Italy, see L. del Panta, *Le epidemie nella storia demografica italiana (secoli XIV–XIX)* (Turin, 1980). On the many uncertainties concerning the impact of the Black Death in late medieval Europe, see D. Williman (ed.), *The Black Death: the impact of the fourteenth-century plague* (Binghamton, NY, 1982), particularly the contributions by Nancy Siraisi (pp. 9–22), and J. M. W. Bean (pp. 23–38).

civic communities towards the Black Death than to the attitudes towards it held by university medical practitioners. Such practitioners were by no means the only healers involved in the battle against the plague; in fact, this battle was waged by *all* the people concerned with health activities: both by those educated in the universities, and by those trained in the 'open' system: ordinary men and women, Jews, Muslims and Christians – and by many who would be classified today as 'quacks'. Yet the record of the participation of university physicians in fighting the plague has been preserved through the works they wrote on the subject. Moreover, these works have the additional interest of reflecting the earliest medical attitudes towards a new disaster which was not to abandon Western Europe until the eighteenth century.[4]

The purpose of this chapter is precisely to explore the earliest perceptions of and reactions to the Black Death during the years 1348 and 1349 among those medical practitioners who lived and worked around the Latin Mediterranean. I mean by this the cultural area of Italy, Provence, Languedoc, the Kingdom of France, and the Crown of Aragon. I shall assume that those practitioners' perceptions and reactions constitute a historical reality in themselves, and therefore have a meaning which can *only* be explained by a non-presentist historical approach. This assumption has for me the following two implications:

First, that it is important to isolate these earliest perceptions and reactions to the Black Death from perceptions and reactions to subsequent plagues, since they represent the *first* responses given by university medical practitioners to this great social disaster, and consequently the first attempts in late medieval Europe to construct it as a disease-entity. The difference between first and later perceptions is clearly seen, for instance by comparing the scanty clinical data given by the medical practitioners who wrote on the Black Death in 1348–9 with the extensive and systematic clinical account of it that Guy de Chauliac, who himself also witnessed it, produced in 1361. This contrast is difficult to explain unless we link Chauliac's account with the wider intellectual perspective and calmness that he was

---

[4] For the attitude of university medical practitioners when faced with the Black Death, see A. M. Campbell, *The Black Death and men of learning* (New York, 1931); D. Palazzotto, 'The Black Death and medicine: a report and analysis of the tractates written between 1348 and 1350', Ph.D. diss. (University of Kansas, 1973); Ziegler, *Black Death*, pp. 63–84; Gottfried, *Black Death*, pp. 104–28. A large number of contemporary medical works on the Black Death and on the subsequent epidemics were discovered and edited during the late nineteenth and early twentieth centuries. Among others see L.-A. J. Michon, *Documents inédits sur la grande peste de 1348 (Consultation de la Faculté de Paris, Consultation d'un practicien de Montpellier, Description de Guillaume de Machaut)* (Paris, 1860); K. Sudhoff, 'Pestschriften aus den ersten 150 Jahren nach der Epidemie des "Schwartzen Todes", 1348', *Archiv für Geschichte der Medizin*, 4 (1910–11), 191–222, 234, 389–424; 5 (1911–12), 36–87, 332–96; 6 (1912–13), 313–79; 7 (1913–14), 57–114; 8 (1914–15), 175–215, 236–89; 9 (1915–16), 53–78, 117–67; 11 (1918–19), 44–92, 121–76; 14 (1922–3), 1–25, 79–105, 129–68; 16 (1924–5), 1–69, 77–188; 17 (1925), 12–139, 241–91; D. W. Singer, 'Some plague tractates (fourteenth and fifteenth centuries)', *Proceedings of the Royal Society of Medicine*, 9 (1915–16), 159–212.

able to acquire in the thirteen years or so which had elapsed between these two dates.[5]

Second, that in looking at the Black Death of 1348 I am deliberately renouncing any attempt at retrospective diagnosis by the criteria of what current Western medicine understands by plague today. For in exploring disease perceptions and reactions by past human societies, we must not forget that the identity of the disease nowadays known as plague, just like the identity of other infectious diseases, relies on an intellectual construction we have inherited from a precise historical and cultural context – that of late nineteenth- and early twentieth-century laboratory medicine and, specifically, from the germ theory. It would therefore be wrong to assume that when we talk about late medieval and early modern plague, we are dealing with the same disease that we recognize as plague today. It is very important to take this into account since, as Andrew Cunningham has pointed out,

the dominance of the laboratory concept of disease has had a significant effect on our understanding of many *pre*-laboratory diseases – leading us to read them as if they were laboratory diseases; hence the coming of the laboratory has led to the *past* of medicine being rewritten to accord with the laboratory model of disease, and it has thereby been misunderstood.[6]

These are the main medical sources used in this paper, listed in chronological order:

Jacme d'Agramont, *Regiment de preservació de pestilència* (Lerida, 24 April 1348).[7]

Gentile da Foligno, *Consilium contra pestilentiam* (Perugia, before 18 June 1348).[8]

---

[5] For Chauliac's account, see Guy de Chauliac, *Chirurgia magna*, tract. II, doct. II, cap. V, *Digressio de mortalitate* (Lyons, 1585; facs. repr. Darmstadt, 1976), pp. 104–6.

[6] Andrew Cunningham, 'Transforming plague: the laboratory and the identity of infectious disease', in Andrew Cunningham and Perry Williams, eds., *The laboratory revolution in medicine* (Cambridge, 1992), pp. 209–44, see p. 209.

[7] For this study I have used a modern edition of the *Regiment*: J. Veny i Clar (ed.), '*Regiment de preservació de pestilència*' *de Jacme d'Agramont (s. XIV). Introducció, transcriptció i estudi lingüistic* (Tarragona, 1971), pp. 47–93 (hereafter, Agramont, *Regiment*). For the scanty available information on Jacme d'Agramont and the medical *studium* of Lerida in the first half of the fourteenth century, see ibid., pp. 21–32; M. R. McVaugh and L. García-Ballester, 'The medical faculty at early fourteenth-century Lérida', *History of Universities*, 8 (1989), 1–25. Agramont's work was commented on by C.-E. A. Winslow and M. L. Duran-Reynals, 'Jacme d'Agramont and the first of the plague tractates', *Bulletin of the History of Medicine*, 22 (1948), 747–65; it was translated into English by M. L. Duran-Reynals and C.-E. A. Winslow, 'Regiment de preservacio a epidimia o pestilencia e mortaldats …', *Bulletin of the History of Medicine*, 23 (1949), 57–89.

[8] For the editions of Gentile's *consilia* used in this study, see Gentile da Foligno, *Consilium contra pestilentiam* (Colle di Valdelsa, c. 1479) (the longest *consilium*: hereafter, Gentile, *Consilium*); Gentile da Foligno, *Consilia* (Pavia, c. 1488), signats. f8v–g2v. Also see Sudhoff, 'Pestschriften', 5 (1911–12), 83–7, 332–5. On Gentile da Foligno and his works see P. Lugano, 'Gentilis Fulginas Speculator e le sue ultime volontà', *Bollettino della Regia Deputazione di Storia Patria per l'Umbria*, 14 (1908), 195–260; G. Sarton, *Introduction to the history of science* (Baltimore, 1927–47), vol. III, part 1, pp. 848–52; L. Thorndike, 'Gentile da Foligno and fourteenth-century medicine', in *History of magic and experimental science* (New York, 1923–58), vol. III, pp. 233–52; Campbell, *Black Death*, pp. 9–13.

Giovanni della Penna, *Consilium in magna pestilentia* (Naples, 1348).[9]

Collegium Facultatis Medicorum Parisius, *Compendium de epidimia* (Paris, October 1348).[10]

Alfonso de Córdoba, *Epistola et regimen de pestilentia* (Montpellier, c. 1348–9).[11]

'Quidam practicus de Montepessulano', *Tractatus de epidemia* (Montpellier, 19 May 1349).[12]

All these works were written at the same critical moment, although they pursued different aims. The *Regiment de preservació de pestilència* of the Catalan physician Jacme d'Agramont seems to have been the earliest medical work written in response to the Black Death of 1348. At the time when Agramont finished writing it, on the eve of the day of St Mark (24 April) 1348, he held a lectureship at the medical *studium* of Lerida in the Crown of Aragon. Apparently, he himself soon fell victim to the *pestilència* he had been writing about. His *Regiment* is just a preventive one, written in Catalan in the form of an *epístola*, addressed to the town councillors of Lerida on hearing the increasingly alarming news about the presence of a mortal epidemic in the regions near Lerida. As Agramont himself indicated, his *Regiment* was intended to help Leridan lay people, not to instruct physicians. This seems to explain why it was written in Catalan, and not in Latin like the other works studied here. It consists of an introduction and two major parts. In the first of these parts, which is quite short and contains two chapters, Agramont's intention seems to have been to supply his readers with rudimentary information about natural philosophy to enable them to understand the rest of the *Regiment*: since the *pestilència* was in the air, lay people had to learn about 'the properties of the air tempered in both its qualities and its substance' (chapter 1), and 'the forms of air change, alteration or distemperance' (chapter 2). The second part deals with the *pestilència*. It contains six major sections on (1) the nature and the name of *pestilència*; (2) the causes of the 'universal pestilence' (*pestilència universal*) deriving from both substantial and qualitative air change, and of the 'particular pestilence' (*pestilència particular*) at a city, a street and a house; (3)

---

[9] Sudhoff, 'Pestschriften', 5 (1911–12), 341–8; and 16 (1922–3), 162–7 (hereafter, Penna, *Consilium*). Only the first manuscript mentioned makes explicit Giovanni's disapproval; for Gentile's text, see Sudhoff, 'Pestschriften', 5 (1911–12), 333.

[10] I use the edition of this work prepared and commented by E. H. Rebouis, *Etude historique et critique sur la peste* (Paris, 1888). The edition of the Paris *Compendium*, along with a French translation, is on pages 70–145 (hereafter, Paris masters, *Compendium*). On this work, see Rebouis' introduction (pp. 1–69); Campbell, *Black Death*, pp. 14–17.

[11] I use the edition of this work published by K. Sudhoff, 'Epistola et regimen Alphontii Cordubensis de pestilentia', *Archiv für Geschichte der Medizin*, 3 (1909–10), 223–6 (hereafter, Alfonso de Córdoba, *Epistola*). On this work and on Alfonso de Córdoba see also Campbell, *Black Death*, pp. 17–18.

[12] I follow the edition of this work prepared and commented by Michon, *Documents inédits*, pp. 71–81 (hereafter, Practicus, *Tractatus*). On this work and on its author, see Campbell, *Black Death*, p. 21.

the signs announcing both the arrival and the presence of *pestilència* deriving from a substantial air change; (4) the effects of the pestilential air, in both its qualities and its substance, upon living beings and humans; (5) the preventive regime against *pestilència* deriving from both a qualitative and a substantial air change; and (6) the nature of 'pestilence morally understood' (*pestilència moralment entesa*).

Gentile da Foligno was a lecturer in the medical faculty of Perugia when the *pestilentia* – which was to cause his own death on 18 June 1348 – began to fall on that Italian city. Gentile wrote a long *Consilium contra pestilentiam*, and three shorter *consilia* are also attributed to him. The major *Consilium* seems to have been written at the request of the university and city of Perugia at the very beginning of the plague. It is divided into four parts, dealing with (1) the causes; (2) the preventive regime; (3) the curative regime; and (4) seventeen *dubia* about plague, which according to him were written to stimulate the wits of medical students, and which evidently kept the *Consilium* free from theoretical discussion. Perhaps the greatest value of Gentile's major *Consilium* consists in its being an actual inventory, both orderly and methodical, of the practical measures used by fourteenth-century university medicine against plague. The other three *consilia* were undoubtedly written after the major one, when the ravages occasioned by the *pestilentia* made Gentile more knowledgeable about the disaster. The earliest one, which is very short, was addressed to the College of Physicians of Genoa. It was followed by another *consilium* with no addressee, in which Gentile mentioned Naples as the city now suffering the 'terrible slaughter'. The last and longest one, which Gentile addressed to the College of Physicians of Perugia, was edited by his son Francesco da Foligno, and seems to have been written just before Gentile's death. This third *consilium* consists of a short preventive regime and ends with three very short *quaestiones* put by the people.

Giovanni della Penna (fl. 1344–87), a lecturer at the medical faculty of Naples, also wrote his *Consilium in magna pestilentia* in 1348, apparently as a reply to that of Gentile da Foligno, and in it he too refers to the presence of *pestilentia* in Naples. Karl Sudhoff collected this work in two fifteenth-century versions which, although completely different in their structure, are very similar in their contents. Giovanni della Penna reproved Gentile's idea that the cause of *pestilentia* was 'a poisonous putrefaction happening near the heart and the lung'. He developed his criticism step by step, dealing with (1) the causes of pestilence; (2) prevention; and (3) treatment.

In October 1348, at the request of King Charles VI of France, the college of masters of the medical faculty of Paris published a long *Compendium de epidimia*, in which they presented their collective opinion about the *epidimia* that was then attacking Paris and the Kingdom of France. This work, which is quite long and written in a rather theoretical and academic style, is divided into two major parts, the first dealing with the causes of pestilence and the second with preventive and curative remedies.

The fifth work of interest to us is the *Epistola et regimen de pestilentia* written by Alfonso de Córdoba. According to this *Epistola* (which is the only piece of information we have about Alfonso de Córdoba), the author was 'master in liberal arts and medicine' and wrote his work in Montpellier. The date of composition is difficult to establish, since from its content the *Epistola* may be dated either 1348 or 1349. Alfonso de Córdoba distinguished three consecutive 'pestilences' occurring from 1348 onwards, each one being due to different causes. He devoted his *Epistola* to the study of the third of these, which he attributed not to natural causes, but to human artifice.

The last work of concern for my discussion is an anonymous one. It is the *Tractatus de epidemia* written by 'a certain practitioner of Montpellier', who addressed his work to both the medical *studium* and the whole University of Paris on St Ivo's day (19 May) 1349. This *Tractatus* seems to be very dependent on the Parisian masters' *Compendium* in its interpretations of the celestial causes of the *epidemia*, but in other respects it differs, insisting that this *epidemia* is particularly transmissible from person to person through the breath and sight of its victims. The 'practitioner of Montpellier' deals extensively with the organic processes involved in this interpersonal transmission of the *epidemia*, and concludes by giving a number of preventive measures.

In the following pages I will try to answer the following questions: How did these medical practitioners perceive what we call the Black Death? Did they perceive it as something new or just one more disaster, along with others like wars, famines and natural catastrophes? To what extent was it perceived as a disease? Was it one of several diseases that were medically labellable? What theories were advanced as to the origin and causes of the Black Death? What medical reactions did it give rise to?

PERCEPTIONS OF THE BLACK DEATH

The identity and name of a new social disaster

The name 'Black Death' to refer to the plague of 1348 did not become popularized in Europe until the eighteenth century. The origin of this name continues to be a minor mystery in the history of plague. *Atra mors* – the Latin expression from which it seems to have derived – was used about plague by Seneca to personify that very epidemic disease.[13] However, Johannes Isaacus Pontanus was in 1631 the first to present it as the name that

---

[13] Seneca, *Oedipus*, 164–70, 180–201 (quoted by S. D'Irsay, 'Notes to the origin of the expression: "Atra Mors"', *Isis*, 8 (1926), 328–32).

mid fourteenth-century Europeans had used.[14] On the other hand, translated into vernacular languages, the expression had already appeared some decades before in Swedish and Danish writings as *swarta döden* (1555) and *den sorte Død* (1601), respectively.[15] Thus, the origin of the name Black Death almost certainly lies in an over-literal translation into the Scandinavian or the English of the Latin *pestis atra* or *atra mors*.[16]

In contemporary chronicles the Black Death first and mainly appears as a very serious disaster which struck different human communities, leaving a trail of death and distress. For the Crown of Aragon, the important set of contemporary documents on the Black Death at the Archivo de la Corona de Aragón, which has been collected and published by Amada López de Meneses, confirms this view. If we look at the names used to refer to the Black Death in these documents, we find that in 105 cases (75 per cent of all the mentions) it is referred to under the substantive *mortalitas/tates*, either alone or with emphatic epithets (*gran, generalis/les, infesta, infinite, ingens, inmense, pestilencialis/les, pestilens, terribilis/les, universalis, valide*); in five cases (4 per cent), under the phrase *mortalitatum clades*.[17] All these names expressively reveal that lay people in the Crown of Aragon perceived the Black Death of 1348 as catastrophic in its mortality. Only later in the century, after the appearance of subsequent epidemic crises, would it receive new names such as *mortalitas prima* and *maxime mortalitates*, characterizing it as the first and highest landmark of a new time characterized by great slaughters,[18] or would it be given a clinical name – that of *glanola / les*.[19] From this same collection of documents it is also obvious that interpretations relating these mortalities to particular conditions in the air were common in the mid fourteenth-century Crown of Aragon; as we will see later on, this seems to reflect a significant social openness towards university learning, both medical and natural-philosophical.[20] It is scarcely

---

[14] J. I. Pontanus, *Rerum Danicarum Historia* (Amsterdam, 1631), p. 476: '... notant chronologi adeo saevam ac diram hoc anno pestem ... grassatam ... Vulgo et ab effectu *atram mortem* vocitabant' (quoted by D'Irsay, 'Notes', p. 328).

[15] I. Reichborn-Kjennerud, 'Black Death', *Journal of the History of Medicine*, 3 (1948), 359–60.

[16] Ziegler, *Black Death*, pp. 17–18.

[17] Other mentions are dominated by *infirmitas/tates* (10 times; along with the adjective *pestifere, pestilenciales, terribiles*, or *valide*), *mortalitatum clades* (5 times), *epidemia* (5), *pestilencia* and *pestilencie* (7 times; along with the adjective *mortalis, infecta, grans*), and *pestis* (2); and other phrases (*egritudo pestifera, malaltia/ties, mortalitatis sevicia*) which are only mentioned once. See A. López de Meneses, 'Documentos acerca de la peste negra en los dominios de la Corona de Aragón', *Estudios de Edad Media de la Corona de Aragón (Sección de Zaragoza)*, 6 (1956), 291–447.

[18] Ibid., docs. nos. 152, 155, and 156.

[19] Ibid., docs. nos. 149, 154, and 157.

[20] There are phrases like 'sterilitates temporum [et] mortalitatum clades'; 'epidemia vel malicia temporis'; 'epidemia et infecta aeris affluencia'; 'generalis epidemia et infecta pestilencia aeris pestilentis'; 'sterilitas temporis et aeris intemperies'; 'mortalitates et aeris intemperies'; 'mortalitates et temporum preteritorum sterilitas'; 'infirmitatum et mortalitatis pestis ac sterilitas temporis'; and 'pestilentialis et corrumptibilis tempus'. See ibid., docs. nos. 19, 25, 29, 71, 73, 77, 90, 111, and 128.

necessary to add that in broad terms what was true about Aragonese lay perceptions towards the Black Death can also be applied to the other southwestern Europeans who were afflicted by it.

How did university medical practitioners in the Latin Mediterranean perceive the Black Death of 1348? One of these practitioners, Jacme d'Agramont, discussed it in terms of an 'epidemic or pestilence and mortalities of people' ('epidímia ho pestilència e mortaldats de gents') which threatened Lerida from 'some parts and regions neighbouring to us' ('algunes partides e regions a nos vehines').[21] Agramont said nothing concerning the term epidímia, but he extensively developed what he meant by pestilència. He gave this latter term a very peculiar etymology, in accordance with a form of knowledge established by Isidore of Seville (570–636) in his Etymologiae, which came to be widely accepted throughout Europe during the Middle Ages.[22] He split the term pestilència up into three syllables, each having a particular meaning: pes (= tempesta: 'storm', 'tempest'), te (= temps: 'time'), and lència (= clardat: 'brightness', 'light'); hence, he concluded, the pestilència was 'the time of tempest caused by light from the stars'.[23] Similarly, another physician, the 'practitioner of Montpellier', stated that the word epidemia came from the Greek epi (= upon) and demos (= containing receptacle or air, according to him). Therefore he concluded that epidemia meant 'plague in the receptacle, i.e. of the air'; and he defined it as 'the corruption of the continent, i.e. of the air, which suddenly kills all the creatures', adding that 'every air corruption has to be reduced to celestial causes'.[24] Other passages of Agramont's Regiment make it possible to clarify the obscure meaning of his etymological approach to the term pestilència. In fact, he distinguished two kinds of 'pestilence': 'pestilence naturally understood' ('pestilència naturalment entesa'), and 'pestilence morally understood' ('pestilència moralment entesa'). The former, to which he devoted his work, was defined as

contra-natural change [mudament] of the air either in its qualities [= alteració] or in its substance [= putrefacció]. This change produces corruptions, sudden deaths,

[21] Agramont, Regiment, p. 47.
[22] See J. Fontaine, Isidore de Séville et la culture classique dans l'Espagne wisigothique, 2 vols. (Paris, 1959); J. Engels, 'La portée de l'étymologie isidorienne', Studi Medievali, 3rd series, 3 (1962), 100–28 (both quoted by D. Jacquart and C. Thomasset, Sexuality and medicine in the Middle Ages (Cambridge, Mass., 1988), pp. 8–16, 198–200).
[23] Agramont, Regiment, p. 55: 'Hon dich que pestilència, segons verdadera enterpretació, vol dir aytant com temps de tempesta que ve de clardat, ço és a saber, de les esteles. Per la primera síl.laba sua, que és .pes., entench "tempesta". E per la segona sil.laba sua, que és .te. entench "temps". E per la terça sil.laba sua, que és .lència'. entench "clardat" car lencos en grech vol aytal dir com "clardat" hon "lum" en latí.'
[24] Practicus, Tractatus, p. 71: 'Videndum est primo quid sit epidemia et quare sic dicitur. Epidemia enim dicitur ab "epi" quod est supra, et "demos" quod est continens, vel aer, qui corruptus est; dicitur pestis in continente, id est in aere: omnes enim corruptiones aeris reducuntur in causas coelestes ... Est autem epidemia corruptio continentis, id est aeris, necans quasi subito creaturas.'

and various diseases, all beyond the ordinary, in the living things of certain regions.[25]

For the definition of 'pestilence morally understood', Agramont paraphrased that of 'natural pestilence':

Pestilence [morally understood] is a contra-natural change (*mudament*) in the spirit and in the thoughts of people, resulting in enmities and rancours, wars and robberies, destructions of places and deaths far beyond the ordinary in certain regions.[26]

From Agramont's discussion of both pestilences, the 'natural' and the 'moral', we may conclude the following. First, that 'moral pestilence' was by no means just a metaphor. Agramont had no doubt about the existence of this kind of 'pestilence', so that his concept of *pestilència* was operative not only in the natural world, but also in the moral one. However, he avoided discussion of the 'moral pestilence', claiming that his understanding was not strong enough, and then he invited 'those whose minds are higher and more subtle' to discuss it instead of him. His insistence on a natural/moral or physical/moral parallelism, jumping at once from the personal to the social, has to be underlined. This viewpoint seems to have been not only shared but also extended by Gentile da Foligno, who found a triple answer to the *quaestio* 'Why do pestilences usually come after wars?': (i) because in wartime human bodies behave in a disorderly way, which makes them generate bad humours susceptible to putrefaction; (ii) because those superior beings who prepare wars, also prepare plagues; and (iii) because the fertility which usually follows on the famine provoked by war, brings about saturation and this saturation causes many obstructions, as a result of which putrefaction and pestilential disease happen.[27] It is obvious that Gentile closely interrelated both orders, the natural and the moral, with regard not only to effects, but also to causes. Both Agramont and Gentile were merely echoing Albumasar's theory of the Great Conjunctions, a very popular doctrine in the late Middle Ages that postulated that some planetary conjunctions cause major political and natural disasters.[28]

Secondly, neither 'natural pestilence' nor 'moral pestilence' was, as might be thought, the *effect* or a contra-natural change – either of the air, in the case of 'natural pestilence', or of the spirit and thoughts of people, in the case of 'moral pestilence' – but properly the change in itself. As we saw above, the 'practitioner of Montpellier' shared the same view with regard to the 'natural' pestilence – the only one he considered. Therefore, accord-

---

[25] Agramont, *Regiment*, p. 52.
[26] Ibid., p. 91.
[27] Gentile, *Consilium*, signat. c4r.
[28] On Albumasar's theory of the planetary conjunctions and its impact in late medieval Europe, see R. Lemay, *Abu Ma'shar and latin Aristotelianism in the twelfth century* (Beirut, 1962); P. Curry (ed.), *Astrology, science and society. Historical essays* (Woodbridge, 1987), passim; R. French this volume.

ing to both Agramont and the Montpellier practitioner the 'pestilence' would not be the disease itself, but the cause of several effects, among which those then and now called diseases are to be counted. However, the concept of *epidimia* held by the medical masters of the University of Paris seems to have been somewhat different since they considered the 'praesens epidimia sive pestis' to be the effect of an air change, not the change in the air itself.[29] It is difficult to evaluate the importance of these contradictory views on the exact meaning of 'pestilence'. In fact, Gentile da Foligno seems to have been inconsistent himself in holding both views at once: he initially agreed with the Paris masters that the *pestilentia* was the disease itself when he said that 'the cause of the *pestilentia* is a certain mutation happening in the air', but he went on to identify the *pestilentia* itself with the mutation in the air, like Agramont and the Montpellier practitioner.[30]

Thirdly, Agramont thought that the 'natural pestilence' consisted in either a qualitative or a 'substantial' change of the air. Gentile recognized these two kinds of change in the air, but held that when the change was qualitative there was just a *mutatio pestilentiosa*, and there was properly the *pestilentia* – with which he intended to deal in his *Consilium* – only when the air change was substantial. A 'substantial' change in the air meant for him the complete corruption of the air as a result of bad vapours that mingled with it right down to its smallest parts, thickening it and macerating it. Gentile illustrated the process by means of two analogies: the substantial change is similar to the putrefaction which happens when stinking water is stirred (taken from Avicenna, although not credited); and the thickening and maceration of the air by bad vapours is similar to the change that occurs in the water used to macerate wheat or linen.[31] Nevertheless, for other physicians like the 'practitioner of Montpellier' and the medical

---

[29] Paris masters, *Compendium*, p. 80: 'credimus autem presentem epidimiam sive pestem *ab aere corrupto in sui substantia, et non solum in qualitatibus alterato*, immediate provenire' (the italics are mine).

[30] Gentile, *Consilium*, signats. a2r–a2v: 'Omissis his dico causam pestilentie esse mutationem quandam in aere factam ... Et hec mutatio est que proprie dicitur pestilentia ...' Although the writings of Caelius Aurelianus were unknown in the Middle Ages and would not be rediscovered until the sixteenth century, they could throw light on the issue of these contradictory views on the concept of 'pestilence' held by the medical practitioners studied here. Indeed, there is a paragraph in the preface of his work *Celerum vel acutarum passionum* (lib. I, Praefatio) where the author attacked Asclepiades and his followers for their use of *metalepsis* in defining a disease – that is, setting forth 'the cause instead of describing the resultant disease itself'. Caelius Aurelianus wanted to illustrate his point precisely with the case of 'plague' (*lues*). He states: 'denique luem diffiniens, "lues", [Asclepiades] inquit, "est qualitas insueta in his ubi est locis consistentium animalium, qua ex communi causa facilibus morbis et infectivis adficiuntur". Etiam nunc luis causam pro effectu sumpsisse perspicitur. Causa etenim luis est qualitas; lues autem declivitas in aegritudinem prona atque celeberrima, communibus antecedentibus causis.' See I. E. Drabkin (ed.), *Caelius Aurelianus. On acute diseases and on chronic diseases* (Chicago, 1950), pp. 8–9.

[31] Gentile, *Consilium*, signats. a2r–a2v. The first analogy comes from the *Canon medicinae* of Avicenna, lib. I, fen 2, doct. 2, cap. 9 (Venice, 1527), fol. 26v.

masters of the University of Paris, 'pestilence' referred only to a substantial change (= corruption) of the air.[32]

And fourthly, Agramont's alleged etymology of the term *pestilència* recognized the 'light from the stars' as the original cause of every 'pestilence'. His view was shared by the Montpellier practitioner, who asserted more generally that 'every air corruption has to be brought down to celestial causes'. To a greater or lesser extent, the celestial causes played a part in all the pestilence tractates studied here, and they will be studied at length in the next section.

Before turning to that, I would like to raise another question: Did medical practitioners perceive the Black Death of 1348 as a different kind of 'pestilence' with respect to the others they knew? Answering this question is not easy. The only practitioner (among those whose writings I have studied) who compared it with any previous 'pestilence', was Gentile da Foligno. He referred to his own experience during a previous epidemic in Padua[33] and to two well-known historical cases: the plague of Athens, which was described by Thucydides and was also mentioned by Galen,[34] and the mysterious plague of the city of Crannon, to which Avenzoar referred.[35] If we look at Gentile's four *consilia* together, it is evident that his perception of the *pestilentia* of 1348 changed as the course of time allowed him to become aware of the actual dimensions of the tragedy. In fact, in his earliest and major *consilium* he referred to it in the following terms: 'this frightening plague, which was around a long time ago, is not yet so malignant as the plague of the city of Crannon ... or that of Thucydides ... although it may reach the same degree [of malignity]'. But in two subsequent *consilia* Gentile changed his mind and labelled 'this pestilence, epidemic, or whatever else it may be called' as very frightening, unheard of, unknown to medical authorities, and much worse than the other two previously mentioned.[36]

The other physicians who wrote on the Black Death of 1348 did not specifically compare it to any previous pestilence. Rather, they seem to have perceived it as just one more (albeit very serious) among those well

---

[32] See notes 24 and 29, above.

[33] Gentile, *Consilium*, signats. b5r, c3v. He was probably referring to the war between Venice and Genoa in 1331–3.

[34] Galen, *De differentiis febrium*, lib. I, cap. IV (Venice, 1490), vol. II, signat. G8va.

[35] Avenzoar, *Liber Theizir*, lib. 3, tract. 3, cap. I (Venice, 1496, fol. 38v).

[36] Gentile, *Consilium*, signat. a1r: '... hanc pestem que diu pullulare videtur multum verenda, licet adhuc non sit tante malitie quante pestis civitatis Craton ... vel quam Thelurides ... quod tamen posset non est dubium ad istum gradum perduci'. Gentile, 'Consilium in epidimia Perusii', *Consilia* (Pavia, 1488), signat. g1v: '... nulla videtur precessisse temporibus memorabilibus pestilentia quam mirabilis sicut pestilentia que nunc est ... famosa enim pestilentia civitatis Craton vel quam scripsit Tolurides vel Galienus vel Zoar non videtur comparabilis in malitia ...'; Sudhoff, 'Pestschriften', 5 (1911–12), 332: '... dicimus quod haec pestilentia sive epidimia sive quo nomine nominetur est multum verenda nec audita nec visa in libris, ita quod pestilentia quam narrat Zoar in Thesir non fuit tantae malitiae ...'.

known and described by previous writers. The peculiar severity and general dissemination of this 'pestilence' caused most of the medical practitioners studied here to attribute its origin to the air, as contrasted with other less serious 'pestilences' that came from water or food. It is not difficult to understand why, since according to the dominant medical doctrine at the time – Latin Galenism – the air-environment was the first and most important of the six non-naturals ('sex res non naturales') because (1) it was the receptacle containing the sublunar world; (2) it was considered as something strictly necessary for the life of all the creatures on the earth, and particularly of humans, according to Galenic doctrine; (3) it moved quickly from one place to another by means of the winds; and (4) it influenced the water and the earth directly. Obviously, any change in the air would entail severe consequences. Indeed, the Paris medical masters stated that 'bad air is more harmful than [bad] food and drink since the former with its evil [*malicia*] soon arrives at the heart and the lung'.[37] On the other hand, Agramont asserted that this *pestilència* affected all beings belonging to the 'three degrees of life' ('tres graus de vida'): (1) trees and plants; (2) beasts; and (3) humans. According to him, apart from the direct effect of the pestilential air upon all creatures, this was the chain process through which these three levels of the *scala naturae* were affected: first, the grain and fruits growing in lands where *pestilència* was or had been present contained a certain *gran infecció* which provoked *corrupcions* in the first degree of life; next, this *gran infecció* acted like 'poison' (*verí*) for every beast consuming the affected products, so that *corrupcions* also afflicted the second degree of life; and, finally, the creatures of the two first degrees usually provided food for humans and normally had 'the property of being of benefit to our body' ('la proprietat d'aprofitar al nostre cors'), but in time of *pestilència* they had 'the property of poisoning and killing' ('han proprietat d'enverinar e de matar').[38] In short, the 'pestilence' affected the basic food chain, and the maintenance source of human energy.

The causes

To a university-trained physician, as to anyone who had pursued the study of the arts at any fourteenth-century European university, it was clear that any universal effect had to be reduced (or brought down) to universal causes, according to certain cosmological conceptions which were unquestionable at that time. (These conceptions had their starting point in

---

[37] Paris masters, *Compendium*, p. 80: 'Quamvis pestilentiales egritudines a corruptione aque et ciborum, sicut accidit tempore famis et sterilitatis, ab aeris tamen corruptione egritudines hujusmodi procedentes periculosiores esse censemus; aer enim malus nocibilior est cibis et potibus, eo quod velociter penetret ad cor et pulmonem cum sui malitia; credimus autem presentem epidimiam sive pestem ab aere corrupto in sui substantia, et non solum in qualitatibus alterato, immediate provenire.'

[38] Agramont, *Regiment*, pp. 52–3.

Aristotle's and Ptolemy's works, they had been reinforced in late antiquity and the Middle Ages by a number of Greek, Arab and Latin authorities, and they still dominated European intellectual life as late as the late sixteenth century).[39] Thus, most of the physicians who wrote on the Black Death of 1348 were compelled to establish a causal chain going from the universal and prime cause to the particular effects of the pestilence. Speaking strictly in terms of medieval Christian cosmology, the prime cause of the pestilence, as of everything else, was God, who permitted it. However, throughout the Middle Ages, thanks particularly to thirteenth-century scholastic philosophy and certain fourteenth-century renewing movements of thought (nominalism and voluntarism), Christian natural philosophers developed the idea of a natural order which, in spite of being presided over by God (the prime cause), was autonomous and – but for some exceptional cases (miracles) – was ruled by natural laws (secondary causes), the knowledge of which was accessible to human reason. Therefore, although the pestilence was always presided over by a supernatural order, it was also part of an autonomous *natural* order ruled by natural causes at two different levels: the level of remote, universal, superior and celestial causes, and that of close, particular, inferior and terrestrial causes – the latter being absolutely dependent upon the former. The role of celestial causes in the plague was a controversial issue, however, which a number of fourteenth-century university physicians chose to ignore, saying that the knowledge of such remote causes was the concern of astrologers, and that astrology little served the aims of the medical art.

This causal model is somewhat simplistic, and, as we shall see, is not entirely applicable to the ideas about the causes of the Black Death held by fourteenth-century university medical practitioners, but it serves nevertheless as a useful guide. Those who followed it most closely were the masters of the Paris medical school and the anonymous practitioner of Montpellier, although each emphasized different points. Gentile da Foligno's position, on the other hand, illustrates very well how some academic physicians did not consider universal causes at any length. Agramont's case is quite particular. In fact, it has been said already that he wrote the *Regiment* with the aim of instructing his fellow citizens on the way to face the pestilence threatening Lerida from neighbouring regions. This compelled him to talk about *pestilència* in a general way and, as a result, to inventory the different causes which could provoke pestilences. In his opinion, they could come from a qualitative air change as well as from a substantial one, nor did he distinguish between celestial and terrestrial causes. Thus it seems impossible

[39] J. E. Grant, 'Medieval and Renaissance scholastic conceptions of the influence of the celestial region on the terrestrial', *Journal of Medieval and Renaissance Studies*, 17 (1987), 1–23; J. D. North, 'Celestial influence – the major premiss of astrology', in P. Zambelli (ed.) *'Astrologi hallucinati': stars and the end of the world in Luther's time* (Berlin and New York, 1986), pp. 45–100; J. D. North, 'Medieval concepts of celestial influence: a survey', in P. Curry (ed.), *Astrology, science, and society*, pp. 5–17.

to know the precise causal interpretation that Agramont would have given to the pestilence that killed him. However, his flexibility in presenting different causal possibilities suggests that he may have held attitudes similar to those of Gentile da Foligno.

To conclude this point, something must be said about the positions held by Giovanni della Penna and Alfonso de Córdoba. Neither of them followed the causal scheme mentioned above, although for different reasons. In the case of della Penna, it was because for him the pestilence took root in the choleric matter of many individuals which had become too heated and corrupted, rather than in any poisonous matter generated near the heart and the lungs as a result of the pestilential air, as Gentile claimed. Della Penna, incidentally, accepted the role of the air in this corruption, and even the influence of 'certain conjunctions' upon this air, but he considered that only an individual's personal constitution determined whether that individual would contract the pestilence or not.[40] Alfonso de Córdoba, for his part, accepted the existence of universal causes for two of the three different pestilences that he distinguished as occurring from 1348 onwards. The first two had been due to celestial and to terrestrial causes, respectively; however, the third, which was the actual subject of his work, was due to a human artifice that had caused the poisoning of food and drink by means of a deliberate corruption of the air.[41]

Was the Black Death the work of God?
Of the six works which are our concern here, two hardly mention the word 'God', two more relegate the prime and supernatural cause to a secondary position, and the remaining two consider divine intervention as a possible cause of 'universal pestilence'. In the first group are the works of Giovanni della Penna and Alfonso de Córdoba, whose attitude on this point was consistent with their respective causal conceptions: neither of them accepted the existence of universal causes for this pestilence.

In the second group are Gentile da Foligno and the anonymous practitioner of Montpellier, both of whom merely mentioned God in the invocations at the beginning and/or the end of their respective works. The practitioner of Montpellier stated at the beginning of his Tractatus that, like whoever else had received the divine grace to know the cause of this epidemia, he felt compelled to investigate it diligently in order to make it possible for 'faithful Christians' to possess a remedy against it.[42] He referred to God twice more when explaining and prognosticating the harmful influence of certain planets in the appearance of epidemics, wars and

---

[40] Penna, Consilium, pp. 342–3, 164–5.
[41] Alfonso de Córdoba, Epistola, p. 224.
[42] Practicus, Tractatus, p. 71: 'Cum enim quilibet secundum gratiam a Deo sibi datam ut cognoscat causam istius epidemiae, debet contemplari diligenter, uti curam christianis fidelibus valeat adhibere, super quod quidam practicus de Montepessulo suam inten- tionem, brevius quam potuit, declaravit . . .'

mortalities, piously recognizing the possibility that the divine will might not permit these evils and could therefore cut short the natural course of these events.[43] Still more sparing in his allusions to God was Gentile da Foligno, who mentioned Him only four times: once at the beginning of his major *Consilium*, when he proclaimed in a syllogistic way the general theological principles which guided the activities of Christian physicians,[44] and three more times in brief invocations to God asking for protection against the pestilence.[45] Gentile's sparingness on this point takes on a greater significance if we consider that in 1480, more than one hundred years after his death, he was accused by a bishop of Foligno of having taken into account only the health of bodies and the preservation of lives, but not the health of souls.[46]

The third group is represented by the writings of the masters of the University of Paris and Jacme d'Agramont. Both of these works considered that the pestilence might occasionally come directly from the divine will. When this happens, the Paris masters said, 'there is no more advice than to humbly turn to Him, although even in such a case medical advice must not be absolutely ignored'.[47] Jacme d'Agramont, on the other hand, thought that God was sometimes behind the appearance of 'universal pestilences'. When this was so, the pestilence must be attributed not only to the 'work of God' ('obra de Déu') but also to 'our merits' ('mèrits nostres') – that is, to 'our sins' ('nostres pecats'). All the examples mentioned by Agramont are commonplaces taken from the Old Testament, from both the Pentateuch and the Book of Kings.[48]

The natural causes

Nearly all the physicians studied here, in discussing the natural causes of the 'pestilence', distinguished the remote, universal, superior and celestial causes from the near, particular, inferior and terrestrial ones. Their thinking here, as was often the case in medieval medical theory, was strongly influenced by Avicenna. Concerning the 'pestilential fevers', Avicenna had distinguished in his *Canon* two groups of causes: the 'remote and first cause', which consisted of the 'forms of the heavens' (or 'celestial figures'),

---

[43] He used the phrases 'nisi Altissimus noluerit' and 'nisi Deus noluerit et Christus'. See ibid., p. 81.

[44] Gentile, *Consilium*, signat. a1r: 'Quoniam gloriosus et excelsus Deus de largitate sua Medicinam produxit, et medicum velut nature refugium creavit, decet eum nil negligentie habere in noscendo sanitatis ingenium, ut Galienus primo de ingenio sanitatis. Immo est de melioribus rebus, et medicus utatur previsione.'

[45] Ibid., signats. b4v, b7r, c4v.

[46] Antonius de Senis, *De divina praeordinatione vitae et mortis humanae* (Rome, c. 1480), cap. XIX (quoted in P. T. Lugano, 'Gentilis Fulginas', pp. 203–4).

[47] Paris masters, *Compendium*, p. 92: 'Amplius pretermittere nolumus, quod quando epidimia a voluntate divina procedit, in quo casu non est aliud consilium nisi quod ad ipsum humiliter recurratur, consilium tamen medici non deserendo.'

[48] Agramont, *Regiment*, pp. 55, 57–8.

and the 'near causes', which were the 'terrestrial dispositions'. In certain conditions, he said, when a synergistic action of both groups, by means of the respective 'celestial agent virtues' and 'terrestrial patient virtues', caused a vehement moistening of the air, then

vapours and fumes rise and spread into the air, and provoke its putrefaction by means of a soft warmth. When air that has undergone such putrefaction arrives at the heart, it rots the complexion of its spirit and then, after surrounding the heart, rots it. An unnatural warmth then spreads all around the body, as a result of which a pestilential fever will appear. It will spread to any human who is susceptible to it.[49]

Celestial causes. The emphasis placed on celestial causes of the 'pestilence' by the different physicians studied here varied quite widely. This was a natural result of the fact that interest in astrology varied among learned people across Europe depending upon their profession and the place where they had studied.[50] Let us compare the opinions on the role of astral causes held by Augustine of Trent and Gentile da Foligno in order to appreciate what different views could be maintained by two academics both lecturing at the *studium* of Perugia, although in different faculties. In 1340 Augustine of Trent, a friar eremite of St Augustine, justified having written a medical and astrological work on a 'pestilence of diseases' happening everywhere in Italy, because of physicians' ignorance about the roots of diseases; this fact was considered by him 'a pestiferous mistake involving many physicians', and he blamed it on their 'ignorance of astronomy'.[51] Almost certainly, Augustine of Trent would have attacked Gentile's attitude towards the celestial causes of the 'pestilence' as a rather lukewarm position. In fact, in his major *Consilium* Gentile made very few, brief and non-specific remarks about this group of causes. On the one hand, he followed the Avicennan scheme mentioned above, to which he added that Avicenna only sometimes ('aliquando') attributed the 'pestilence' to the action of 'celestial bodies which move the inferior agents to cause it'.[52] On the other hand, Gentile seems to have kept a distance with respect of the

[49] Avicenna, *Canon*, lib. IV, fen i, tract. 4, cap. 1 (Venice, 1527, fol. 325v).

[50] To the best of my knowledge, medical astrology in late medieval Europe is a topic much neglected by historians. In a recent collection of papers on the history of medieval and Renaissance astrology in Europe whose editor, Patrick Curry, underlines the lack of historical studies on this topic, scarcely four pages are devoted to medical astrology. See P. Curry (ed.), *Astrology, science and society*; and for classical studies on the history of astrology, see the bibliography. For medical astrology in twelfth-century Europe, see Roger French's paper in the present volume.

[51] L. Thorndike, 'A pest tractate before the Black Death', *Sudhoff's Archiv*, 23 (1930), 346–56: 'Determinavi infrascripta in universitate studii Perusii propter ignorantiam infirmitatis. Nam in ista pestilentia infirmitatum medici Florentie Perusii Rome atque in ceteris regionibus Ytalie tribuebant unam medicinam omnibus humoribus, ut scriptum fuit mihi, ignorantes radices infirmitatum. Et accidit error iste pestiferus multis medicis propter ignorantiam astronomie' (p. 349).

[52] Gentile, *Consilium*, signat. a1v.

precise role of these remote causes: he dealt with them in the third person, under the clause *Astrologi dixerunt* which introduced a literal quotation from Pietro d'Abano, relating star eclipses and planet conjunctions to the induction of 'bad constitutions in the seasons by means of their mutations in their essence and nature'.[53]

Works from other geographical areas assigned a more relevant role to celestial causes in the genesis of the 'pestilence'. Most of them identified these celestial causes with harmful planet conjunctions. The *Compendium* of the Paris masters – and along with it the *Tractatus* of the anonymous practitioner of Montepellier, which appears dependent upon it on this point[54] – illustrates this conception perhaps better than any other work. According to the Paris masters, the conjunction of three major planets (Saturn, Mars and Jupiter) in Aquarius on 20 March 1345 at one o'clock in the afternoon was, 'along with other conjunctions and eclipses', the remote origin of a 'deadly corruption of the surrounding air', which brought 'mortality and famine', in addition to other effects which were not their current concern.[55] They based their argument on the authority of *De causis proprietatum elementorum* – then attributed to Aristotle, but actually a pseudo-Aristotelian work – and on Albert the Great's commentary on this work. According to this pseudo-Aristotle, the conjunction of Saturn and Jupiter caused 'great mortalities and depopulation of kingdoms'.[56] Albert the Great's commentary added that the conjunction of Mars and Jupiter provokes 'a great pestilence in the air, particularly when it happens in a warm and humid sign of the zodiac, as is the case now'. This was the result of the combined effect of the actions of both planets since 'Jupiter, a warm and humid planet, elevates bad vapours from earth and water, while Mars, an intemperately warm and dry planet, ignites the elevated vapours thus causing the multiplication in the air of lightnings, sparks, pestiferous vapours and fires.'[57] The Paris masters concluded their astrological dissertation by emphasizing that the peculiar situation of 'wicked Mars' during late 1347 and early 1348 only served to intensify the always frightening effects of this planet.[58]

---

[53] Ibid., signat. a1v–a2r. Gentile made other mentions of celestial causes in the *dubia* ending his *Consilium* (see signats. c2v, c3r, c4r), although their tone did not differ from that in the commented paragraphs. For the quotation from Pietro d'Abano, see his *Conciliator*, diff. 94 (Venice, 1564, fol. 142v).

[54] Practicus, *Tractatus*, pp. 71–2.

[55] Paris masters, *Compendium*, p. 76.

[56] Ibid., p. 76. For the text of the Pseudo-Aristotelian *De causis proprietatum elementorum*, see the critical edition prepared by P. Hossfeld, in W. Kubel (ed.), *Alberti Magni Opera omnia* (Münster, 1980), vol. v, pars ii, p. 63.

[57] Paris masters, *Compendium*, p. 78. For the text of this work of Albert the Great (*De causis proprietatum elementorum*, lib. 2, tract. 2, cap. 1), see the critical edition prepared by P. Hossfeld, p. 96.

[58] Paris masters, *Compendium*, pp. 78, 80: '... presertim quia Mars, planeta malivolus, coleram generans atque guerras, a sexta die octobris, anni XLVII, usque in finem Maii anni presentis, fuit in Leone una cum capite Draconis; que omnia, quia sunt calida, multos

Alfonso de Córdoba, on the other hand, related to celestial causes only the earliest of the three 'pestilences' that he distinguished, mentioning an unspecified 'constellation of unfortunate planets'; he gave most importance, however, to a lunar eclipse which had happened (according to him) in the sign of Leo, shortly before the beginning of that 'pestilence'.[59]

Finally, Jacme d'Agramont considered astral causes in his discussion of the 'universal pestilence', only where they had the same level of importance as other possible causes. But he always referred to planetary influences. In the 'pestilences' due to a qualitative air change, certain unspecified planets provoke these qualitative changes (heat, cold) depending on season changes or on the variable distance between those planets and the sun, or both. In the 'pestilences' due to a substantial air change, Agramont referred to planetary conjunctions and to the frightening 'glance' ('esguardament') or aspect of some of them. With respect to the 'pestilence' due to a substantial air change, Agramont – who quoted the same paragraph of Albert the Great as the Paris masters – stated that the origin of this celestial influence was an 'occult property ['proprietat amagada'] without a proper name' that came from a 'specific virtue' ('vertut specíffica').[60]

Terrestrial causes. There is no better work to illustrate the standard causal scheme we have been discussing than that of the Paris masters. They affirmed in a very mechanistic way that during the period of the planetary conjunctions which they referred to, 'many corrupted vapours' ('multi vapores corrupti') rose from earth and water, and multiplied and spread into the air. These vapours, helped by the frequent blast of southerly winds, rotted the air in its substance. The Paris masters warned everyone against the harmful character of southern winds since

because of their impetus they carry or have carried to us bad, putrid, and poisonous vapours from other places, such as marshes, lakes, deep valleys, and from corpses which have been neither buried nor burned.[61]

Gentile da Foligno, by contrast, after referring to universal causes (as mentioned above), inventoried the terrestrial causes of the 'pestilence' as follows:

vapores attraxerunt, et ob hoc hyemps non fuit frigida, ut deberet. Mars etiam, quia fuit reterogradus, plures a terra et aqua vapores atraxit qui aeri commixti ipsius substantiam corrumpunt: et etiam quia Jovem aspexit, aspectu malo, scilicet 4°, ideo dispositionem seu qualitatem malam in ipso anime nostre inimicam et repugnantem causaverunt. Exinde generati sunt venti validi, quia, secundum Albertum, libro quarto meteorum, Jupiter habet a proprietate sua elevare materiam ventorum fortium qui, ut plurimum meridionales existentes, caliditatem et humiditatem superfluas in istis inferioribus induxerunt. Humiditas tamen in nostra regione caliditatem superavit.'

59 Alfonso de Córdoba, *Epistola*, p. 224.
60 Agramont, *Regiment*, pp. 59–60.
61 Paris masters, *Compendium*, p. 82.

The particular and manifest causes are the perceptible corruptions which are present at a place or carried in from distant places by means of winds (above all, by southerly ones), as happens from either the opening of wells and caverns that have been long closed; the unventilated and constricted air within walls and ceilings; small lakes and pools (as Galen said); or animal dung, corpses, and other stinking putrefactions etc. . . .[62]

It is obvious that both these passages take their authority from Avicenna, although he is not mentioned in either.[63] Nevertheless, they differ somewhat in approach: while the Paris masters mechanistically related a particular and near cause to the universal and remote one, Gentile merely mentioned an extensive range of possible manifest causes which could give rise to the 'pestilence' according to current academic learning.

Agramont seems to have thought along the same lines as Gentile, since he mentioned very similar terrestrial causes (winds, putrefying corpses, putrid waters and the bowels of the earth). To him the winds could cause either of the two kinds of 'universal pestilence' that he considered. So, on the one hand, the *tramontana* (north wind) and the *migjorn* (south wind), depending on their intensity and the season of the year, could alter the air quality and bring about a 'pestilence'.[64] And, on the other hand, the 'pestilence' due to a substantial change of the air could happen when warm and moist winds blew, since these winds 'produce great humidity in the air, and humidity is the mother of putrefaction'.[65] This Catalan physician also noted that sometimes a 'universal pestilence' could happen when after a battle or a long siege a number of human and horse corpses lay without being buried, 'because a great infection and corruption of the air follows the putrefaction of dead things' – not to mention the generation of 'flies and very poisonous horseflies'.[66] According to Agramont, rotten waters could also cause 'universal pestilences' owing to a substantial change of the air. He explained that this process could happen when 'many vapours rise from putrid water as a result of the sun's heat', and he stressed that 'these vapours are much more pernicious and harmful than the putrid water itself, because they are more thin and acute so that they mix with the air, corrupt it and rot it in its substance'.[67] Remarkably, while other works such as that of the Paris masters mentioned the important causal role of rotten water in

---

[62] Gentile, *Consilium*, signat. a2r.
[63] Avicenna, *Canon*, lib. IV, fen I, tract. IV, cap. I (Venice, 1527), fol. 325v. For the quotation, see p. 252 above.
[64] Agramont, *Regiment*, p. 56.
[65] Ibid., p. 60.
[66] Ibid., p. 60: 'Encara més en altra manera se pot fer, car a vegades per bataylla ho en gran setge moren gran moltitut de gents e de cavalls, los quals no.s sotarren, per què.s segueix de la putrefacció dels cosses morts gran infecció e corrompiment en l'àer. Encara dels cosses podrits s'engenren mosques e tavans molt verinoses . . .'
[67] Ibid., p. 62.

the appearance of less malignant and diffused 'pestilential diseases', they did not relate it to 'universal pestilences'.[68]

Agramont also defended the telluric origin of some 'pestilences', the appearance of which was related to the terrestrial 'exhalations of fumes' that provoked earthquakes. These fumes caused a substantial air change through the same process as those from putrid waters.[69] Two more of the works studied here also echoed the same idea, namely those of Alfonso de Córdoba and of the Paris masters. The latter attributed the origin of some pestilences to 'putrefactions constricted in the bowels of the earth'.[70]

The artificial causes

During the Black Death of 1348 the charge that some minorities – mainly Jews and lepers – had been the actual causers of this disaster was frequent in certain parts of Europe, among them Languedoc, Provence and Catalonia.[71] Jacme d'Agramont and Alfonso de Córdoba seem to have echoed this charge, although without explicitly identifying the culprits. Indeed, Agramont restricted himself to considering it very likely that the 'pestilence' that was causing so many deaths in north Catalonia, Languedoc and Provence in 1348 could actually have consisted of a deliberate poisoning provoked by 'wicked men, sons of the devil, who, by means of very false ingenuity and wicked skill, corrupt foods with various poisons and medicines'.[72] Doubtless Agramont was just echoing the information that he had received from these trans-Pyrenean regions, but in doing so he also encouraged the charge against the minorities, especially since he ruled out the possibility that this kind of 'pestilence' could be identified with any 'universal pestilence' owing to a substantial change of the air. Shortly after he wrote his *Regiment*, the pogroms that were happening in these regions began to take place in Catalonia as well.[73]

According to Agramont the barony of Montpellier was one of the regions where these deliberate poisonings were occurring in 1348. The

---

[68] See note 37.

[69] Agramont, *Regiment*, p. 61.

[70] Paris masters, *Compendium*, pp. 82, 84. Alfonso de Córdoba, *Epistola*, p. 224.

[71] On this question see S. Guerchberg, 'La controverse sur les prétendus semeurs de la 'Peste Noire' d'après les traités de peste de l'époque', *Revue des Etudes Juives*, 108 (1948), 3–40; English translation: 'The controversy over the alleged sowers of the Black Death in the contemporary treatises on plague', in S. Thrupp (ed.), *Change in medieval society. Europe north of the Alps, 1050–1500* (London, 1965), pp. 208–24.

[72] Agramont, *Regiment*, p. 58: 'Per altra rahó pot venir mortaldat e pestilència en les gents, ço és a saber, per malvats hòmens fiylls del diable qui ab metzines e verins diverses corrompen les viandes ab molt fals engiynn e malvada maestria, ja sie ço que pròpriament parlan, aytal mortalitat de gents no és pestilència de la qual acì parlam, mas he.n volguda fer menció per ço car ara tenim temps en lo qual s'a[n] seguides moltes morts en alcunes regions prop d'acì axí como en Cobliure, en Carcassès, en Narbonès e en la baronia de Montpesler e a Avinyó e en tota Proença.'

[73] A. López de Meneses, 'Una consecuencia de la Peste Negra en Cataluña: el pogrom de 1348', *Sefarad*, 19 (1959), 92–131, 321–64.

epistola of Alfonso de Córdoba suggests that practitioners presumably close to the Montpellier university community were receptive to the idea that the 'pestilence' was in fact artificially provoked by wicked men. As has already been said, Alfonso de Córdoba distinguished three successive 'pestilences' within the year 1348, each being attributable to different causes, although it was the last one which actually concerned him. He denied that this one had been caused by 'any constellation, and thus it is not the result of any natural infection of the elements'; on the contrary, he attributed its origin to a practice or artifice which he described as deriving 'from the depths of an evil discovered through the most subtle practice of profound iniquity'. He added that against this artifice, which above all victimized Christians, the advice of 'learned physicians' was utterly useless.[74] He was referring to an artificial and deliberate infection of the air, which then passed through waters (mainly standing water) and affected foods, drink, and in general all life-giving things. Later in his work, with regard to the utility of some 'pestilential pills', Alfonso de Córdoba explained the way to produce this artificial pestilence and to infect any place with it:

... air can be infected by means of artifice, as when a preparation is made in a glass amphora. When this preparation is well fermented, whoever wishes to produce this evil [*illum malum*] will wait for a strong and steady wind coming from any world region. Then he will walk against the wind, and will put his amphora near a stony place opposite the city or town which he wishes to infect. Going back against the wind, so as not to be infected by the vapour, with the amphora neck covered up, he will throw the amphora with violence against the stones. As soon as the amphora is broken, the vapour will spread out and disperse in the air. Whoever is touched by this vapour will die very soon as if he were touched by the pestilential air.[75]

Thus, Alfonso de Córdoba was absolutely convinced that provoking the 'pestilence' artificially was possible at any time and place. The procedure he described consisted of a controlled diffusion of pestilential vapours which had been artificially made, and fermentation was the key process involved.

---

[74] Alfonso de Córdoba, *Epistola*, p. 224: 'Et est alia causa quam naturalis et propter hoc et propter compassionem fidelium, quae praecipue patiuntur, descripsi istam epistolam et regimen cum medicinis ne pii et boni tot periculis subiciiantur et sciant sibi praecavere de tantis periculis et malis imminentibus praecipue christianis in ista pestilentia. Ante omnia praecavendum est ab omni cibo et potu quae infici possunt et intoxicari ab aquis praecipue non fluentibus, quia ista potissime possunt infici. Experientia docuit quod ista pestilentia non vadit ex constellatione aliqua et per consequens nullam naturalem infectionem elementorum, sed vadit ex profundo malitiae per artificium subtilissimum profundae iniquitatis inventae, quare consilium sapientium medicorum non proficit nec iuvat illos detentos isto pessimo crudeli et pernicioso morbo ...' The idea of a primary infection of the air is not present here, but it is easily inferred from further paragraphs of the same work (see next footnote).

[75] Ibid., pp. 244–5: '... aer potest et infici per artificium, ut quando praeparetur quaedam confectio in amphora de vitriaco et quando fuerit illa confectio bene fermentata, ille qui illud malum velit facere, exspectat quando fuerit ventus fortis et lentus ab aliqua mundi plaga, tunc vadat contra ventum et locat amphoram suam iuxta lapides contra civitatem vel villam quam velit inficere et zona longa alligata recedendo contra ventum ne eum

Fermentation – the process as well as the idea – was a commonplace in the Western Middle Ages. Since time immemorial its empiric basis had been provided by the observation of facts well known to everyone. Around these facts various technologies developed, some of them as old as those of making wine, vinegar and cheese. The idea of fermentation came from the ancient world and spread throughout medieval Europe in at least two ways. On the one hand, the idea of metallurgical 'ferment' passed from ancient literature into the alchemy of the Arabs, and in the early fourteenth century into the Latin alchemical *corpus*. On the other hand, Aristotle doubtless had in mind a fermentative process when, in explaining the formation of the foetus, he compared analogically the formative role of semen upon the material basis of menstrual blood with the effect that rennet produces when acting upon milk. Albert the Great was expressing something very similar when he wrote that 'eggs grow into embryos because their wetness is like the wetness of yeast'.[76] Again, Avicenna applied the idea of 'fermentation' to pharmacology. He emphasized that each pharmacological compound contained not only the sum of the properties (*virtutes*) of the simples constituting it, but also other unique and specific properties that derived from its 'specific form' and which appeared as a result of a 'fermentation'. The 'specific form' of any compound could be learned only through experience. Avicenna also thought that the *virtus* of any fermented product became doubled, which implied that the intensity of its expected effect doubled too.[77]

Alfonso de Córdoba probably took this important idea from Avicenna, for as a result of his claimed status of 'master in liberal arts and medicine' he would have been well acquainted with Avicenna's pharmacological doctrine. Certainly, the traces of Avicennan thought in Alfonso's discussion are unmistakable. Nevertheless, this does not reduce the significance of this discussion occurring in mid fourteenth-century Europe: indeed, Alfonso de Córdoba was to my knowledge the only physician dealing at this time with such a question in a plague treatise. On the other hand, his remarks did not refer just to the poisoning of food and drink – perfectly possible, and in fact common at the time – but to that of the air on a large scale, and with the

inficeret vapor, trahat fortiter amphoram super lapides et amphora fracta se vapor effunditur et dispargitur in aere et quemcunque tetigerit ille vapor, ille morietur tanquam de aere pestilentico et citius'.

[76] J. Needham et al., *Science and civilisation in China*. Vol. V: *Chemistry and chemical technology. Part V: Spagyrical discovery and invention: apparatus, theories and gifts* (Cambridge, 1980), pp. 366–7.

[77] Avicenna, *Canon medicinae*, lib. v, Tractatus scientialis, De qualitate compositionis (Venice, 1527), fols. 391r–391v; Avicenna, *De viribus cordis*, tract. II, cap. IV (De differentibus laetificandi et confortandi repertis in medicinis) (in *Canon*, fol. 427v). Also see M. R. McVaugh, *Arnaldi de Villanova opera medica omnia*. Vol. II: *Aphorismi de gradibus* (Granada and Barcelona, 1975), pp. 18–19; J. M. Riddle and J. A. Mulholland, 'Albert on stones and minerals', in J. A. Weisheipl (ed.), *Albertus Magnus and the sciences. Commemorative essays 1980* (Toronto, 1980), pp. 203–34, at pp. 206, 208.

purpose of provoking a 'pestilence'. To his contemporaries, this view meant firstly a significant affirmation of human power over nature, since he stated that the natural conditions that caused a 'pestilence' could be reproduced through human artifice; secondly, the legitimation of natural philosophy as a useful instrument by which to attain this power over nature (this might explain why kings and other rulers were interested in alchemy, natural philosophy, and whatever other knowledge could be used by them as an instrument to get or to increase their political power). And, thirdly, it meant the possibility of using medical and natural philosophical knowledge in a double direction (good–evil): in order to achieve health and the public good, or to cause destruction and death. In addition, Alfonso de Córdoba's work could well provide a rational interpretative basis for the charge that Jews had caused the 'pestilence', since he mentioned the Christians as being its main victims and, when describing the artifice causing this 'pestilence', he made use of an aggressive tone including phrases like 'evil' and 'the most subtle practice of profound iniquity', which might be culturally significant among fourteenth-century Christians when referring to Jews.[78]

The immediate cause and the spread of the Black Death
Historians have often tended to consider the explanatory views on the diffusion of pestilence held by people in late medieval and early modern Europe in terms of two opposite sets of positions, which they have conceptualized as 'aerist' (also sometimes called 'miasmist') and 'contagionist' theories, the former imputing the spread of plague to the corruption of the air, the latter to spread by contact. According to these historiographic conceptions, university physicians were (generally speaking) more attached to aerist theories, while lay people were more concerned about contagion. Thus the new health measures emerging in Europe at the time would seem to have been promoted by the city health boards as a result of empirical experience which allowed the communities to establish more and more sophisticated and effective ways of preventing plague and other pestilences. University physicians usually turned away from these developments and supposedly maintained their loyalty to the ancient medical texts which held that the pestilence came from the air. This historiographical interpretation often includes the thesis that it was only through Girolamo Fracastoro's alleged theory of the 'living contagion' that in the second third of the sixteenth century university physicians fully integrated into their discourse the empirical assumptions lying behind the decisive health developments which the most advanced European communities had been putting into practice for a long time.[79]

[78] J. Arrizabalaga, L. García-Ballester and Ll. Cifuentes, '"Pestis manufacta": how to make plague by human artifice' (article in preparation).
[79] For a recent instance of this very common approach, see the otherwise excellent work by A. Carmichael, *Plague and the poor in Renaissance Florence* (Cambridge, 1986), particularly pp. 2, 3, 110–11, 112, 114, 128–31.

I assume that air spread and contagion can no longer be considered as opposite views of the diffusion of pestilence, but rather as referring to two successive stages of its dissemination, the air being in addition the place where pestilence is generated. Recently Vivian Nutton has shown that the idea of contagion was foreign neither to Galen nor to sixteenth-century Galenism, and that Fracastoro's merit consisted not in the alleged original-ity of his theory, but in his habit of systematizing the ideas on contagion contained in the Galenic works and reformulating them in the framework of sixteenth-century Galenism.[80] However, two major questions have not yet received an absolutely satisfactory answer: (1) how did university physicians deal with the concept of contagion during the late Middle Ages?; and (2) what relationship (if any) existed between university physi-cians and lay communities during this period, with respect to the concept and the avoidance of contagion? This brings us back to the standard causal system that we are following.

As said above, 'pestilence' could start when a substantial corruption occurred in the air as a result of the joint action between two groups of causes, celestial and terrestrial. According to Gentile da Foligno, this air corruption became apparent through 'perceptible corruptions' (corruptiones sensibiles) which could enter the human bodies in contact with this air through two main routes: (1) via the air inhaled through the respiratory tract, and (2) via the air perspired via the pores of the skin. While some bodies could resist the attack of this corruption, others could not (these individual differences, which were interpreted by means of the Galenic theory of the constitution, were unanimously recognized among late medieval university physicians).[81] When the 'perceptible corruptions' entered a susceptible body, a 'poisonous matter' was generated near the heart and the lung. This matter did not act by means of its qualities, but through its poisonousness – that is, through its specific property of being poisonous ('per proprietatem venenositatis'). Gentile explained how this 'poisonous matter', even when only a small amount, could eventually infect the whole body and, like Alfonso de Córdoba, he stressed the power of self-multiplication of this 'poison', which in contact with the 'humidities of our body' acted in the same way as other poisons, and turned what it touched into its similar so that it spread by continuity all around the body. When the poison reached and touched the heart, it turned it into poison, so that the vital spirit lying in the heart yielded to the poison form and

---

[80] V. Nutton, 'The seeds of disease: an explanation of contagion and infection from the Greeks to the Renaissance', Medical History, 27 (1983), 1–34; Nutton, 'The reception of Fracastoro's theory of contagion: the seed that fell among thorns?', Osiris, 6 (1990), 196–234.

[81] To these individual peculiarities which made some bodies resistant to the corruption and others liable to suffer damage Gentile dedicated five different dubia (nos. 5, 6, 10, 11, 12) plus one more (no. 9) to show 'why men die from the pestilence while oxen and other beasts do not'. See Gentile, Consilium, signats. c1v–c2v, c3r–c4r.

abandoned the heart, leaving it and the body without movement – that is, dead.[82] Agramont, who did not mention this poisonous matter, gave an alternative explanation of how corruption spread through the human body. According to him, after the 'corrupt and putrid air' had gone straight into the heart, it rotted both the arterial blood, which was engendered in the cells of the heart, and the vital spirits; this rotten blood, which corrupted and decayed the rest of the blood by its presence, then passed via the arteries to the other parts of the body.[83] In one way or another, all three (Gentile da Foligno, Alfonso de Córdoba, and Jacme d'Agramont) seem to have resorted to the theory of the 'multiplication of species' to explain how corruption spread into bodies.[84]

Gentile's idea that the cause of *pestilentia* was a 'poisonous matter' generated near the heart and the lung as a result of pestilential air was far from being widely accepted at the time. Most of the physicians studied here seem to have ignored it; Giovanni della Penna even denied it. He claimed, by contrast, that the 'pestilence' affected only those individuals whose choleric matter had become too heated and corrupted. Thus, it was their personal constitution that eventually made it possible for the 'pestilence' to take root in their 'choleric matter'.[85] To some extent, della Penna's view could be identified with what Agramont called 'pestilence' caused by air overheating[86] – a qualitative air change which we will deal with later on.

The 'poisonous vapours' shed by the infected body, according to Gentile da Foligno, were communicated to others through the breath and the skin. As a result, the 'pestilence' spread rapidly by means of contagion ('per contagionem'), passing from one person to another and from one place to

---

[82] Gentile, *Consilium*, signats. c4r–c4v: '[Quomodo aer infectus a corde trahitur] ... hoc contingit ex multitudine veneni vel aeris venenosi pestilentialis que se ipsa multiplicat inficiendo humiditates nostri corporis qua venenositate multiplicata augetur illa mala qualitas. Nam, ut dicitur in geometria, quantitas augmentat virtutem. Unde ex modico veneno assumpto convertente quod tangit ad suum simile augetur virtus et multiplicatur, ita quod de facili per modum continui corporis extrema se tangunt, et attingit parum in quantitate venenum ipsum cor, et quod contagit convertit ad venenum, et ex eo tunc spiritus vitalis non habens debitum organum in quo resideat cedit forme veneni, et egrediens de corde dimittit cor et corpus sine motu et hec est mors, cuius signum est, ut ait Conciliator, si tale comedatur efficitur venenum comedenti.'

[83] Agramont, *Regiment*, p. 74: 'Encara més, aquest àer corromput e podrit, alendan e respiran entre sens tot migà al cor. Per què podrix e corromp la sanch arterial que.s fa e s'engendre dins les çelles del cor. Corromp encara e podrix los espirits vitals, lo qual sanch corrumput va del cor per les venes que polsen, les quals són apelades artèries, als altres membres. E la damontdita putrefacció ho corrupció de sanch per vicinitat corromp e podrix l'altre sanch.'

[84] On the theory of the 'multiplication of species', see A. C. Crombie, *Robert Grosseteste and the origins of experimental science, 1100–1700* (Oxford, 1953), pp. 86, 109–10, 112, 114–15, 117–18, 137–8, 140, 144–9, passim; D. C. Lindberg, *Theories of vision from Al-Kindi to Kepler* (Chicago and London, 1976), pp. 19, 98, 113–16, 223, 254–5, passim; and also the bibliography given by these authors.

[85] Penna, *Consilium*, pp. 341–2.

[86] Agramont, *Regiment*, p. 72.

another.[87] At this point Gentile echoed two significant Galenic paragraphs taken from De differentiis febrium: the first referred to 'certain seeds of the pestilence' which were thrown off from the pestilent body into the surrounding air through the two routes mentioned above; the second talked about the 'remains of warmth' which were present in the air long after the 'pestilence' had gone, and which infected like a 'ferment' in a bread oven.[88]

Most of the medical doctors who wrote on the 'pestilence' of 1348 seem to have distinguished a major and a minor level of dissemination, the former consisting of transmission between different places, the latter involving interpersonal transmission. With respect to transmission from one place to another, Agramont – seemingly the most explicit in this respect – accepted up to three different reasons for the spread of 'pestilence': (1) because of contiguity; (2) because of eating wheat and other foods coming from a 'pestilential region'; and (3) because of winds.[89]

The interpersonal transmission of plague was dealt with in all the works studied here. In brief, they seem to have taken into consideration three different avenues of transmission: breath, skin perspiratio, and gaze. On the first two of these something has already been said with regard to Gentile's views. Agramont said that 'association with a sufferer from a pestilential disease' ('participació ab malalt de malaltia pestilencial') caused this disease to be communicated from one person to another, and so on 'like a wild fire' unless God protected one against it with His grace. After having listed several diseases transmitted in this way, the Catalan master ended by stressing that in general terms 'every disease that originates from pestilence in the air' was liable to be communicated from one person to another.[90] However, he added, in agreement with the Galenic theory of the constitution, that individual differences in temperament and way of life caused some people to catch a disease and other people not to catch it, and some to catch it more easily and sooner than others. Thus, the people more likely to contract a pestilential disease were those who (1) had in their bodies a superabundance of humours, particularly if these were corrupted and rotten; (2) had eaten and drunk too much during the previous year; (3) had too many sexual relationships with women; and (4) had enlarged body

---

[87] Gentile, Consilium, signat. a2r.
[88] Ibid., signat. a3v: 'Inquit [Galenus] enim [?] circundantem nos aerem inferri quedam pestilentie semina'; idem, signat. a3r: 'Manent enim reliquie caliditatis, ut in clibano, que velut fermentum inficiunt . . .'
[89] Agramont, Regiment, pp. 53–4.
[90] Ibid., p. 65: 'Altra rahó [de pestilència particular] és participació ab malalt de malaltia pestilencial, car d'u se pega en altre axí com a foch salvatge e d'aquell en altre. E axí s'estén als altres si Déus misericordiós no y tramet la sua sancta gràcia. E si algú me demane quals són les malalties que.s peguen d'u en altre, dich que aquellas són axí com lebrositat ho meseleria e roynna e tisiguea e lagaynna, febre pestilencial, pigota e sarampió e tiynna. E universalment tota malaltia que.s fa per pestilència de l'àer.'

pores, either by nature or artificially (due to the effects of baths).[91] Similar views were held by the other physicians studied here. The Paris masters, for example, considered that among others who were particularly susceptible to the pestilence were those who were hot and humid, those who had many bad humours and were constipated, and those following a bad regime.[92]

The anonymous practitioner of Montpellier, whose ideas echoed Agramont's, insisted on the high risk to all those present of massive interpersonal transmission of pestilence through the effect of the breath of sufferers dying from the *epidemia*.[93] On the other hand, he was the only one who referred to the gaze as another mode of interpersonal transmission. He perceived this mode of transmission as extremely dangerous:

However, the most virulent moment of this *epidemia*, which causes an almost sudden death, is when the air spirit emitted from the sick person's eyes, particularly when he is dying, strikes the eye of a healthy man nearby who looks closely at him; then the poisonous nature of this member [the eye] passes from one to another, killing the healthy individual.[94]

The Montpellier practitioner explained the harmful influence of a dying patient by appealing to the authority of Euclid. Actually, he referred to the pseudo-Euclidean book entitled *Catoptrica*. The Montepellier practitioner claimed that Euclid could naturally set on fire buildings, houses, army camps and trees by means of his well-known burning mirrors.[95] Something analogous to this happened, according to the Montpellier practitioner, when the *epidemia* was transmitted through the gaze of a dying patient. When the poisonous humidity of the 'epidemic' had ascended to the patient's brain, sometimes it was expelled through the optical nerves up to the eyes. There the first windiness generated received the surprising property of continuously producing a toxic spirit that looked for a place of any nature in which to rest. If a healthy person then looked at this invisible spirit, he would receive an impression of the pestilential disease. This impression was stronger than that provoked by the inhalation of a sick

---

[91] Ibid., pp. 65–6.

[92] Paris masters, *Compendium*, pp. 90, 92.

[93] Practicus, *Tractatus*, p. 72: 'Cum igitur haec epidemia secundum aliquos habeat solo aere, solo flatu, sola conversatione contra aegros, plures occidere dicunt, quod aere inspirato infirmis et a sanis circumstantibus aspirato, ipsos laedi et necari maxime illo tunc quando sunt in agone; sed non subito, sed per intervallum, et paulatim illa necatio posset esse.'

[94] Ibid., pp. 72–3: '... sed major fortitudo hujus epidemiae, et quasi subito interficiens, est quando spiritus aerius egrediens ab oculis aegroti repercusserit ad oculum sani hominis circumstantis, et ipsum aegrum respicientis, maxime quando sunt in agone: tunc enim illa natura venenosa illius membri transit de una in alia, occidendo alium'.

[95] Ibid., p. 73. The *Catoptrica*, which in fact contains a mixture of Euclidean and post-Euclidean theory, was compiled by Theon of Alexandria (fl. second half of the fourth century). The Byzantine Neoplatonist Proclus (fifth century) is generally blamed for the misattribution to Euclid. See C. C. Gillispie (ed.), *Dictionary of scientific biography*, 16 vols. (New York, 1970–1980), vol. IV, p. 430; vol. XIII, pp. 322–3.

man's breath, 'since this diaphanous poison [penetrates] deeply faster than thick air does'.[96] Two additional analogies were suggested by the Montpellier practitioner to illustrate how the poison could act through the gaze of someone infected with the plague: that of the mythological animal called the basilisk, and that of the so-called 'Venomous Virgin'. The story of the basilisk, which dates back at least to Pliny, had a long written tradition in ancient and medieval Western culture. In the thirteenth century the analogy between the gaze of the basilisk and that of a menstruating woman became widespread through the *De secretis mulierum* by pseudo-Albert the Great; these and other elements appeared together in a well-known story, that of the 'Venomous Virgin', which spread all over Europe at the end of the century, and which was one of the most important examples of the gynophobic tradition in the Middle Ages.[97] The analogy that the Montpellier practitioner drew between the gaze of a patient dying from the 'pestilence' and the maleficent gaze of the 'Venomous Virgin' reveals how seriously he considered this manner of 'pestilence' transmission.

The signs

Most of the late medieval and early modern medical works concerning plague and pestilences referred to two kinds of signs or signals: those announcing the coming of the disaster, and those revealing its presence at a particular place and time. Both of these were phenomena observable in the natural environment – but while the former were used to forecast the outbreak of a pestilence at a certain place in a more or less close future, the latter were used to establish the presence *de facto* of the pestilence.

While the Paris masters and Gentile da Foligno referred to these signs to a greater or lesser extent,[98] it was Agramont who dealt most with this question.[99] After stating that he did not consider it necessary to deal with the signs of a pestilence due to a qualitative change in the air 'because they are clear and manifest to all those who can distinguish the difference between hot and cold', he systematically referred to the signals of a pestilence due to a substantial corruption in the air. Concerning the signs or signals announcing the imminent arrival of the pestilence, Agramont affirmed that the causes that gave rise to pestilence were also signs of the

[96] Ibid., p. 75: 'et aliquando cerebrum expellit hanc ventosam et venenosam materiam, per nervos opticos, concavos ad oculos, et tunc aeger est in agone, tenens oculos quasi non possent moveri de loco ad locum, et ibi prima ventositas recipit proprietatem mirabilem, quae sic stans et permanens, continuo fit spiritus ille toxicus, et quaerit habitaculum in aliqua natura in quam possit intrare, et quiescere. Et quem spiritum visibilem si quis sanus aspexerit, suscipit impressionem morbi pestilentialis, et intoxicatur homo citius quam aere aegroti abstracto, quod illud venenum diaphanum citius in profundo quam aer grossus.'

[97] Ibid., pp. 75–6. On both stories and their transmission, see Jacquart and Thomasset, *Sexuality*, pp. 74–6, 191–2, 211–12, 232.

[98] Paris masters, *Compendium*, pp. 84, 86, 88, 90; Gentile, *Consilium*, signat. c3r.

[99] Agramont, *Regiment*, pp. 69–72.

pestilence itself since 'all the things that produce the pestilence in the air and in the people can be called signs, whether they be constellations or winds or other things'. Nevertheless, the Paris masters warned that 'the constellations and other celestial causes of pestilence, as well as astrologers' judgements according to Ptolemy, have to be placed between the necessary and the possible'.[100]

Among the signs announcing the coming of the pestilence Agramont stressed what he called the 'inflammations [fiery bodies?] appearing in the sky', some of which were apparently fixed, like the 'comal star' (*estela comada*), while others were mobile and of several kinds according to their shape and size. Among the latter he referred to a very large one called *drach* (flying dragon?), such as

the one seen in Lerida by many notable persons worthy of belief in the year 1345 on the last day of February just before sunrise. Its width was larger than a great shaft of a lance, and according to trustworthy estimates it was twenty lance-lengths long. And it had greater brilliancy than any lamp. So there was great fright among all who saw it.[101]

These 'inflammations' were more or less frequent in accordance with the 'multitude of exhalations from the earth into the regions of the air as a result of the virtues of both the sun and the conjunctions of some planets'.[102] However, Agramont did not rule out that God might sometimes, because of the evil conduct of people, 'have sent the fire from the sky, or created it anew from the earth so that it would burn and destroy all those people'.[103]

Concerning the signs revealing pestilence already present in the air, Agramont enumerated several kinds of signs, all of which consisted of abnormal phenomena in the natural world. Some of them were in the air itself, as when there was cloudiness in the air the whole air was filled with dust, or it had no colour and yet it seemed as if it were yellow or greenish. Others were unusual changes in the vegetable and animal world, as when fruit was blighted, or the grain harvest would not keep and had a strange smell. Certain beasts – snakes, lizards, other reptiles, and frogs – were present in abundance and came forth from the corners of the earth, and from the water more than usual; birds fled from their nests and abandoned their eggs.[104] Some of these changes in animal behaviour were used by Gentile da Foligno to determine whether the pestilence was to be attributed to superior or inferior causes: for example, when worms and snakes came

---

[100] Paris masters, *Compendium*, pp. 86, 88.
[101] Agramont, *Regiment*, p. 69.
[102] Ibid., p. 70.
[103] Ibid., p. 70: 'Emperò no contrast que Déus tot poderós per la malvestat de les gents d'aquella no pogués aver tramès foch del cel ho creat de nou en la terra qui cremàs e dissipàs tota aquella gent ...'
[104] Ibid., p. 71.

out of the earth, and birds escaped to high places, then the causes of pestilence were inferior.[105] Finally, according to Agramont, in such a time diseases were very deceptive and many pestilential fevers prevailed, accompanied by 'bad tumours and apostemata, such as anthraces or *mala busaynna*, "smallpox" and worms, and other malignant maladies'.[106] According to him, the development and multiplication of these fevers and such accompanying maladies were the most decisive signs indicating that there was putrefaction and corruption in the substance of the air. (Later, when dealing with the prevention of the Black Death, I will explore how Agramont, like any Galenist physician, considered stink as a sure sign of putrefaction.)

The effects

In looking at how the Black Death of 1348 was perceived by university medical practitioners in Latin Mediterranean Europe, I have already pointed out that to Jacme d'Agramont, as to the Montpellier practitioner (and to some extent also to Gentile da Foligno), the 'pestilence' was the air change in itself, not its consequences. Agramont distinguished between 'moral' and 'natural' pestilence, each of which caused the outbreak of a number of effects. The 'moral pestilence', which he did not deal with, provoked enmities, rancours, wars, robberies, destructions of places and deaths; the 'natural' one caused corruptions, sudden deaths and various diseases, among which Agramont mentioned as typical of the 'time of epidemic or pestilence' ('temps de epidímia ho de pestilència') various pestilential fevers, tumours, apostemata under the armpits, in the groin and in other parts of the human body, *pigota* ('smallpox'), worms, and other very dangerous and mortal malignant diseases.[107]

Agramont dedicated the fourth section of his *Regiment* to a detailed discussion of the effects of the *àer pestilencial* as well as to the way in which these were generated.[108] Ostensibly, most of these effects were also mentioned by him as signs revealing pestilence already present in the air, but he did not make this relationship explicit. The effects varied according to whether the air was pestilential in its qualities or in its substance. In both cases not only human bodies were affected but also vegetables (plants and trees in the qualitative change, grains and fruits in the substantial one). In

---

[105] Gentile, *Consilium*, signat. c3r.

[106] Agramont, *Regiment*, p. 71: :'... males exidures e apostemacions, axí com àntrachs ho mala busaynna, pigota e cuchs e altres malvades malalties'.

[107] Ibid., pp. 51–2: '... no.s deu negun hom maraveyllar si l'àer a vegades és rahó que les gents muyren sobtanament, ho que diverses febres pestilencials regnen, ho exidures, ho apostemacions se facen sots la exella ho en l'angonal ho en altres lochs, ho que regne pigota ho cuchs ho altres males malauties fort periylloses e mortals. E aytal temps pot ésser dit temps de epidímia ho de pestilència'.

[108] Ibid., pp. 72–4.

the first case all the effects derived from changes in the qualities of cold and heat, presumably the pair whose alterations were most evident. Thus, overheating made cholera burn and 'dominate the remaining humours', as a result of which 'every disease generating itself from cholera' could happen.[109] And overcooling could provoke 'apoplexy, which is an apostema of the brain', 'epilepsy' or 'falling sickness', 'paralysis, and twisting of the face, the eyes, and the mouth' – and death, if it were extreme.[110] On the other hand, air pestilential in its substance could cause several diseases, although in all of them there was 'always continuous fever of one or more humours according to the manner in which these humours receive the impression or putrefaction of the pestilential air'. When blood rotted within the substance of the heart, it generated a heart *apostema* which was sometimes transmitted by nature to the armpits, where it eventually reproduced. On other occasions an *apostema* appeared in the liver, from which it could travel to the groin. When rotten blood bubbled like must, it could generate *pigota e sarampió* (smallpox and measles). Lastly, when the humour most affected by putrefaction was phlegm, 'worms' (*cuchs*) of different kinds were generated.[111] Without explicitly mentioning the *apostema* (although this can be inferred), Gentile da Foligno briefly referred to the back of the ears, the left armpit, and the right groin as the usual places where 'signs' (*signum*) appear indicating 'lesion' of the three principal members – brain, heart and liver – which were the seats of the three souls in Greek-based natural philosophy.[112] I will return to this question later on in dealing with the theory of the emunctories.

In contrast to Agramont's sophisticated classification of the effects of pestilence, the Montpellier practitioner epitomized them in just one general effect: the sudden death of living beings.[113] Nevertheless, the more clinical character of Agramont's work does not mean that death was not also for him the pestilence effect of greater concern. It could not be otherwise since pestilence was now, as we have already seen, nearly synonymous with death. In addition, as Agramont stressed at the very beginning of his *Regiment* when explaining why he had written it, 'while all death is universally held very terrible, sudden death [like that caused by the *pestilència*] is particularly dangerous, especially to the soul', and 'still more terrible when it is also accompanied by very terrible accidents'.[114] Hence, the high risk which the people of Lerida faced was not only that of a

[109] Ibid., p. 72.
[110] Ibid., p. 73.
[111] Ibid., p. 74.
[112] Gentile, *Consilium*, signat. a2v: 'Et pro evidentia nota quod cum leditur cor, signum apparet sub ascella sinistra, aut cerebrum post aures, quando epar in inguine dextro'.
[113] Practicus, *Tractatus*, p. 71 (see note 24).
[114] Agramont, *Regiment*, p. 47: 'E ja sie açò que universalment tota mort sie molt terrible, emperò mort sobtana és molt periyllosa specialment quant a la ànima. Es encara molt terrible en aytant com la acompaynnen molt terribles accidents.'

terrible disease almost certain to bring about death in very dramatic conditions, but also that of eternal condemnation as a result of a quick death without spiritual relief.

However, the likelihood of death frequently carried with it the necessity to determine whether in doubtful cases it had indeed occurred. Agramont did not neglect this question. In mentioning *apoplexia* – which he identified with brain *apostema* – as one of the effects of a pestilential air by overcooling, he said that it brought about a 'sudden loss of movement and of feeling which renders men so inert that one can hardly know, either by the pulse or by the breath, whether they are dead or living'.[115] For this purpose he suggested to the readers of the *Regiment* two simple proofs that he agreed to describe in detail only because of his urge to serve the common good. The first one consisted of observing whether a very thin shred of wool, held near the nostrils or the mouth of someone supposedly deceased, moves as a result of the air passing in and out with the breath. The second consisted of seeing whether water in a glass put on the chest near the heart moves as a result of the heartbeat.[116] Agramont insisted that this question was not at all trivial now, for 'it is certain that many men and women who suffer from this disease [*apoplexia*] are thought to be dead by the common people and many are buried alive'. Therefore, it was advisable that 'all those who are subject suddenly to such accident [sudden death] be carefully watched and examined by physicians before they are buried'. Failing this, Agramont recommended that, in accord with Avicenna's counsel, a period of seventy-two hours be allowed to elapse before the burial of the deceased.[117]

REACTIONS TO THE BLACK DEATH

To all the physicians whose works have been studied here the prevention and cure of the pestilence and of its effects were not only desirable, but also possible. The most evident of their alleged motivations in pursuing both goals was their desire to promote the common good. In this section I will concentrate on those who dealt at greatest length with the prevention and cure of the pestilence – namely Jacme d'Agramont, Gentile da Foligno and

---

[115] Ibid., p. 73.

[116] Ibid., p. 73: 'Per què a provar si són morts ho vius pren hom .1. floch de lana fort prima e fort sobtil e pose-la'ls hom prop los forats del nas ho a la bocha e si poch ni molt alenden, la lana se mou per l'àer que ix e entre per los forats del nas e de la bocha. Encara.n fa hom altra prova, ço és a saber, que.ls pose hom un gubell plen vertent d'aygua sobre.l pits, endret lo cor. E si per aventura lo cor ha degun moviment, veu hom moure l'aygua. E si per aventura no.s mou, liurar pots lo pacient als capelans.'

[117] Ibid., p. 73: 'E ja sie açò que posar aquests seynals, sie exir de nostre propòsit, emperò jo.ls é volgut posar per proffit comú. Car çert so que mols hòmens e moltes dones a qui esdevé aquesta malautia se cuyden los vulgàs que sien morts e molts ne sotarren qui són vius. Per què conseyllaria que aytals a qui ve aytal accident soptosament ffossen guardats e esprovats per bons metges diligentment enans que hom los soterràs. Ho que hi fos observat almeyns lo conseyll d'Avicenna qui vol que aytals sien esperats a soterrar almenys per LXX e dues hores que són III dies naturals entegres e complits.'

the Paris masters – all of whom were at one in stressing at the very beginning of their works that they were pursuing this aim.

In fact, Agramont, after indicating that he had written his epistle as a sign of gratitude towards the city and citizens who had so much honoured and benefited him, stated that with the help of his scanty knowledge, he wished 'to get and to secure some benefit, and to avoid every damage to the above-mentioned city [Lerida] and to its individuals, with the aim of preventing men and women from getting sick during the pestilential times'.[118] He added that he had written his *Regiment* 'for the benefit of the people, not for the instruction of physicians',[119] and concluded his declaration of intentions by asking the town councillors of Lerida to distribute a copy of his work to everyone wanting it since 'it has been written for common and public utility'.[120] Similarly, Gentile da Foligno stated in the foreword of his major *Consilium* that he had written it 'to preserve and to honour this university [that of Perugia], moved by affection as much as by the praise of many citizens', and later added: 'All that I know about his problem, I have written down in this "counsel" [*consilio*] for the common benefit of all.'[121] The Paris masters, on the other hand, indicated that they had written their *compendium* about the causes of, and the best remedies for, the 'epidemic', because of their obedience to the royal authority of Philip VI of France – although they were 'equally desirous of serving the common good'.[122]

The question of the common good – that is, the responsibility of every organized society to supply all of its members with what they need for their welfare and happiness as citizens – had already been formulated long before by Aristotle in his *Politics*. It was taken up again and developed by scholastic philosophers, particularly by Thomas of Aquinas, who affirmed that every human society had two kinds of aims that were not at all incompatible,

---

[118] Agramont, *Regiment*, pp. 47–8: '... volén da ma pocha sciència fer e procurar alcun profit e esquivar tot damnatge a la ciutat damont dita e als singulars d'aquella, per preservar cascú e cascuna d'esser malaut ho malauta per temps pestilencial'.

[119] Ibid., p. 48: '... car lo tractat aquest es feyt principalment a profit del poble e no a instrucció dels metges ...'.

[120] Ibid., p. 48: 'E com lo damontdit tractat, segons que ja he dit, sie feyt a utilitat comuna e publica, plàcie-us, seynnors, de donar-ne treslat a tot hom qui.n vuylle còpia'.

[121] Gentile, *Consilium*, signat. a1r: 'Ymo in tantum quidem ex eius malicia pestilentie ad preservationem, et tutellam, ac honorem huius alme universitatis, tam ex affectione quam multorum civium precatu me ad ipsorum precepta paratum redidi. Et que in re ipsa sentiam, in communi utilitate omnium hoc consilio redigam.'

[122] Paris masters, *Compendium*, pp. 70, 72: 'Verum, quia ex ipsorum declaratione adhuc plurima dubitationis materia exurgebat, idcirco nos omnes et singuli Magistri de Collegio Facultatis medicorum Parisius, ad mandatum Illustrissimi Principis et domini nostri serenissimi domini Philippi, Francorum Regis, incitati, utilitati etiam publice intendere cupientes, causas epidimie universales et remotas, particulares et propinquas, necnon et salubriora remedia, quantum ipsius rei natura humano intellectui se subjicit, clarissimorum philosophorum antiquorum dictis, ac etiam modernorum sapientum, tam astronomorum quam medicorum, certioribus sententiis utentes, Deo nobis ministrante, proposuimus sub brevi compendio declarare.'

namely, its own or natural aims, and spiritual ones. An adequate relationship between the common good and the supreme good had always to be sought so that neither need be sacrificed to the other.[123] In the thirteenth century the common good emerged throughout Europe as a social value of increasing importance. In addition, in the late thirteenth century, and during the fourteenth century, health came to be considered a public value.[124] It cannot be surprising, then, that the common good of preserving the citizens from the pestilence, and of curing it, was the leitmotiv for the three physicians mentioned above.

As was usual in later medieval Galenism, the practical section of all the works studied here included a preventive regime, and following it a curative one (though the latter is not always present). Intentional reasons rather than epistemological ones explain the absence of the latter element in Agramont's *Regiment*. As we have seen, his purpose was the benefit of the people, not the instruction of physicians. To the Catalan master, his *Regiment* offered all his fellow citizens adequate information to keep them from falling ill during the pestilential time. He insisted that all the measures he suggested could be safely followed without medical help, which was not possible in the case of a curative regime.[125] Thus indirectly Agramont was affirming that the cure of pestilence belonged only to physicians. Apparently, Agramont's was the only medical work written on the occasion of the Black Death of 1348 that was addressed to the general citizenry. Apart from the *Compendium* that the medical masters of the University of Paris wrote for the King of France, the other works studied here seem to have had as their primary addressees other medical professionals, although natural philosophers and other members of the university elites were also potential readers. The existence of all these works, and many other contemporary ones devoted to the plague of 1348, has an obvious significance which need not be underlined here, although it may at least be formulated: it reveals that scholastic medicine responded – and did so quite unanimously, in different geographical areas – to the challenge presented by the outbreak of a catastrophical disease. Otherwise, it is not possible to understand how Gentile could suggest in the minor *Consilium* that he addressed

---

[123] Thomas of Aquinas, *De regimine principum*, lib. I, cap. I and 14, in L. Carbonero y Sol, *El gobierno monárquico, o sea el libro 'De regimine principum', escrito por Santo Tomás de Aquino. Texto latino y traducción castellana* (Seville, 1861), pp. 2–13, 85–93; Thomas of Aquinas, *Summa Theologiae*, I–II, q. 90, art. 2 and 3, q. 92, art. I; I–II, q. 39, art. 2, q. 47, art. 10, q. 58, art. 5, q. 61, art. I (Madrid, 1951–2), vol. II, pp. 612–14, 622–4, vol. III, pp. 280–2, 332–3, 393–4, 414–15.

[124] L. García-Ballester, 'Changes in the *Regimina sanitatis*: the role of the Jewish physicians', in Sheila Campbell, Bert Hall and David Klausner (eds.), *Health, disease and healing in medieval culture* (Basingstoke and London, 1992), pp. 119–131.

[125] Agramont, *Regiment*, p. 48: 'E de regiment de preservació pot tot hom usar ab aquest present tractat sens de metge, sens tot periyll. Mas lo regiment de curació és apropriat al metge en lo qual cascú sens de la art medicina porie leugeramant errar. Perquè a esquivar aquest periyll, del regiment damontdit no he volgut fer menció'.

to the College of Physicians of Perugia, that 'the college should advise landlords to designate some good men to meet with physicians, and to follow their instructions in order to make the necessary arrangements for preserving the health of people in the city'.[126]

But, beyond this general conclusion, the Paris masters' and Agramont's works allow us to estimate to what degree university medicine had spread and achieved social prestige in mid fourteenth-century Latin Europe. In the one case the lecturers at the medical faculty of Paris responded as an expert group to the request for a report about plague, its causes and its remedies, made by the King of France. In the other, a medical master at the University of Lerida communicated to the town councillors of the city all the practical knowledge that they could use to keep people safe from the threatening pestilence. Agramont's *Regiment* represents a noticeable effort to spread, beyond the limits of a circle of initiates, a new medical knowledge structured according to scholastic medicine and natural philosophy, and full of abstruse technical terms. He made this popularizing effort (which to the best of my knowledge was novel at that time), by means of both translating this new knowledge into the vernacular of his fellow citizens, and putting the conceptually and formally complex language of scholastic medicine and natural philosophy into a simple and direct form.[127]

The preventive and curative measures that these authors proposed were determined by three major elements: namely, their conceptions of the causes of the plague; the limits placed on their activities by the existence of other professions concerned with human diseases, particularly priests; and – in the case of Agramont – his already mentioned purpose of benefiting ordinary people, rather than of instructing physicians. With respect to the second element it is important to stress that the measures proposed by physicians were concerned only with the care of the body, as was clearly established by Gentile when he entitled the preventive chapter of his major *Consilium*, 'Regime to preserve bodies from the pestilential air, with the addition of some special remedies'.[128] Doubtless the regime of the soul was also present in the minds of all late medieval Christian physicians, and its adequate care was a *conditio sine qua non* in order for every regime of the

---

[126] Gentile, 'Consilium in epidemia Perusii', in *Consilia* [Pavia, 1488], signat. g2r: 'Consulitur autem per collegium [magistrorum de Perusio], quod domini terrarum ordinent aliquos bonos homines qui coloquia habeant cum medicis, et secundum eorum ordinationem disponant civitatem in quantum pertinet ad sanitatem hominum'. In Sudhoff's edition: 'dominus, cui cura est de ipso, ordinet', instead of 'domini ... ordinent'; 'informationes', instead of 'ordinationem'; and 'securitatem', instead of 'sanitatem' (see Sudhoff, 'Pestschriften', 5 (1911–12), 86).

[127] On the use of technical terms in works written by and addressed to laymen, see the documents mentioned in notes 17 and 20, above. Part of the ideas expressed here are the result of talks with Luis García-Ballester (who is working with Michael McVaugh on this topic), and have not yet been published. See the Introduction to this volume

[128] Gentile, *Consilium*, signat. a2v: 'Capitulum secundum. Regimen corporum preservandorum ab aere pestilentiali narrat quasdam medicinas speciales addendo.'

body to have the desired effect, although it was not their job but that of the Church. (I have already mentioned that 140 years after his death Gentile was accused by a bishop of Foligno of having taken into account only the health of bodies and the preservation of lives, but not the health of souls.)[129] If, as we have seen, Agramont stressed the question of sudden death, it was only because the high risk of dying without spiritual assistance required a medical expert to give his opinion on this contingency, not because the physician was there to give such assistance.

A new nuance was given to this question when the possibility that epidemics came directly from the divine will was contemplated, as it was by Jacme d'Agramont and the Paris masters. What attitude did the physician take in this case? When this happens, the Paris masters said (as we have seen), 'there is no more advice than to humbly praise Him, although even in such a case medical advice must not be absolutely ignored'.[130] It seems that, although they were respectful toward their God, the Paris masters were not prepared to renounce their monopolistic practice over human physical health, even when the *pestilentia* had been caused by Him. They defended their position through an argument taken from Ecclesiasticus (38: 1–15) – a Biblical book whose authority was often resorted to by late medieval physicians to justify their profession: God created medicine, and He is the only one able to cure us, but He has not forgotten to teach God-fearing people the true art of curing.[131] In contrast to the Paris masters, Agramont emphatically affirmed that 'if corruption or putrefaction of the air is due to our sins or faults the remedies of the medical art are useless, since only He who tied can untie'. To this Catalan master, to whom invocations to the saints were also useless in this case, the best remedy was to recognize, to repent, and to confess our sins before the holy Roman Church and its representatives, as well as to do penance.[132]

---

[129] See note 46.

[130] See note 47.

[131] Paris masters, *Compendium*, p. 92: 'Altissimus enim de terra creavit medicinam; unde sanat solus langores Deus qui de fragilitatis solo producit in largitate sua medicinam. Benedictus Deus, gloriosus et excelsus qui, auxiliari non desinens, certam curandi doctrinam timentibus explicavit'. Gentile da Foligno started his major *Consilium* with a very similar discussion (Gentile, *Consilium*, signat. a1r) (for quotation see note 44).

[132] Agramont, *Regiment*, pp. 78–9; '... car si la corrupció ho putreffacció de l'àer és venguda per nostres peccats ho per nostres mèrits poch valen en aquest cas los remeys de la art de medicina, car aquell qui ligue ha a desligar. E a açò a confermar se pot enduyr.I. test de la Sancta Escriptura, lo qual és estat allegat dessús en lo segon article lo qual és escrit *Deuteronomii, XXVIII capitulo*, honse die axí: "*Percutiat te Dominus ulcere Egipti et partem corporis, per quam stercora egeruntur, scabie quoque prurrigine, ita ut curari nequeas*".

Diu-se encara vulgarment que can Déus no vol, sants no poden, car no és degú que a la mà ni al poder de Déu pugue contrastar. Emperò lo major remey que en aquest cas podem aver, si és que regonegam nostres pecats e nostres deffalliments avén cordial contricció e vocal confessió d'obra e de feyt, satisfacció a Déu per verdadera penitència e ab lo prohisme, retén e donan a quascú, ço del seu, lo qual regiment nos fo figurat *Regnum .III., capitulo octavo*, hon se diu axí: "*ffames si aborta fuerit in terra . . . si quis cognoverit plagam cordis sui*", (habendo veram contriccionem) "*et expanderit manus suas in domo hac*" (hoc est habendo recursum ad sacrosanctam Romanam Ecclesiam et ad eius vicarios humiliter petendo veniam de obmissis) "*Tu exaudies in celo . . . super faciem terre quam dedisti patribus nostris*".'

Prevention

All the preventive measures against pestilence suggested by the physicians studied here were structured around the six non-naturals (*sex res non naturales*). This is not surprising when we consider that the work that was the source of this topic, the *Isagoge* of Johannitius, had a wide diffusion in late medieval Europe. In fact, the *Isagoge* was a constant component of the *Articella*, which constituted the basis of medieval medical teaching after the thirteenth century. It is interesting that Agramont, in accordance with his distinction between 'air pestilential in its qualities' and 'in its substance', developed two parallel preventive regimes with two different lines of advice about the six non-naturals.[133]

Given that to all these physicians the immediate origin of the pestilence lay in the air, this element which constituted the first non-natural was the first priority in their preventive measures, followed by those concerning the remaining five non-naturals. In order to strengthen the effect of these measures all the authors suggested adding certain medicines, and even practising phlebotomy. The place where these enhancing measures appear in the works being studied here varies widely: sometimes they are discussed along with the six non-naturals, and sometimes in a separate section. However, for the sake of convenience, I will study first the measures concerning the six non-naturals and then those reinforcing them.

The six non-naturals (*sex res non naturales*)

It is easily observable in all the medical works studied here that the adequate management of the six non-naturals exerted an almost hegemonic control over the life-regime specified by physicians to preserve individuals from the pestilence. It is also evident that in all of them the concept of the 'middle term' (*mesotes*), which was spread into the medieval world by Aristotle's *Nichomachean Ethics*, dominated the six non-naturals. This Aristotelian concept was applied as much to the natural order as to the moral one, since both orders were regulated by the six non-naturals, by means of which scholastic physicians aimed to regulate the *whole* of human life. Therefore it is not surprising that Gentile da Foligno, in insisting on the importance of following the preservative regime he put forward, wrote at the beginning of it that, according to Galen, 'if someone works moderately and leads a decorous life, he will be able to remain untouched [by the pestilence]'.[134]

---

[133] Agramont, *Regiment*, pp. 74–89.

[134] Gentile, *Consilium*, signat. a3r: 'Et est sane huic sequenti regimini insistendum, nam si quis moderatis laboribus et vita decora utatur, omnino impassibilis perseverat, ut Galienus *De differentiis febrium* capitulo primo [*sic*]'. Gentile's reference to Galen is wrong. Actually it comes from Galen, *De morbo et accidenti*, lib. 2 (*De causis morborum*), cap. 5 (*Opera*, Venice, 1490, vol. II, signat. o7v).

Air and environment. Air was a matter of major concern in these medical works. Because of its very close link to life it constituted the first and most important non-natural, and was the basis of Galenic vitalism. Of its role Gentile asserted,

among all the things surrounding the human body, there is nothing that changes it so intensely as the air; after being inspired through the mouth, the nose, or the arteries, air reaches the heart keeping (presumably) its qualities, and then is combined within the arteries with the spirits of the body by means of which all the bodily actions of life are performed.[135]

Although some historians have caricatured the preventive measures specified by late medieval and early modern physicians against the pestilence by reducing them to the practical advice 'fugere cito, longe, et tarde reverti' (flee quickly and far, return slowly), they actually were sophisticated and complex. Not to understand them means not to understand the basic model of mid fourteenth-century medical thought. These preventive measures were actually aimed towards three practical goals: (1) choosing a place protected from the pestilential air, (2) correcting or purifying the adulterated air, and (3) avoiding every risk of contact with infected people.[136]

Within the first group of measures Gentile, as well as the Paris masters, echoed and recommended first the popular counsel of fleeing from every air bringing the 'poisonousness' of the pestilence.[137] Significantly, Gentile also insisted at the very end of the curative chapter of his major *Consilium* that 'fleeing is the best choice in every plague' since it is 'the most venomous of all the poisons, that infects and stains everyone with its irradiation'.[138] However, neither he nor the Paris masters paused to gloss this advice. On the contrary, both works went on to describe a large number of measures to be taken by those who did not abandon the places where pestilential air reigned, and mentioned some of the reasons which might prevent a person from leaving. While the Paris masters simply talked about the impossibility of leaving, Gentile considered two more situations: when the move would be uncomfortable, and the presence of a 'universal pestilence' which made any move useless.[139]

Choosing a suitable place to stay during times of pestilence involved

---

[135] Gentile, *Consilium*, signat. a3r: '. . . inter hec que humano corpore approximantur nihil est quod mutet ipsum fortius quam aer, qui per os nares et arterias ad cor inspirando provenit cum qualitatibus suis utputa aer, quoniam per omnes arterias miscetur spiritibus corporis, per quos omnes actiones vite corporales perficiuntur'.

[136] Paris masters, *Compendium*, pp. 94, 96.

[137] Gentile, *Consilium*, signat. a3r: Paris masters, *Compendium*, p. 96.

[138] Gentile, *Consilium*, signat. b7r: 'Possem prolongare materiam, sed quia gaudent brevitate moderni, reassumendo summaliter concludo quod fugere, ut dixi, est optimum in peste particulari. Est enim hec passio venenorum venenosissima, nam sua irradiatione et macula cunctos inficit'.

[139] Paris masters, *Compendium*, p. 96; Gentile, *Consilium*, signat. a3v.

questions not only about the geographical area, but also about one's house and even a particular room, the position and ventilation of which had to be carefully studied – all of these being considerations framed within a Latin Galenism that significantly conditioned medieval urbanism from the fourteenth century onwards. The Paris masters advised moving one's house away from every place where putrefactions were copiously generated, such as 'marshy, muddy, and stinking places, stagnant waters and ditches', ventilating it through windows open to northerly winds (as long as these did not pass through putrid and infected places), and protecting it from southerly ones because these were the usual carriers of pestilential air.[140] With respect to the correction of the adulterated air with which those remaining at an infected place unavoidably came into contact, both Gentile da Foligno and the Paris masters suggested that all the rooms of a house should be fumigated with fumes from aromatic plants to purify the air, and that dry and aromatic logs should be burned in these rooms to eliminate the 'venomous vapours' that transported the pestilence. Both works listed various plant species for this task, depending upon the season and the social condition of those using the plants. With respect to the season, the reigning principle was the Hippocratic *contraria contrariis*, which obliged one to look for plants and logs with primary qualities moderately opposed to those of the current season. Concerning the social groups to whom these measures were directed, while neither work specified the social condition of the intended addressees of most of these measures, at the end of the relevant section Gentile dedicated a short paragraph to measures directed to the 'poor' (*pauperes*), for whom, apart from contraindicating the eating of certain vegetables, he recommended two remedies, namely the very cheap one in a Mediterranean country of smelling aromatic herbs such as marjoram, savory and mint, and the very expeditious one of making oneself perform universal evacuations. The Paris masters also recommended that 'the rich and the powerful' should use three substances which were then very expensive, namely wood of aloes, amber and musk.[141]

Among other measures for purifying the pestilential air Gentile stressed the value to the public of lighting fires in the streets to remove the stink from houses and cities.[142] To any Galenist physician the link between stink and putrefaction was as obvious as that between putrefaction and pestilence. And in fact the lack of stink – and still better the presence of a pleasant smell in the environment – was a definitive sign that putrefaction had disappeared and that the air had become purified. Therefore, stink perceived through the sense of smell played a central role in the semiology of pestilence in the same way that a pleasant smell was a sign of health. This

---

[140] Paris masters, *Compendium*, p. 96.
[141] Gentile, *Consilium*, signats. a3v–a4v; Paris masters, *Compendium*, pp. 98, 100.
[142] Gentile, *Consilium*, signat. a4r: 'unum debet fieri quod toti populo est utile facere ignem accendi in stratis cum emundatione omnium fetorum domorum et civitatum'.

idea, originally Aristotelian, underlay all the above-mentioned air purification measures suggested for the interior of houses. What is noteworthy about Gentile's suggestion is the fact that he was the only one of the three physicians studied here to propose applying these measures to the public spaces of cities. Although this idea is already present in the pseudo-Galenic work *De commoditate theriacae*,[143] its adoption by Gentile might be related to the increasing concern for the physical environment that appeared all around the Mediterranean during the fourteenth century. In fact, from 1300 onwards, more and more reports appear from different communities of the area which connect an adequate and clean air with the preservation of collective health and, reciprocally, connect a stinking air – and therefore a putrid one – with the appearance of diseases. In Catalonia reports showing the social applicability of this idea appear in non-medical documents from as early as the first third of the fourteenth century. For instance, in 1330 the *veguer* of Barcelona responded to neighbourhood complaints about the stink (*fetores*) from the uncontrolled openings of drains, sewers and latrines which emerged from the Jewish quarter into the open air through a hole opened in the old wall. As a result of these stinks an *infectio* occurred 'that could cause diseases not only in this neighbourhood but also in other parts of the city'. The *veguer* ordered the hole to be shut because of the harm it caused to the public health (*publicam valitudinem*).[144]

Agramont was well aware of the association of stink and disease since he said that in cities like Paris, Avignon, and Lerida itself a 'local pestilence' restricted to each city had appeared as a result of their 'dirtiness' (*sutzea*). Indeed, he recommended avoiding (1) the throwing out of entrails and refuse of beasts or dead beasts near the town; (2) the placing of manure heaps next to the town; (3) the deposit or throwing of excrements inside

---

[143] *De commoditate theriacae*, cap. VI (Venice, 1490, vol. I, signat. qq7vb): 'Quo circa laudo mirabilissimum Ypocratem quoniam pestilentiam illam que de poemia ad ellines attinxit non aliter curavit nisi vertens aerem et alterans ut non attraheretur per respirationem talis existens. Invenerit enim per civitatem totam accendi ignem non simplicem unctionis materiam hebentem, sed serta et florum odorabilissimos et hec consulebat esse nutrimentum ignis et superinfundere in ipso que pigmentorum pinguissima et delectabilem odorem habentia ut sit purissimum effectum respiret permutatum aerem.' *De commoditate theriacae*, actually a fragmentary Latin translation from the Greek original made by Niccolò da Reggio in the first half of the fourteenth century, circulated at the time as a work attributed to Galen. In 1531 Johannes Guinter of Andernach edited a complete retranslation of it under the title *De theriaca ad Pisonem*. For the question of the problematic authorship of this text, see Nutton, 'The seeds', p. 6. For the fourteenth-century Latin translation of this work, see M. R. McVaugh, *Arnaldi de Villanova opera medica omnia*. Vol. III: *De amore heroico. De dosi tyriacalium medicinarum* (Barcelona, 1985), pp. 57, 65.

[144] L. García-Ballester, *La medicina medieval a València* (Valencia, 1988), p. 104. The document mentioned by García-Ballester comes from the Archivo de la Corona de Aragón (Barcelona), Reg. 437, fol. 1015. Among other things it says: '[Judei] fecissent cloacas, alblones et latrinas in eorum hospitiis ... ex quibus comitebantur fetores per quoddam foramen muri veteris ipsius civitatis ad carreriam publicam ... necminus infectio veris propterea emergebat ex quo possent infirmitates nodum in ipso convicinio, immo alibi in pluribus civitatis eiusdem vigere.'

the town either in the daytime or at night; (4) the keeping of skins to be soaked for tanning inside the town; and (5) the killing of cattle and other beasts. Agramont ended this section by saying that 'from all such procedures great infection of the air occurs'.[145] On the other hand, Agramont's preventive measures for dealing with the air in a 'universal pestilence' present some peculiar features which need to be examined. For 'air pestilential in its qualities' he recommended compensating for excess heat or cold by wearing lightweight or warm clothing and by remaining in places that were naturally or artificially kept cold or hot. For 'air pestilential in its substance' the situation was more complex. Indeed, Agramont distinguished up to three lines of action, according to the different causes involved in the 'putrefaction of air': (1) repentance and confession, when pestilence was due to the divine will because of our sins; (2) moving to high areas and mountains, when putrefaction of the air came from water or earth; and (3) moving to low areas, keeping windows and peepholes shut, and remaining (if necessary) under the earth when the pestilence came from any planetary conjunction or from the 'glance' ('esguardament') or aspect of a planet.[146] Agramont agreed with Gentile and the Paris masters in stressing the great efficacy of fire in purifying air that was substantially corrupted; and, like them, he distinguished between the preventive measures within the reach only of 'great lords' ('grans seynnors'), and the cheaper ones ('de bon mercat') which had to be resorted to by the 'common people' ('gent comina').[147]

To illustrate the third group of preventive measures – that is, the avoidance of every risk of contact with people infected with plague – we have only the evidence given by Gentile da Foligno, who recommended that 'political meetings should be avoided as much as possible, since they allow infected people to intermingle with those not infected'. (Given that no mention was made of any other kind of meetings, such as religious ones, it is appropriate to wonder to what extent Gentile's medical discourse meshed at this point with the wishes of the Perugian authorities to control the city population, highly anxious as they would have been as a result of the threat of plague.)[148]

Eating and drinking. As was usual in most late medieval *sanitatis regimina*, this section is the most extensive of the preventive measures against pestilence recommended by the physicians studied here.[149] As the Paris masters emphasized, the general role was 'to avoid every superfluous

---

[145] Agramont, *Regiment*, p. 64.
[146] Ibid., pp. 78–80.
[147] Ibid., pp. 79–80.
[148] Gentile, *Consilium*, signat. a4v: 'Et nota quod evitande sunt conversationes politice quantum plus possibile est, ne fiat confusio et permixtio de infectis ad non infectos.'
[149] Agramont, *Regiment*, pp. 80–3; Gentile, *Consilium*, signats. a4v–a6v; Paris masters, *Compendium*, pp. 102, 104, 106, 108, 110, 112.

food and drink as well as every humid one, since this predisposes one to the epidemic', while making liberal use of 'fine foods, which are easily digestible, and which generate good blood'.[150] All these works reviewed the food and drinks usually consumed, starting naturally with bread – the basis of the diet at the time. According to Gentile this should contain a little bran, should not have an 'accidental bad disposition', and should not be eaten until three days after it is baked.[151] Next came two basic drinks: (1) water, which has to be running, clean, and transparent; and (2) wine, which is very useful because in multiplying the spirits and in drying the superfluities it strengthens the natural heat, but which should be either just moderately hot or watered to reduce its heat.[152] Then followed a long list of both recommended and contraindicated foods of every kind (vegetables, meats, eggs, milk, fish and fruits) with instructions and comments on their properties and, for those recommended, on the way they should be consumed. Some of the authors also referred to the utility of various condiments, among which (following Avicenna) they emphasized those of a sour nature, particularly vinegar.[153]

Exercise and rest. All the recorded statements on the value of exercise are similar and correspond to commonplaces in late medieval Galenism. The authors recommended the practice of moderate exercise during times of pestilence, since in activating the natural heat it caused the dissolution of superfluities and facilitated their elimination from the body. In contrast, they counselled against any violent exercise because this elevated the body heat excessively and provoked the attraction of a great deal of air to the heart; since, as Agramont said, this air was 'corrupted and poisoned, it rots the body, its blood, and its spirits', and it originated the 'impressions' typical of the pestilence.[154]

Along with their recommendations about exercise the Paris masters also echoed those on baths, which Agramont placed among the measures concerning repletion and emptying. The Paris masters disapproved of hot baths because of their moisturizing and rarefying effect on the body; nevertheless, they considered that hot baths could be used (though only infrequently) by those who were used to them, and by those whose body contained an excess of thick and compact humours in order to soften them and to favour their ejection.[155] Agramont, on the contrary, condemned all baths, arguing that 'a bath opens the pores of body through which the

---

[150] Paris masters, *Compendium*, pp. 102, 104.
[151] Gentile, *Consilium*, signat. a4v; Paris masters, *Compendium*, p. 104.
[152] Gentile, *Consilium*, signats. a4v–a5r; Paris masters, *Compendium*, pp. 108, 110, 112.
[153] Agramont, *Regiment*, p. 81, Gentile, *Consilium*, signat. a6v.
[154] Agramont, *Regiment*, p. 80; Gentile, *Consilium*, signats. a6v–a7r; Paris masters, *Compendium*, pp. 100, 102.
[155] Paris masters, *Compendium*, p. 102.

corrupted air comes into the body, and provokes a strong impression on it or on its humours'.[156]

Sleep and wake. Our physicians discussed the fourth non-natural only briefly, merely transmitting commonplaces of contemporary university medical learning: (1) sleeping is very healthy, although sleeping too much is not good; (2) one must sleep at night because doing so in the daytime is very dangerous, particularly after eating before digestion has been accomplished, except for those who are accustomed to taking a short nap; (3) one should not sleep in a supine position because of the risk that superfluities will rise to the brain and cause very serious diseases; (4) while sleeping one must periodically change position, alternately leaning on the right side and on the left side, in order to prevent the liver from becoming overheated by the stomach.[157]

Inanition and repletion. Again, the comments and suggestions on this topic in all the works studied here were commonplaces in Galenic and Galenist dietetics. As Gentile pointed out, the bodies most inclined to putrefaction were 'those full of superfluities and those of inactive men, copious eaters and drinkers, indulging in immoderate venereal activities'.[158] Therefore, keeping the body clean and pure by decreasing the plethora was recommended in order to avoid contracting the pestilence. This could be achieved by means of: (1) a desiccative regime; (2) a moderate ingestion of food and drink; (3) the active maintenance of all the ways to evacuate excreta (digestive, urinary, epidermal) by either natural or artificial means; and (4) the practice of blood-letting for those with sanguinary plethora.[159]

At the end of this section none of the physicians forgot to counsel males not to have sexual relations during the time of pestilence. Such practices were mentioned under generic expressions like 'to lie lusty with a female' ('jaure carnalment ab fembra') and 'venereal acts' ('actus venerei'), or in more precise terms, as in the case of Gentile who pointed out that 'no one should induce his wife to do it, nor try to win other women' during the pestilence. According to all the writers this prohibition should be absolute since sexual relations at such times represented a 'serious risk for the body'.[160]

Accidents of the soul. According to both Galenic doctrine and medieval Galenism, 'the body' – as the Paris masters pointed out at the beginning of their brief comments on this sixth non-natural – 'could sometimes fall ill

---

[156] Agramont, *Regiment*, p. 85.
[157] Gentile, *Consilium*, signats. a6v–a7r; Paris masters, *Compendium*, p. 112.
[158] Gentile, *Consilium*, signat. a7r.
[159] Agramont, *Regiment*, pp. 84–5; Gentile, *Consilium*, signats. a7r–a8v; Paris masters, *Compendium*, pp. 112, 114.
[160] Agramont, *Regiment*, p. 85; Gentile, *Consilium*, signat. a8v: '... nullus debet uxores ducere pro tunc nec procurare novas venationes mulierum'; Paris masters, *Compendium*, p. 114.

as a result of accidents of the soul'.[161] Therefore, all were advised (1) to avoid rage, sadness and solitude, because these accidents of the soul negatively influenced the bodily complexion and favoured the appearance of diseases; (2) to seek joy and delight by means of 'melodies, songs, stories and other similar pleasures',[162] since 'pleasure, although it sometimes moistens the body, strengthens the spirit and the heart'.[163] More restrictively, Agramont insisted that enjoyment was beneficial during times of pestilence only whenever 'no bad regime of diet, of lechery, or of other things' intermingled accidentally with it.[164]

The physicians also stressed, in accordance with Aristotle, Galen and Avicenna, the important role played by autosuggestion (*ymaginatio, ymaginació*) in keeping oneself healthy as much as in falling ill. If individuals keep themselves quiet and hopeful they will have more chance of preserving themselves from the pestilence; if, on the contrary, they feel frightened of becoming ill and of dying, almost surely they will get sick and die.[165] With the purpose of neutralizing the adverse effects of fear, the Paris masters recommended the addressees of their *compendium* 'to make peace with God, because in doing so they will be less fearful of death'.[166] Meanwhile, Agramont insisted that 'in such times [of the pestilence] no chimes and bells should toll in the case of death because the sick are subject to evil imaginings when they hear the death bells'.[167]

Additional preventive measures

I indicated at the beginning of this part that the life-regime according to the six non-naturals needed the reinforcement of other measures which help to strengthen the resistance of human bodies to the pestilence. The importance of these additional measures within the literary genre of the *regimina sanitatis* increased over the course of time. The significance of this fact seems clear, since it reflected (1) the increasing technical power of the physician over nature (though of course the physician was always the servant of nature); (2) the increasing control of community health by health professionals, namely physicians, surgeons and apothecaries; and (3) the

---

[161] Paris masters, *Compendium*, p. 114. On the role of accidents of the soul in Galen's medical doctrine, see L. G. García-Ballester, 'Soul and body, disease of the soul and disease of the body in Galen's medical thought', in P. Manuli and Mario Vegetti (eds.), *Le opere psichologiche di Galeno. Atti del Terzo Colloquio Galenico Internazionale (Pavia, 10–12 settembre 1986)* (Naples, 1988), pp. 117–52.

[162] Gentile, *Consilium*, signat. b1r.

[163] Paris masters, *Compendium*, p. 114.

[164] Agramont, *Regiment*, p. 85.

[165] Agramont, *Regiment*, pp. 85–7; Gentile, *Consilium*, signat. b1r; Paris masters, *Compendium*, p. 114.

[166] Paris masters, *Compendium*, p. 114: '... cum Deo faciant pacem, quia inde mortem minus timebunt ...'.

[167] Agramont, *Regiment*, pp. 86–7: 'Per què conseyll que en aytal temps per degun mort no sie sonat seynn ni campana car molt ne prenen mala ymaginació los malalts can hoen sonar los seynns.'

increasing economic gains of all of these professionals, which at the same time reinforced their social position.[168]

I have also pointed out that the positioning of these auxiliary measures within the discussion of health preservation was not the same in all the works being studied here. Gentile da Foligno, for example, although he briefly mentioned some of them when dealing with the fifth non-natural, put all of them together after the six non-naturals, and defined them as 'certain special medicines' that 'strengthen the act of prevention so that we gain power to defend ourselves against plague'.[169] Agramont, on the other hand, introduced these measures in two different sections: some were included within two of the non-naturals – the second (food and drink), and the fifth (inanition and repletion); and other measures such as cauterization, cupping glasses and blood-letting appeared along with simple and compound medicines.[170] Finally, the Paris masters placed these auxiliary measures in a section entitled 'On cure and prevention by means of medicines', where phlebotomy was also referred to.[171]

All the authors gave a long list of remedies that were to be taken according to several guidelines and combined since they pursued various purposes.[172] Some of them, like vinegar, garlic and sour milk, were considered to be at once both foods and drugs; others were thought of only as medicines. Some of the latter, like Armenian bolus, *terra sigillata*, and agaric were simples; others such as theriac, mithridate (*mithridatium*), emerald, and pills of aloes, saffron and myrrh, were compounds, sometimes made up of tens of simples. Nearly all these drugs produced more than one effect. However, according to the number of desired effects, they constitute three groups: (1) those that moisturized and desiccated, the effect of which was to cleanse the body of superfluities by dissolving and/or purging them; (2) cordials which invigorated all the three main members (heart, brain, and liver); and (3) antidotes which neutralized the effects of the pestilential poison. Nearly all the drugs appearing in the works we are studying here, both simples and compounds, were taken from medical authorities, mainly Galen, Rhazes, Avenzoar, Averroes, Avicenna and Pietro d'Abano.

The group of antidotes was easily the largest and most highly valued. Except for small differences, all the authors used the same list of simple and

---

[168] On this point, see L. García-Ballester, M. R. McVaugh, and A. Rubio-Vela, *Medical licensing and learning in fourteenth-century Valencia* (Philadelphia, 1989), *Transactions of the American Philosophical Society*, vol. LXXIX, part 6, and Michael McVaugh's paper in the present volume.

[169] Gentile, *Consilium*, signats. a1v ('quasdam medicinas speciales'), b1v ('quedam medicinalia facientia ad actum previsissimum ut valeamus nos a peste defendere').

[170] Agramont, *Regiment*, pp. 81–3, 84–5.

[171] Paris masters, *Compendium*, p. 74: '... de remediis curativis et preservativis per medicinalia'.

[172] Agramont, *Regiment*, pp. 76, 77–8, 79–83, 84–5; Gentile, *Consilium*, signats. b1v–b4v; Paris masters, *Compendium*, p. 114.

compound drugs. These drugs were thought to produce marvellous effects, for they blocked and/or eliminated the poison of pestilence, and prevented the pestilence from causing putrefaction inside the body. Almost all the remedies had a long tradition of use in the ancient and medieval world. The most historically well known were theriac and mithridate, which were already famous in Galen's time; others were Armenian bolus, *terra sigillata*, powdered emerald, the 'seven herbs', the pills of aloes, saffron and myrrh, and other sophisticated magistral preparations which had to be administered under different forms (electuaries, troches and pomades, among others). In general, all operated by means of their 'specific form', which allowed them to resist the poison of pestilence so that they strongly repelled the very venomous putrefaction of pestilence. Antidotes were endowed with this 'specific virtue', sometimes naturally, at other times under the influence of certain celestial constellations. Most of these antidotes brought high prices in the market, according to their fame and to the value of their ingredients.[173] Thus, it is not surprising that the Paris masters advised men who were 'strong and robust, eating roughly, living near bad waters, and drinking little or no wine, to eat garlic from time to time, mainly in winter', since garlic was 'a theriac against every kind of poison'. On the other hand, they contraindicated its use by those 'who often suffer from headaches, living delicately or feeling slightly ill, since garlic develops every disease which the body is inclined to'.[174]

Phlebotomy was unanimously considered too as another preventive measure at the same level as pharmacological ones. Jacme d'Agramont and Gentile da Foligno recommended it as something which should be used by all during the time of pestilence. The latter emphasized that multiplying the number of small blood-lettings was preferable to extracting large amounts of blood at one time – something that scholastic physicians almost constantly indicated for every pathological process affecting the body complexion. The Paris masters, however, were less enthusiastic about this practice, which they said should be performed only on those whose bodies were sufficiently humid and whose blood moved swiftly. They recommended more specifically that 'men of the people and farmers who do not enjoy a delicate life' should seek to be bled from the median vein ([*vena*] *mediana*).[175]

Last, but not least relevant, Gentile da Foligno and Jacme d'Agramont mentioned several preventive measures against the appearance of worms

---

[173] On the history of theriac and mithridatium in general, see G. Watson, *Theriac and mithridatium. A study in therapeutics* (London, 1966).
[174] Paris masters, *Compendium*, p. 122.
[175] Agramont, *Regiment*, p. 85; Gentile, *Consilium*, signat. a8r; Paris masters, *Compendium*, p. 116. On the role of phlebotomy in scholastic medicine, see Pedro Gil-Sotres' long introductory study to L. Demaitre (ed.), *Arnaldi de Villanova opera medica omnia'*, Vol. IV: *Tractatus de consideracionibus operis medicine sive de flebotomia* (Barcelona, 1988), pp. 7–120; and P. Gil-Sotres's chapter in the present volume.

(*vermes*). They agreed in emphasizing this condition, which according to Agramont caused 'fevers and sudden deaths', as being very frequent in pestilential times. Gentile attributed it to the presence of a 'great corruption' during the time of pestilence. He restricted himself to prescribing an 'ointment very effective against worms' with which the stomach and navel, the parts of the back corresponding in a straight line to these members, and the hollow of the back had to be anointed.[176] Agramont, for his part, established a whole regime to avoid the appearance of 'worms and "lombrichs"', and to facilitate ridding the body of dead ones. This regime included: (1) the recommendation of some foods (garlic, vinegar), and the contraindication of others (milk, sweet fruits, vegetables and, in general, every phlegmatic and viscous food); (2) the prescription of *gerapigra Galieni*, which killed and ejected the worms from the body, and of other purgatives that eliminated phlegm – the humour which facilitated the generation of worms; and (3) the application of several plasters and ointments to anoint the bellies of different social groups – bourgeoisie, 'common people' (*gent communa*), children – with the purpose of preventing the appearance of worms.[177]

Cure

The measures that Gentile and the Paris masters put forward to cure the victims of pestilence (for Agramont considered only the preventive regime) were to a large extent the same as those recommended to healthy individuals in order to keep themselves healthy. Thus the Paris masters, after dedicating a whole section of their preventive regime to the six non-naturals, included both preventive and curative medicinal remedies in the next section. The medicines were grouped into three chapters: universal remedies, particular ones, and antidotes.[178] Except for changes of order, the guidelines for the curative regime appearing in all the *regimina* were very similar, mainly because all the regimes followed a conception of disease (the Galenist one) which all the physicians shared. According to this conception, as we have already seen, the poison transmitting the pestilence was in the air, and entered the human body through mouth, nostrils, skin pores and, according to the Montpellier practitioner, also through the gaze (we leave aside for the moment the peculiar ideas of Alfonso de Córdoba). When an individual body was incapable of destroying it, the poison borne by the air spread throughout the body and provoked putrefactions and the functional failure of its main organs. The individual then fell seriously ill and died unless he or she received an adequate treatment to re-establish the natural

---

[176] Gentile, *Consilium*, signats. b2r–b2v.
[177] Agramont, *Regiment*, pp. 87–9.
[178] Paris masters, *Compendium*, p. 74.

virtues and allow them to destroy the poison of the pestilence and reverse its effects before the body was completely ruined by the poison.

This is why Gentile, as well as the Paris masters, said that after having established that a sick person was a victim of the pestilence, and having verified the condition of his or her nature, the practitioner should phlebotomize every patient right away. Gentile insisted, based on his own experience, that in order to save the patient from death, bleeding had to continue until the patient lost consciousness.[179] *Apostemata* were signs revealing damage in the different bodily members, and indicated the emunctories (*emunctoria*) where superfluities coming from these members were evacuated; their location thus determined which vein had to be bled in each patient. The purpose of this bleeding was to provide an exit for the collected venomous matter in order to avoid the continued putrefaction in the relevant member and to prevent the poison from reaching the heart. Gentile listed as many as six different veins to be bled according to the position of the *apostema*. Of all the possible locations of *apostemata* the most worrying to him were three – namely, under the left armpit, behind the ears, and in the right groin, because these corresponded to damage in the three main bodily members: heart, brain and liver, respectively.[180]

It sometimes happened that an *apostema* would gradually disappear after the bleeding, but then others would appear perhaps several days later, as a result of the lingering disease. In such cases, Gentile recommended resorting without delay to a new phlebotomy, accompanied by a diet allowing the patient a quick recovery. In addition to this he suggested a direct treatment to break the *apostemata* and to attract and to evacuate the poisonous matter collected in them. This consisted in either deep scarification and the application of cupping glasses over the *apostemata*, or cauterizing them and applying plasters to dissolve and attract the poisonous matter. Gentile preferred 'actual' cauteries (red-hot iron) to 'potential' ones (burning medicines), although he did not rule out the use of the latter; he did not specify the composition of solvent and attractive plasters, 'since they are well known by surgeons'. After an *apostema* had been broken, and its poisonous matter extracted, Gentile recommended the topical use of various medicines to cleanse and moisturize the region.[181]

In general, *apostema* was the only symptom referred to by the physicians in their discussion of curative measures against pestilence. Gentile was the only writer who also mentioned (though very briefly) 'anthrax or carbuncle' (*antracem vel carbunculum*), a symptom which later medical works on plague would deal with at length – probably as a result of the clinical

---

[179] Gentile, *Consilium*, signats. b4r–b5r; 'Et credendum est quod ille flebothomie liberant hominem a morte, sed debent fieri usque ad sincopim recuperabilem quam lipothomiam medici vocant idest animi defectionem.'

[180] Ibid., signats. a2v, b4v–b5r.

[181] Ibid., signats. b5r–b5v.

experience of the disease which physicians gradually gathered. Gentile merely indicated that according to some people a carbuncle quickly softened if a potion of root of *palma Christi* was administered to the patient.[182]

Along with all these measures for the cure of *apostemata*, Gentile listed some more general treatments: (1) strong enemas, if the condition of the patient permitted their use; (2) cupping glasses applied to strategic places to avoid the afflux of poisonous matter to the main bodily members; (3) cordial preparations to strengthen the functioning of these main members; (4) different special foods to resist dissolution; (5) a regime following the six non-naturals, with particular attention to the air environment of the patient's room; and (6) antidotes (the same ones recommended for the preventive regime) because they had curative properties as well as preventive ones.[183]

Two aspects of point five in the above list merit attention before concluding this discussion. First, the Paris masters strongly stressed that improving the quality of the atmosphere in the patient's room by means of aromatic products which could be burned, fumigated, sprinkled, or simply breathed in was imperative in order both to make all the remaining therapeutic measures effective and to avoid the spread of pestilence.[184] This shows clearly the extent to which the association between good smell and pure air (that is, air free of pestilence), as well as the opposite association of stink and putrefaction (characteristic of times of pestilence), operated in their minds as a major criterion of therapeutical efficacy. Secondly, both Gentile da Foligno and the Paris masters in their curative regimes offered a range of therapeutic preparations directed to different social groups. The most significant example of this may be the potion that Gentile suggested to those who were 'rich and wealthy enough': it consisted of barley water which had to be boiled with a gold straw (*virga auri*) before serving as the basis for preparing various dishes (*fercula*).[185]

CONCLUSIONS

In the previous pages I have explored the earliest perceptions and reactions that the so-called Black Death raised among Latin Mediterranean medical practitioners during the years 1348 and 1349, through six contemporary medical works.

More than a disease-entity, the Black Death was for all these physicians a social disaster, one which they scarcely characterized from a clinical point of view, but which they did not hesitate to confront with the help of their intellectual tools – namely, their university training within the conceptual

---

[182] Ibid., signat. b7r.
[183] Ibid., signats. b5v–b7r.
[184] Paris masters, *Compendium*, pp. 128, 130, 132. See also Gentile, *Consilium*, signat. b6r.
[185] Gentile, *Consilium*, signat. b6v.

framework of late medieval Latin Galenism, their clinical experience in previous pestilences, and the support of the Greek, Roman, Arabic and Latin medical authorities to whom they had access. Their interpretations of the nature and causes of the Black Death, as well as the measures they suggested to keep their fellow citizens healthy and the (very few) remedies to cure those who were taken ill with pestilence, represent the earliest responses made by professionals trained at the rising university medical faculties to a scourge which would not leave Western Europe until the eighteenth century, as well as the first steps towards the construction of this disaster as a disease-entity. The writings in which these physicians expressed their thoughts and practical advice on the pestilence represent the beginning of a new medical literary genre – that of the plague *regimina* – which notably developed in late medieval and early modern Europe.[186]

Most of the physicians whose works have been studied here conceived of the *pestilentia* as a universal air condition and attributed it to celestial causes, although the emphasis which each one placed on these causes differed according to geographical variations. While Albumasar's theory of constellations was their major reference point in explaining the relationship between macrocosm and microcosm,[187] the concept of corruption which Aristotle developed and applied to the whole sublunar world was the common basis of all their interpretations concerning how the pestilence broke out and spread.[188] And given that they believed that air was the most basic element of life, it was no surprise to them that the effects of the pestilence were very widespread. According to the thinking of the time, the process of corruption, and the resultant putrefaction, could be detected through the stink perceptible to the sense of smell.

Although the outbreak of any pestilence as a result of the corruption of live matter was essentially unpredictable, the greater the amount of live matter involved in this process the higher was the risk of pestilence. Once the pestilence had started as a result of the process of corruption on a large scale, the disaster easily spread from one place to another through the air, helped by natural atmospheric phenomena; at the same time it could pass from a sick person to a healthy one through the breath, through skin pores, and, according to the Montpellier practitioner, also through the gaze. Since to most of the physicians studied here the outbreak of any pestilence was brought about by macrocosmic powers, it was beyond the control of humans, who could only protect themselves from it. The one exception to this rule was the university master Alfonso de Córdoba, whose *Epistola et regimen de pestilentia* reveals that sectors of opinion close to the University of Montpellier were adding fuel and even intellectual support to the serious

---

[186] On the important changes in the *Regimina sanitatis* during the second half of the fourteenth century, see García-Ballester, 'Changes', pp. 119–125.

[187] Lemay, *Abu Ma'shar*.

[188] See Aristotle, *De generatione et corruptione*, particularly Book II, chs. 9 to 11.

charge that the pestilence had been caused by wicked men. Although Alfonso de Córdoba did not point directly at a specific social group or minority, the anti-Jewish pogroms then taking place in various parts of Languedoc and Provence give us a possible clue to the identity of the culprits he had in mind.

Owing to the causal ideas held by most of these physicians, the preventive measures they suggested were oriented in three different and complementary ways. First, impeding and/or halting the process of corruption in the air – the place where the pestilence lay – by keeping rooms, houses, and, in general, the whole city well ventilated and clear of filth, particularly of offal and of manure which could easily cause this process; and also strengthening the resistance of the air to corruption by means of aromatic herbs and vinegar fumigations. Secondly, keeping the human body resistant to the corruption which brought about the pestilence, by means of a regime based on the adequate management of the six non-naturals, together with some specific antidotes whose efficacy had been proved. And thirdly, once the pestilence had broken out, avoiding any occasion on which interpersonal transmission could occur.

All this leads us to conclude, in opposition to the widespread historiographical view, that there is no reason at all to continue separating into two different and disconnected worlds the measures against the pestilence which were established by the European civil communities and those which university physicians suggested. On the contrary, they were closely interrelated. None of the health measures taken by western Mediterranean civic communities in 1348 went beyond the theoretical framework delineated by contemporary university medicine,[189] while the most relevant works studied here – those of Jacme d'Agramont, Gentile da Foligno and the Paris masters – were actually addressed to the political authorities, and showed a clear concern for the health of the community as a whole. Furthermore, the concept of contagion as a means of pestilence transmission from one person to another is present in most of these works, in clear disproof of the widely accepted historical assumption that this idea and its development in the late Middle Ages were achievements of the city laymen's 'healthy' empiricism opposed to the aerist and miasmatic views held by university physicians. As said above, air spread and contagion can no longer be considered as contradictory views of the diffusion of pestilence, but rather as referring to two different and successive stages of its dissemination, the air being in addition the place where pestilence is first generated. In these circumstances we have to conclude that the health measures taken by these communities were largely influenced by the thinking of university physicians.

---

[189] On this point, see also J. Henderson, 'Epidemics in Renaissance Florence: medical theory and government response', in *Maladie et societé (XIIe–XVIIIe siècles). Actes du colloque de Bielefeld* (Paris, 1989), pp. 165–86, and his forthcoming book *Death in Florence: the impact of plague, 1348–1631* (New Haven).

Therefore, the perceptions of and reactions to the Black Death among Latin Mediterranean medical practitioners during the years 1348 and 1349 offer an excellent example of how widely university medical and natural philosophical learning had become accepted in Latin Mediterranean Europe by the mid fourteenth century – and, more generally, of how deeply scholastic thought as developed in the universities had penetrated into Latin Mediterranean civil society.

ACKNOWLEDGEMENTS

I am deeply indebted to Luis García-Ballester for his valuable suggestions and remarks at many stages of this paper. I also wish to thank Michael McVaugh for his useful comments, and Julia McVaugh for her great care in revising my text and in dramatically improving its English style. I am grateful too to Andrew Cunningham for his revision of an earlier version of this paper, and to José Martínez-Gázquez for his help in accurately translating the quotations from Alfonso de Córdoba.

9

John of Arderne and the Mediterranean tradition of scholastic surgery[1]

PETER MURRAY JONES

Scholastic surgery originated in the milieu of the north Italian medical schools, and was successfully exported to other Mediterranean environments in the thirteenth and fourteenth centuries. In this study I hope to show that its impact was felt outside the Mediterranean world too, although this impact was a very different one in an environment where there were no schools of surgery in university cities. The character of scholastic surgery made this inevitable. While scholastic surgery had its origin in the earlier translation and reception of Arabic writings on practical medicine and surgery, its evolution into a true *scientia* on the model of other scholastic sciences came at the hands of Italian master surgeons like Guglielmo da Saliceto and Dino del Garbo. They succeeded in giving scholastic form to the teaching of surgery, which had previously been largely a matter of craft training in which the master instructed his *familiares* in the secrets of his *ministerium*. The learned surgeon was now expected to combine *ministerium* with *magisterium*, and to be able to put down his secrets in written form, following an organized scholastic model of exposition. The role of practical experience and learning by watching was not eliminated, but instead was accommodated within the scholastic model as a procedure of verification and exemplification of the surgical *scientia*.[2] The elaboration and refinement of this scholastic model of surgery went hand in hand with its export from north Italy to France and the Crown of Aragon.

The differences between the scholastic institutions of Italy and those of France were such that the claims of surgery to the status of a true *scientia* never achieved recognition at the University of Paris. Instead the College

[1] I should like to thank Professor Linda Ehrsam Voigts and Dr Faye Getz for reading a first draft of this paper and making many valuable suggestions and corrections. All remaining errors are of course my own.

[2] See Jole Agrimi and Chiara Crisciani, *Edocere medicos: medicina scolastica nei secoli XIII–XV* (Milan and Naples, 1988), and essays by Nancy Siraisi, Jole Agrimi and Chiara Crisciani in this volume.

of Saint Cosmas was set up as a rival institution for surgeons. Nevertheless
this did not mean that these claims were abandoned – rather the opposite.
The case for surgery as a science was stated still more emphatically by the
master surgeons in their own defence, in the face of attempts by the
physicians to dismiss their claim to recognition. The learned surgeons
presented themselves as a closed elite with an intellectual training as
rigorous as that of the physicians, and distanced themselves from unlearned
surgeons, who had at best a craft training to fall back on. The master
surgeons claimed a monopoly on rational surgery because they had access
to the Latin surgical tradition, dismissing other practitioners as blind
empirics with no understanding of the reasons for the procedures they
followed. By divorcing themselves from the empirics, the learned surgeons
hoped to establish credentials equivalent to those of the learned physicians.[3]
The surgeries of Lanfranco of Milan and Henri de Mondeville, both
written in the Parisian milieu, state the case for scholastic surgery in its most
fully elaborated form, and represent the culmination of the genre. Even if
surgery had failed to find a place within this northern university, a body of
doctrina had evolved which was fully scholastic in form, and which could be
used as a basis for exposition and disputation.

The continuities between scholastic surgery in the Mediterranean world
and Paris in terms of personnel, doctrine and methods of exposition are
striking, but a fundamental discontinuity emerged when the tradition
crossed the English Channel. One of the significant differences between the
reception of scholastic surgery in Paris and in England was the fact that the
English universities, Oxford and Cambridge, in organization and teaching
methods really satellites of Paris, were not metropolitan universities. Not
only was there little scope for surgery within the university medical
curriculum, but there was no chance of a corporation like the College of
Saint Cosmas establishing itself alongside the English universities. There
were no courts at Oxford and Cambridge, and the cities were not large
enough to sustain a community of surgeons combining teaching with
practice on the Mediterranean model. *Magisterium* and *ministerium* could
not go hand in hand, and as a consequence we know of no surgeons
practising in England in the fourteenth century who had a university
background, not even Englishmen who had received a training at one of
the continental schools of surgery.[4]

---

[3] See Cornelius O'Boyle in this volume. See also a number of studies on professionalization
in medicine by Vern L. Bullough: 'Medical study at Mediaeval Oxford', *Speculum*, 36
(1961), 600–12; 'The mediaeval medical school at Cambridge', *Mediaeval Studies*, 24 (1962),
161–8; *The development of medicine as a profession* (Basle and New York, 1966); 'Achieve-
ment, professionalization and the universities', in Jozef Ijsewijn and Jacques Paquet (eds.),
The universities in the late Middle Ages (Leuwen, 1978).

[4] I base this on a search of the biographical details of surgeons given in C. H. Talbot and
E. A. Hammond, *The medical practitioners in medieval England: a biographical register*
(London, 1965). Of the 91 names of surgeons and barber-surgeons listed as practising in
England in the fourteenth century, 30 are given the title of master surgeon (*magister*), and

Despite this significant institutional difference between Oxford and Cambridge on the one hand and the Mediterranean university towns on the other, scholastic surgery nevertheless did cross the English channel in the course of the fourteenth century. It crossed not as from Italy to France in the persons of the surgical masters themselves, but in the form of manuscripts of the scholastic texts. Unfortunately few data are available to throw light on the circulation of scholastic surgical texts in England in this period, so our understanding of this process is necessarily limited.[5] One surgical book probably written in England in the early fourteenth century contains the Glosses of the Four Masters to the surgery of Roger Frugard of Parma, and the surgeries of Johannes Jamerius, Lanfranco, and Henri de Mondeville, as well as other texts. Who owned it is unknown. But this means that the works of Lanfranco and Mondeville may have been known in England quite soon after their date of composition. Another such book, probably written in Italy, containing the surgery of Rolando (Rolandino) of Parma, the Glosses of the Four Masters, the surgeries of Guglielmo da Saliceto, Bruno Longoburgo, Albucasis and Jamerius, was owned by William Rede, and given by him to Merton College Oxford in 1385.[6]

But if the scholastic surgeries had been known only to academics like Rede, and not to practising surgeons, their impact necessarily would have been limited. At least one of these surgeries – that of Roger Frugard – was, however, known in England in an Anglo-Norman translation by the middle of the thirteenth century.[7] Two manuscripts of this translation are beautifully illustrated, suggesting that whoever commissioned them had unacademic tastes but also wealth enough not to have to practise surgery for a living. There is no evidence as yet that the availability of a surgical text in Anglo-Norman made any impact on practising English surgeons,

another 8 are entered as barber-surgeons. Barbers not specifically identified as surgeons are not included. None of the 91 has been found in university records, although 4 were resident in Oxford, and 1 in Cambridge. The statistics on surgeons given in Robert S. Gottfried, 'English medical practitioners, 1340–1530', *Bulletin of the History of Medicine*, 58 (1984), 164–82, are not always reliable; Stuart Jenks, 'Medizinische Fachkräfte in England zur Zeit Heinrichs VI (1428/9–1460/1)', *Sudhoffs Archiv*, 69 (1985), 214–27, supplies a necessary corrective to Gottfried's assumptions, though Jenks provides new data on surgeons for a small part of the fifteenth century only.

5 A systematic search of the manuscript catalogues of British libraries and foreign libraries holding British manuscripts might give some indication of the availability of surgical texts in England in the fourteenth century, and this might in time be supplemented by information from the developing corpus of British medieval library catalogues.

6 The manuscript containing texts of Lanfranco and Mondeville is London, Royal College of Physicians, MS 227a (N. R. Ker, *Medieval manuscripts in British libraries*, vol. I (Oxford, 1969), pp. 199–201); the Rede MS is Oxford, Bodleian Library, MS e Museo 19 (Bodleian *Summary catalogue*, vol. II, part 2, no. 3500 (Oxford, 1951, repr. 1980)). See also F. M. Powicke, *The medieval books of Merton College* (Oxford, 1931), pp. 166–7.

7 See Johan Vising, *Anglo-Norman language and literature* (London, 1923), no. 315, for the translations of Roger; also Paul Meyer, 'Manuscrits médicaux en français', *Romania*, 44 (1915–17), 161–214, esp. 163–72, 191–4. Further references are provided by Linda Ehrsam Voigts, 'Medical prose', in A. S. G. Edwards (ed.), *Middle English prose: a critical guide to major authors and genres* (New Brunswick, 1984), pp. 315–35.

though more surgeons may have been able to read in Anglo-Norman or French than in Latin. Similarly, the vernacular French versions of Lanfranco, or Henri de Mondeville have left no visible trace on English surgery. That there was, however, a larger potential audience in England for vernacular surgical texts in the fourteenth century is shown by the fact that by the end of the century the first Middle English translations of these works were under way.[8]

On the other hand our knowledge of the personnel of English fourteenth-century surgery is unfortunately too sketchy to allow generalizations about the extent to which English surgeons may have had direct knowledge of the scholastic surgeries.[9] Only one of the surgeons listed in Talbot and Hammond can be shown to have read these texts, and it would be easy to infer that English surgeons all fall into the category of empirics, at least as defined by the Parisian masters. But one fourteenth-century English surgeon at least not only read these surgeries but wrote Latin treatises on surgery and practical medicine for the use of his fellow surgeons. By examining this one case in more detail we can learn enough to

[8] London, Wellcome MS 564 contains a translation of Henri de Mondeville and what appears to be an original surgery written in Middle English and dated to 1392. Both have been edited by Richard Grothé, 'Le ms. Wellcome 564: deux traités de chirurgie en moyen-anglais', Ph.D. diss. (University of Montreal, 1982). Linda Ehrsam Voigts, 'Scientific and medical books', in *Book production and publishing in Britain, 1375–1475* (Cambridge, 1989), pp. 345–402, provides a valuable survey of surgical and other medical book production. A French translation of Lanfranco's *Chirurgia parva* is found in a number of different versions in manuscripts of the fourteenth century, and some of these versions were certainly owned by practising surgeons. See Claude de Tovar, 'Les versions françaises de la *Chirurgia parva* de Lanfranc de Milan', *Revue d'Histoire des Textes*, 12–13 (1982–3), 195–262. The German translations of Lanfranco's works are surveyed in Kurt Ruh et al. (eds.), *Die deutsche Literatur des Mittelalters: Verfasserlexikon*, vol. v (Berlin, 1985), s.v. Lanfrank von Mailand, with further references to modern studies of these translations as examples of *Fachprosa*.

[9] R. Theodore Beck, *The cutting edge: early history of the surgeons of London* (London, 1974) provides biographical records for a number of English medieval surgeons, including extracts from wills, where found. Seven surgeons are known to have left books on surgery, the earliest will dating from 1462, the latest 1501. Four left only one book, identified in three cases as the surgery of Guy de Chauliac. John Dagville left 'all my bokes bilongyng to my crafte of sirurgie & also all bokes of phisik, as well tho bokes that be written in Englissch as tho that be written in Latyn', in a will dated 26 September 1477. No surgeons are listed in Susan H. Cavanaugh, 'A study of books privately owned in England: 1300–1450', Ph.D. diss. (University of Pennsylvania, 1980). We know rather more about books owned in the fourteenth century by Italian and Catalan surgeons. Those owned by Pasquale de Villorba, *c.*1375, included several manuscripts of Bruno da Longoburgo, and others by Guglielmo da Saliceto, Albucasis, Roger of Parma (or possibly Roger Baron), and Rolando Cappelluti. Guglielmino da Trevisa owned before 24 September 1351 manuscripts of Rhazes (*Ad Almansorem*), Rolando, Guglielmo da Saliceto, and Dino del Garbo (*Receptarium in Cyrurgia*). These inventories are printed in Luciano Gargan, *Cultura e arte nel Veneto al tempo del Petrarca*, Studi sul Petrarca, 5 (Padua, 1978), pp. 198–203. See also the article by Pesenti Marangon (note 77 below). Bernat Serra, surgeon of Jaume II, Count of Catalunya, owned before 17 November 1387 works by Teodorico, Rolando, Rhazes (*Ad Almansorem*), Roger, Bruno, and Lanfranco. See Societat de Cirurgia de Catalunya, *Tres Treballs Premiats en el concurs d'homenatge a Gimbernat* (Masnou, 1936), pp. 21–2 (I owe this reference to Michael McVaugh).

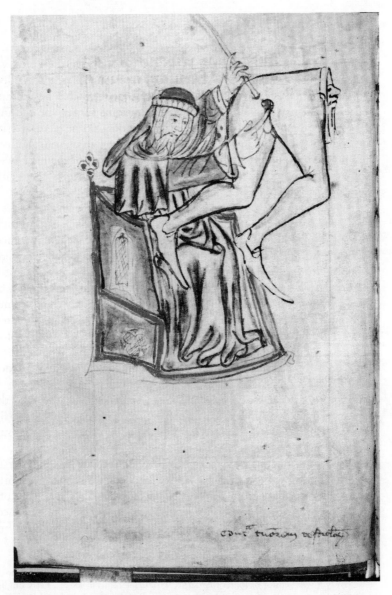

Figure 7   Master John of Arderne probing a fistulous hole to see if it perforates the rectum.

be cautious of assuming that scholastic surgery could be of use or interest only to a learned elite of surgeons who combined *magisterium* and *ministerium*, or at the very least had been educated in the university schools of surgery.

JOHN OF ARDERNE

John of Arderne, who practised surgery in Newark, a market town in the English Midlands from 1349 to 1370, and at London in the 1370s, wrote a *Practica* of fistula-in-ano, and a number of other smaller treatises collected as a *Liber medicinarum*. Case studies in his writings show that he attempted to put into practice in Newark a concept of rational surgery he had imbibed from his reading of the Latin scholastic surgeries. Yet he seems to have had no contact with the continental schools of surgery in person, and his name has not been found in any university register. Most of the little we know for certain about the career of John of Arderne comes from his own writings.

He was born in 1307, since he declares himself to be seventy years old in 1377, the date of one of his works.[10] At the beginning of the *Practica* of fistula-in-ano, his major work, he tells us that he began to practise in Newark, in the county of Nottinghamshire, in 1349, and transferred to London in 1370. Apart from these details, many of the mentions of a John of Arderne in documents might plausibly be linked to our surgeon, but the name was a very common one in the fourteenth century. No certainty can attach itself to claims that he bought a small estate in Mitcham, in Surrey, in 1347–8, and that he moved to Newark after the death of his wife of plague in 1349.[11] The date of his death, put variously by different authorities as 1380 and 1392, is likewise inferred from mentions of a John of Arderne in charters, and cannot be relied on. He may have been a member of the distinguished Warwickshire family of Ardernes, but the fact that he practised in the Midlands is hardly sufficient to prove it, and his social status as a surgeon, albeit he described himself as a master surgeon, rather suggests the opposite.

With no evidence that Arderne had any connection with universities in England and elsewhere, there has been a tendency for modern authorities to claim for him a background in battlefield surgery.[12] In the absence of royal or other warrants for his service in military campaigns, the evidence once again depends on references to such campaigns in his writings. Unfortu-

---

[10] *De cura oculi*, as found in British Library, Sloane MS 75, fol. 146.

[11] *Pace* C. H. Talbot, *Medicine in medieval England* (London, 1967), p. 121, who follows D'Arcy Power, editor of John of Arderne, *Treatises of fistula in ano . . .*, Early English Text Society, no. 139 (London, 1910), pp. x–xiv, in his account of Arderne's career. Huling E. Ussery, *Chaucer's physician: medicine and literature in fourteenth-century England*, Tulane Studies in English, 19 (New Orleans, 1971), pp. 62–9, corrects a number of other statements made about Arderne's career on flimsy evidence.

[12] In particular Robert S. Gottfried, *Doctors and medicine in medieval England 1340–1530* (Princeton, 1986) would like to see all English surgeons as relying on experience by contrast with the academic physicians, and attempts to make Arderne fit this picture by referring to his campaign experience; Gottfried inexplicably claims (pp. 138–9): 'About a quarter of his [Arderne's] surgical and general medical manuals deal with military medicine.'

nately these references are far from solid evidence for Arderne having battlefield experience, although there is a possibility that he served in the entourage of Henry, Earl of Derby and first Duke of Lancaster between 1338 and 1347. Arderne shows some familiarity with details of English campaigns in Gascony and Spain, but the references are hardly conclusive evidence. They may indicate that he had heard stories from others rather than handled these cases himself.[13] The most circumstantial passage concerns Adam, second Baron Everingham, a prominent soldier, of whom Arderne says:

Lord Adam was in Gascony with Lord Henry, then Earl of Derby, and afterwards Duke of Lancaster, a most vigorous leader. Lord Adam suffered from fistula-in-ano, and he consulted all the physicians and surgeons he could find in Gascony, at Bordeaux, Bergerac, Toulouse, Narbonne, and Poitiers, and many other places; they all gave him up as incurable. Learning this Adam hastened to return to England, and when he got home he put off all his military gear and put on mourning clothes, in order to await his imminent death. However I, John Arderne, was called in and came to see him, and we agreed terms on a cure, which I undertook. With God's help I cured him perfectly within six months. Afterwards he stayed sound and healthy for thirty years or more, and enjoyed a pleasant existence. From this case I gained great honour and praise throughout England.[14]

This passage suggests not that Arderne was on campaign with Adam of Everingham but that he treated him only after Adam had made his return to England. Since we know that the second Baron Everingham, to whom this passage must refer, died as late as 1387/8, and that the *Practica* was written in 1376, the thirty years or more lived by Adam after his fistula operation at the time of writing would put his return to England at a point within Derby's campaigns of 1345–7 in Gascony. Since Everingham's home was at Laxton, some ten miles north-west of Newark, it would appear that Arderne was already in the Newark area before he began practice in 1349 there, on the basis of the reputation gained by the Everingham case. There are very few references to battlefield wounds within Arderne's writings, far fewer for instance that in the writings of his

---

[13] This point is made by Ussery, note 11 above.

[14] ' . . dominus Adam fuit in gasconia cum domino henrico tunc comite de darby nominato & postea factus est dux lancastrie strenuissimus domino vero Adam predicto fistulam in ano paciente omnes medicos & sirurgicos vasconie quos invenire poterat consulere fecit apud Burdewes & Brigerake Narebone Poyters & multis aliis locis & omnes eum pro incurabili reliquerunt / Quo viso & audito dictus Adam reperare festinavit & cum domum venerat disposuit omnia vestimenta sua militaria & induit vestes lugubres in proposito expectandi corporis dissolucionem sibi iam eminentem / Tandem requisitus ego dictus Johannes Arderne ad illum veni & pacto inito curam meam ei peregi & domino mediante infra dimidium annum illum perfecte curavi Et postea sanus & incolinus per triginta annos & plus vitam letam duxit pro qua cura magnum honorem & laudem per totam Angliam adeptus sum' (Sloane MS 56, fol. 38–38v). Here, and henceforth, readings in this MS have been collated with those in Sloane MS 335 and Glasgow, Hunterian MS 112.

contemporaries Guy de Chauliac or Thomas Scellinck. Most of the injuries he describes are incurred as a result of accidents in the home or the street.

The best evidence for the nature of Arderne's practice comes from the particular passage at the beginning of his *Practica* of fistula-in-ano which includes the mention of Adam of Everingham. The *Practica* of John of Arderne is unique amongst works of practical medicine and surgery in beginning with a list of cures undertaken by Arderne. Other such works may of course contain names of those cured amongst *consilia* (written consultations) or as part of the information contained in *experimenta* (illustrative case histories).[15] But none of them have a comparable list of cures, nor do they focus on one particular ailment in the way that Arderne's list does.[16] On looking more closely at the list itself, it is apparent that the status of the patients was important to Arderne. Twenty-one male patients are named, eleven cured while Arderne was practising in Newark, and ten more in London after 1370. The list includes two peers, the treasurer of the Black Prince's household, the custody of the Franciscans in York, and three secular clergy, all cured in the Newark period; the mayor of Northampton, a London fishmonger, and four Dominicans cured after Arderne's move to London.[17] The first cure mentioned is that of Sir Adam Everingham, a noted soldier in the retinue of Henry Earl of Derby, whose case is described above.[18] The background to Everingham's cure is described in more detail than the others, and, as we have seen, Everingham's case was the foundation of Arderne's successful career as a surgeon who could cure fistula-in-ano.

The picture that Arderne gives of his fistula-in-ano practice is of an exalted clientele, which fits in with the charges he recommends for the operation. For a patient *nobili* and *magno*, Arderne suggests charging between 100 marks and 40 pounds, with robes, fees (*feoda*) and an annuity of 100 shillings for the patient's lifetime. For *minoribus* Arderne recommends between 40 pounds and 40 marks without any fees, and says that he

---

[15] '*Consilia* convey a good deal about the social context of the professional practice of learned physicians, since the name, rank or occupation, place of residence, age, and sex of the patient are quite frequently included. Thus, out of the approximately seventy-five *consilia* by Taddeo that consist of more than just recipes, one or more of the above facts is found in thirty-four cases': Nancy G. Siraisi, *Taddeo Alderotti and his pupils: two generations of Italian medical learning* (Princeton, NJ, 1981), p. 276. See Michael R. McVaugh, 'The *Experimenta* of Arnald of Villanova', *Journal of Medieval and Renaissance Studies*, 1 (1972), 107–18, for use of this term to describe illustrative case histories, sometimes with details of individual patients.

[16] The only close parallel known to me is the list of cures in British Library Harley MS 2558, written out by Thomas Fayreford, who seems to have practised in north Devon in the first half of the fifteenth century. I am working on a study of this list and its relation to his surgical compendium. See Talbot and Hammond, *Medical practitioners*, p. 343.

[17] The following have been identified from other sources (although no independent confirmation of their having suffered from fistula-in-ano is available): Adam, 2nd Baron Everingham (c.1307–1387/8); Reynold, 4th Baron Grey of Wilton (1311–70); Henry Blakburn, treasurer of the Black Prince's household; John le Colier, mayor of Northampton 1326–7, 1339–40; John Haket, B.Th. (fl. 1368–97), Dominican author.

[18] See p. 295.

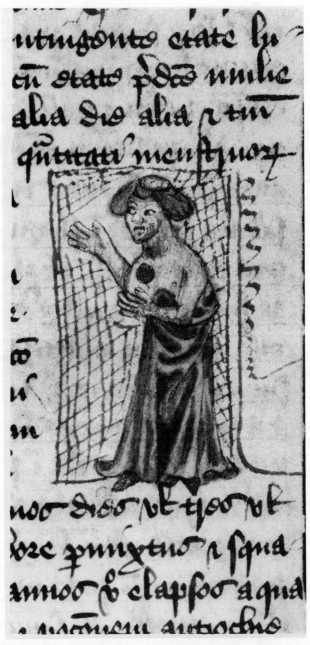

Figure 8 A chaplain from Colston with a sore on his breast.

never took on a cure without agreeing a charge of at the very least 100 shillings beforehand.[19] These figures suggest that Arderne charged as much as any medical practitioner of the period, despite his identifying himself as a mere *chirurgicus*.[20] The difficulty of the cure and the fact that he considered himself the only practitioner able to perform it no doubt determined his policy of charging as much as the medical market-place would allow.

Arderne's practice was not entirely devoted to fistula-in-ano of course. Outside the *Practica*, some idea of his experience with other types of surgery can be gained by looking at his case histories. The largest group of these occurs at the end of the longer manuscripts, and Arderne refers to these as his *curae* or *experimenta*, although others occur randomly where they are used to illustrate various therapies which Arderne recommends on the basis of his own experience. The *curae* at the end of the manuscripts number eighteen, but only twelve of these mention Arderne's own involvement with the patient. The remaining six are represented as stories told to Arderne about the experience of other practitioners, including a *sirurgicus expertus*, a *maister*, and two Franciscans.[21] The stories Arderne has to tell reveal quite a lot about how Arderne saw himself in relation to other medical practitioners, and his patients, as well as about the types of cures he undertook.

One of the most interesting *curae* is not in fact the story of a cure at all, nor does it feature Arderne himself. It shows the patient taking his ailment to three different types of medical practitioner, two of whom recommend ineffective or positively dangerous treatments, while the hero of the story is a *sirurgicus expertus* whose contribution is to warn of the danger of such treatments rather than to offer a cure:

A chaplain from Colston near Byngham developed within the skin of his nipple on his right breast a little nodule rather like a pea, which made him itch. And in the course of time the nodule grew to the size of a hen's egg, in the shape of a spinning top. He was troubled by pain for two, three, or more days each month. Its colour was livid and flecked with red, and hard and scaly to the touch. After two years had passed he was taught by a certain lady to apply plasters and he drank Antioch potion for a long period. At length he saw that the medicines were doing him no good, and went to the town of Nottingham to be let blood. A barber who saw the

[19] Sloane MS 56, fol.40v. At one point in the *Liber medicinarum* Arderne recalls a case of a genital ailment successfully treated, for which he charged 40 shillings, and another 20 shillings for treatment of scabies (Power, *Treatises of fistula in ano*, p. 111).

[20] For a discussion of fees charged see E. A. Hammond, 'Incomes of medieval English doctors', *Journal of the History of Medicine*, 15 (1960), 154–69; D'Arcy Power, 'The fees of our ancestors', *Janus*, 14 (1909), 287–93; repr. in D'Arcy Power, *Selected writings* (Oxford, 1931), pp. 95–102. It would seem that fees and annuities averaged much less than those claimed by Arderne. In a valuable recent study, Carole Rawcliffe, 'The profits of practice: the wealth and status of medical men in later medieval England', *Social History of Medicine*, 1 (1988), 61–78, has emphasized the range of financial rewards which both physicians and surgeons could expect from the patronage of influential people, but also the difficulty in collecting fees which went with this patronage.

[21] Sloane MS 56, fols. 84r, 88r, 92v, 93r, 93v, 94r, 94v.

nodule asked him if he wanted to be helped, claiming that he knew how to cure this ailment. The chaplain told him that he wanted to be cured but that he wanted to take advice as to whether the suggested cure would work. In the same town there was an experienced surgeon of whom the chaplain was informed. He went to him and sought his advice as to whether it was curable by incision, corrosives or medicines of this type. The doctor warned him not at any cost to place corrosives or other violent medicines on the sore, or to allow himself to be operated upon. He was warned that if he experienced any of these things he ran the risk of contracting an illness from which he would not recover but die.[22]

There is good reason to think that the lady and the barber-surgeon mentioned in this case are meant to show up two kinds of medical practitioner whom Arderne sees as (ineffective) rivals to the *sirurgicus expertus*, with whom Arderne identifies. A *domina* is mentioned in three other cures, and she is always characterized as using ineffectual plasters or pills, and the drink of Antioch.[23] Barber-surgeons are not mentioned among the other cures, but occur several times elsewhere in Arderne's writings, always attempting radical and dangerous cures.[24] Arderne's own interventions are portrayed as rescue missions which deliver the patient from the ministrations of other medical practitioners. The other feature of this story which deserves notice is the way in which patients move from practitioner to practitioner in search of a cure, often beginning with a *domina*, and moving on to other *medici*. This suggests that Arderne saw himself as at the top of a hierarchy of medical practitioners, and that the patient began by consulting women who dispensed medicines as part of their responsibilities for the household.

Rather less is said about the patients in Arderne's cures. Many of them appear as *quidam*, 'someone' (8 of 18), with a *quaedam* and a *puella*. One is a

---

[22] 'Cuidam capellano de Colston iuxta Byngham supervenit in dextra mamilla infra coreum super caput mamille quidam parvus nodulus in modo cuiusdam pise cum pruritu / Et crescente vero nodulo predicto per tempus aliquot tandem ad magnitudinem ovi galline pervenit formam habens unius troci .i. a toppe Et cum qualibet in neomenia illum dolore infestavit per duos dies vel tres vel plures / Color illius fuit lividus rubore permixtus & squamosus tactuique durus Post duos annos vero elapsos a quadam domina edoctus emplastrata apponere & pocionem antiochie bibit per longum tempus Tandem percipiente medicinas predictas sibi nil valere ivit ad villam de Notyngham ut sanguinem minueret / Barbitonsor vero cum perciperet nodum predictum inquisivit ab illo si de illo nodo vellet auxiliari asserens se scire curam talis infirmitatis / Capellanus vero dixit se velle curari sed tamen dixit se velle consulere si iam fieri posset quod sibi dixit in eadem vero villa fuit quidam sirurgicus expertus de quo idem capellanus habuit noticiam ad illumque perrexit & consilium illius petit si iam curabilis esset aut si inscicionem vel corrosionem vel huiusmodi medicinas pateretur Medicus ille vero sibi inhibuit ne ullo modo predicto fico corrosivas vel alias violentas medicinas apponeret seu inscidi permitteret.
Quod si faceret permisit se usque ad mortem ipsius langorem irrecuperabilem incurrere etc.' (Sloane MS 56, fol. 84r.)

[23] See Power, *Treatises of fistula in ano*, p. 120 for the makeup of the drink of Antioch.

[24] See, for example, the case of a fishmonger in London injured in the arm by a knife, and treated by a barber-surgeon who inserted tents into the wound unsuccessfully (Power, *Treatises of fistula in ano*, p. 100).

baby. Four of them are clergy, two chaplains, a rector, and a canon. At opposite ends of the economic scale are the *dives* and the gardener. Finally, there is the son of Sir Thomas Newmark, born with a wen on his head. But none of the last three is treated by Arderne himself. Of those treated by Arderne, only in the case of the rector and the canon is the status specifically mentioned. This reinforces the impression given by the list of cures at the beginning of the *Practica* that the clergy, both seculars and regulars, may have comprised a substantial part of Arderne's clientele.

The ailments mentioned in the cures are those that we would expect of a surgeon rather than a physician, since all of them (bar perhaps one) are diagnosed by external appearances. Seven are swellings or apostemes, two fistulae, five excrescences of one sort or another, and four wounds. The only doubtfully surgical case is a chaplain whose chest swelled up after being urinated on by a *rato*, which D'Arcy Power believes to be a case of hysteria or neurasthenia rather than a physical ailment.[25] Eleven of the ailments affected the limbs of the patient, three the penis, and two the head, and the canon with the *nodulus* on his breast is the only other case where the trunk of the patient was involved. On the basis of this sample we may tentatively assume that much of Arderne's practice was taken up with the visible ailments affecting the limbs of his patients, while the number of cases affecting the male genitalia hint at something of a specialism.

What we know of Arderne's practice suggests therefore that he dealt with all sorts of surgical cases, but had a bias towards the treatment of fistula and genito-urinary problems. When not treating fistula-in-ano he treated both men and women, though his most profitable cases were those brought to him by the clergy, wealthy merchants, and the knightly class. Although he is not named as one of the sworn master-surgeons of the city of London after his move there in 1370, it is probable that he considered himself their equal in terms of prestige and professional accomplishment. His use of the term master-surgeon to describe his own status indicates this. It is the fact that he wrote about surgery that distinguishes him from the others.

ARDERNE'S WRITINGS

The *Extracta emoroydarum*

Arderne's best-known work is the *Practica* of fistula-in-ano, which was composed in the 1370s after his move to London. It has the very recogniz-able *incipit*: 'Ego Iohannes predictus a prima pestilentia ...'. This text is present in all manuscripts of his works, usually in conjunction with a number of other texts.

---

[25] D'Arcy Power, 'The lesser writings of John Arderne', *Seventeenth International Congress of Medicine* (London, 1913), section XXII, History of Medicine, pp. 127–8.

The difficulty of characterizing these other writings, which include sections on a variety of apparently unrelated medical topics, led D'Arcy Power, the editor of one of the four Middle English translations of Arderne, to lump them together at one point under the heading *Liber medicinarum sive receptorum liber medicinalium*, while in another place he described them as a succession of small treatises on a variety of subjects. One of these shorter treatises is headed *Extracta emoroydarum*, and is dated to 1376 – the same year as the *Practica*. While all the shorter texts are usually found in the same order in different manuscripts, the point at which the sequence begins varies between manuscripts. In the case of at least one of these texts, the *Speculum fleobotomiae*, it is not even certain that the work is attributable to Arderne. Other texts deal with medicinal simples, eye problems, gynaecology, diseases of the kidneys and the genito-urinary tract. Whether these were all conceived as part of a single work originally or not is a question still unresolved, but it is impossible to reassemble them to make a compendium of practical medicine on the scholastic model, like that of Arderne's English contemporary John of Mirfield.[26] The *Practica* of fistula-in-ano is most often found embedded within this complex of texts called by Power the *Liber medicinarum*, although it relates in subject matter only to the *Extracta emoroydarum*.

Even in these shorter works of Arderne there are plentiful signs of his reading of scholastic texts. Two of them are given titles which announce them as extracts from named works by others, the *Extracta de libro qui dicitur liber virtutum*, and the *Extracta emoroydarum*. The first is based on John of St Paul's *De simplicium medicinarum virtutibus*.[27] The full title of the second is worth quoting at length because it reveals the breadth of Ardernes's reading, and his concern for accuracy of citation:

Extracts on haemorrhoids taken from Lanfranco of Milan, the most learned master who served the King of France, who composed two books of surgery, viz. the minor which begins 'Attendens venerabilis amice Bernarde componere librum etc.', and the major which begins 'Protector in se sperancium deus excelsus et gloriosus cuius nomen sit benedictum in secula etc.

Omne quod investigari potest uno trium modorum investigari potest aut per eius nomen etc.' Also extracts on haemorrhoids from master Bernard de Gordon in his book composed at Montpellier in 1303, in the twentieth year of his lecturing there, which begins 'Interrogatus a quodam Socrates quomodo possit optime

---

[26] Author of the *Breviarium Bartholomei*. See *Johannes de Mirfeld of St Bartholomew's Smithfield: his life and works*, ed. P. H.-S. Hartley and H. R. Aldridge (Cambridge, 1936); James B. Colton, transl., *John of Mirfield (d.1407) Surgery: A translation of his Breviarium Bartholomei, part ix* (New York, 1969). See also Faye Getz, 'John Mirfield and the *Breviarium Bartholomei*; the medical writings of a clerk at St Bartholomew's Hospital in the later fourteenth century', *Society for the Social History of Medicine Bulletin*, 37 (1985), 24–6. I am at present in the process of editing Arderne's writings, and hope to throw more light on the complicated textual history behind them.

[27] Lynn Thorndike and Pearl Kibre, *A catalogue of incipits of mediaeval scientific writings in Latin*, 2nd edn (London, 1963), col. 230.

dicere Respondit si nichil dixeris nisi quod optime sciveris nichil autem optime scimus nisi quod a nobis frequenter dictum est et quod ab omnibus receptum est.' Also extracts from the Passionarius of master Bartholomew which begins 'Assiduis peticionibus mi karissime compendiose morborum signa causas et curas inscriptis redigere cogitis etc.' Also extracts from the Micrologus of the excellent master Ricardus Anglicus, diligently compiled, and from the book of master Rolando and of master Guy de gracia pauperum, and from the Practica of Roger Baron, and of Roger, and of master Johannes Jamarcius, and of Gilbertinus, and of many other experienced surgeons whose writings I have examined. The fruits of experience I have discovered by practice should become known through this little book with God's help. Also Ricardus Anglicus whose treatise begins 'si quid agam preter solitum veniam date cuncti', Rolando, Roger Baron, Rogerinus, Johannes Jamarcus, Guy, and Gilbertinus[28]

As Power suggests, this is an impressive record of Arderne's reading, and important evidence for the texts available to him. All of the *incipits* given in this list can today be identified with the aid of Thorndike and Kibre, a fact which speaks also for his concern for bibliographical accuracy (although the text he calls the *Passionarius* of master Bartholomew is in fact the *Breviarium* or *Practica* of John of St Paul). Yet there is surely a hint here too in the extraordinary thoroughness of this list that Arderne may not have expected his readers to be able to identify and find these texts easily, and consequently felt he had to provide more than the sort of brief reference appropriate to a reader with a background in the schools. Arderne himself was evidently acquainted with most of the principal Latin sources for information on haemorrhoids, though he does not include any Arabic

---

[28] 'Extracta emoroidarum secundum Lanfrancum bononensem (*sic*) discretissimum magistrum Regis francie qui duos libros cirurgie composuit viz minorem qui incipit sic Attendens venerabilis amice Bernarde componere librum etc Majorem vero qui incipit sic Protector in se sperancium deus excelsus et gloriosus cuius nomen sit benedictum in secula etc

Omne quod investigari potest uno trium modorum investigari potest aut per eius nomen etc.

Item extracta emoroidarum secundum magistrum bernardum de Gordon in suo libro quem librum composuit dictus Bernardus apud Montem Pessulanum .i. Montpelers anno domini millesimo ccc iii et anno lecture sue xx qui sic incipit Interrogatus a quodam Socrates quomodo possit optime dicere Respondit si nichil dixeris nisi quod optime sciveris nichil autem optime scimus nisi quod a nobis frequenter dictum est et quod ab omnibus receptum est

Item extracta a passionario Magistri Bartholomei qui sic incipit Assiduis peticionibus mi karissime compendiose morborum signa causas et curas inscriptis redigere cogitis etc.

Item extracta a micrologo Magistri Ricardi excellentis industrie et a libro Magistri Rolandi et a libro Magistri Gwidonis de gracia pauperum et a practica Rogera Baron Et a practica Rogeri et a practica Magistri Johannis Jamaracii et Gilbertini ac aliorum plurium expertorum quorum doctrinam inspexi et practizando que experciora reperi in hoc libello domino mediante innotescent

Ricardus qui incipit Si quid agam preter solitum veniam date cuncti

Rolandus Rogerus Baron Rogerinus Johannes Jamarcus Gwidon Gilbertinus (A Latin transcription by Miss E. M. Thompson is provided in Power, *Treatises of fistula in ano*, p. 122. My transcription from Sloane MS 56, fol. 65r–v differs only in minor details.)

authors, as might have been expected.[29] Nor does he seem to have been aware of the *Regimen sanitatis* for King Jaume II of Aragon by Arnau de Vilanova, which includes a long final chapter on haemorrhoids. Not surprisingly, Arderne makes more use of the surgical authors on this subject than the medical, though he does include John of St Paul, Ricardus Anglicus, Roger Baron, and Gilbertus Anglicus. But his principal sources were Lanfranco and Bernard de Gordon, as can be confirmed by the quotation of passages from them in the body of the text.[30] The other surgeons, Roger of Parma, Rolando, Jamerius, Bruno and Guy (de Chauliac?), play a less vital role, though Arderne borrows his definition of haemorrhoids from Roger (beginning 'Emoroys apud grecos dicitur fluxus sanguis ...').

The technique of compiling excerpts from other authors on specific medical and surgical topics was of course a development of scholastic education, allied to the literary *florilegium*. Guy de Chauliac's *Inventarium seu collectorium cyrurgie* purports to be excerpted in this way, and Gilbertus Anglicus describes his *Compendium* as 'ab omnibus auctoribus et practicis magistrorum extractus et excerptus'.[31] The student had in his hands a convenient summary of the opinions of the masters on different topics, assembled into scholastic order (usually head to toe in the case of *Practicae*). The *aggregator* was of course free to declare his opinion on disputed matters, or resolve apparent contradictions between authorities. Arderne's *Extracta emoroydarum* belongs recognizably to this genre, although it deals only with haemorrhoids, and does not fit within the frame of a larger compendium. His quotations are not generally attributed to authorities, and vary in length from a phrase to whole paragraphs.

There are also passages in the *Extracta emorydarum* where it is clear that Arderne is not relying directly on other authorities but offering opinions of his own. Thus, having defined haemorrhoids after Roger of Parma, Arderne goes on to say that the term haemorrhoids has been used indiscriminately by the *vulgi* to cover any ailment of the backside involving suffusion with blood, itching or smarting, and that the *laici* and *inexperti* have also other words for haemorrhoids – the French call them *fics* and the Londoners *piles*. Despite the local reference, it is clear that here Arderne is lining up with his learned authorities as opposed to the *vulgi, laici* and *inexperti*. Arderne also intrudes on the exposition to make use of his own experience in diagnosis and cure. He describes the making of the

---

[29] This feature was pointed out to me by Danielle Jacquart. In other parts of the *Liber medicinarum*, by comparison, Arderne does cite Rhazes, Albucasis, and Haly Abbas.

[30] See, for instance, the passage beginning 'in causa ergo frigida predicta dentur ea que calefaciunt ... ' (Sloane MS 56, fol. 69v), which can be found in Bernard de Gordon, *Lilium medicinae* (Lyons, 1550), p. 620.

[31] *Liber morborum tam universalium quam particularium a magistro Gilberto Anglico editus ... qui Compendium medicine intitulatur* (Lyons, 1510). See Agrimi and Crisciani, *Edocere medicos*, ch. 6, for an analysis of this aggregative habit.

medicament *tapsivalencia* 'hec est medicina quam ego Johannes de Ardern composui quam nunquam carere volui quod omnem inflacionem emoroidibus dolorem ac puncturam cum ardore mirifice mitigat' ('which I John of Arderne composed, and which I wish always to have by me and which mitigates all painful swellings and burning sensations in haemorrhoids marvellously').[32]

In the *Extracta emoroydarum*, John of Arderne shows his respect for scholastic authorities by making detailed reference to a number of relevant authors and texts, in a way that would enable his readers to find and study these texts for themselves. He follows the conventions of an established genre of scholastic treatise based on extracting and reconciling authorities, while appealing occasionally to the lessons of his own practical experience. Yet there are also passages in which Arderne moves outside the language and conceptual framework of the scholastic authorities. In these passages we find vivid and personal descriptions of the practice of surgery in language which is both more immediate and more homely, and suggestive of the difficulties involved in practical application. References to other practitioners and to the circumstances in which the surgeon operates also occur. The following is one such passage:

> If indeed the doctor sees any patients having circular excrescences around the anus, on the summit of which appear things like black spots, as depicted here, then he knows for certain that black blood has coagulated in them. Knowing this the doctor applies poultices and ointments two or three times, and then afterwards he should not delay in laying open with a lancet the excrescence at the place where it began to grow, without forewarning the patient. Once opened up, the doctor can press out the coagulated blood with his finger and he should do so boldly so that the patient will feel no pain. I have proved this cure works many times, and I have seen many cured very swiftly and permanently this way. The doctor should be careful in case any of the bystanders see how it is done as the excrescences are opened up. Since once the barbers grasped the method they would usurp this cure for themselves to the considerable shame and harm of the master surgeons.[33]

This passage is illustrated with a picture of the *macule nigre* in schematic form, breaking with the conventions of scholastic discourse (writings on surgery were occasionally illustrated with diagrams of instruments but

---

[32] Sloane MS 56, fol.72r. See *Pharmacopoeia Londinensis* ... (London, 1618), pp. 160–1, for *tapsivalencia* and two other remedies attributed to Arderne, called there *Chyrurgus excercitatissimus*. Also Power, *Treatises of fistula in ano*, pp. xxxi, 69.

[33] 'Si vero viderit medicus aliquos habentes circa anum exterius tumbrositates rotundas in quarum summitatibus apparent quasi macule nigre sicut hic depingitur tunc sciat pro certo quod in illis est sanguis niger coagulatus Quo igitur cognito post fomentaciones factas & uncciones etc bis vel ter postea non tardet medicus predictas tumbrositates in loco ingredinis cum lancete paciente nesciente aperire quibus apertis cum digito potest exprimere sanguinem coagulatum & hoc faciat audacter quia paciens inde gravamen non senciet . probavi enim pluries & hec curacio quam plures imperpetuum sanare vidi & hoc valde cito / Et caveat medicus quod nemo astancium percipiat quando huiusmodi

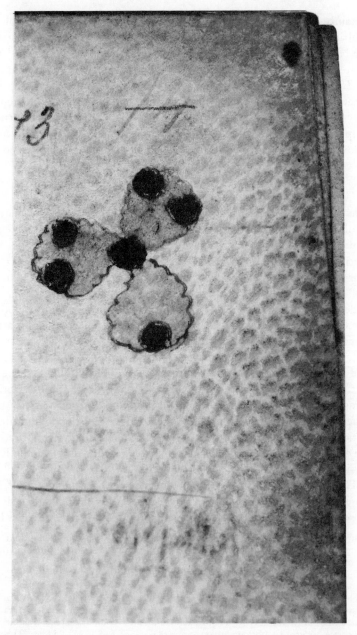

Figure 9 *Macule nigre*: a form of haemorrhoids.

certainly never with illustrations of *signa* or symptoms, least of all in propaedeutic exercises like collections of *extracta*).[34] Arderne's worry that the barber-surgeons might usurp the operation properly reserved to the master-surgeons is very apparent here. The consequence would be *dedecus ac dampnum* to the fellowship of master-surgeons, shame presumably because the barber-surgeons would bring the operation into disrepute as they would not understand the reasons for the procedure but perform it by simply aping the manual technique of the master surgeon. Harm too to the fellowship since this could diminish their business and their prestige.

The *Practica*

The use of the term *Practica* for Arderne's better-known treatise on fistula-in-ano brings us up immediately against the question of its relationship to the *Practicae* of the scholastic tradition. Although the earlier works given this name vary in their overall structure, they share two basic characteristics – the fact that they deal with surgery of all parts of the body, and the fact that they deal with these parts in a head-to-toe order.[35] Arderne's *Practica* differs in dealing with only one zone of the body and consequently in eschewing head-to-toe order. It differs just as sharply in that its structure is hardly articulated by the standards of scholastic surgery. Instead of a hierarchical structure of books, *distinctiones*, and chapters, we find no clear division even into chapters. The best witnesses to the Latin text do not have any divisions in the text at all, except for a scattering of paragraph marks, and there are no indications that the text as Arderne conceived it had such divisions. D'Arcy Power has supplied a numerical sectional structure for his edition of the Middle English text, elaborating on the chapters provided by the translator of one of the four Middle English versions.[36]

There is, however, a narrative structure implicit in the text itself, in the sense that the order in which Arderne tackles his subject proceeds from those things that it is necessary for the surgeon to know and discover before

tumbrositates cum lanceta vel huismodi aperiat. Quia si barbitonsores istud factum cognoscerent curam istam sibi usurpando appropriarent in dedecus ac dampnum magistorum non modicum' (Sloane MS 56, fols.72v–73r).

[34] Björn Wallner, 'Drawings of surgical instruments in MS Bibl. Nat. Angl. 25', *English Studies*, 45 (1965), 182–6.

[35] The medieval *practica* and attempts made by Renaissance writers to 'humanize' it are discussed by Andrew Wear, 'Explorations in Renaissance writings on the practice of medicine', in A. Wear, R. K. French, and I. M. Lonie (eds.), *The medical renaissance of the sixteenth century* (Cambridge, 1985), pp. 118–45. See also J. M. Riddle, 'Theory and practice in medieval medicine', *Viator*, 5 (1974), 157–84; Luke Demaitre, 'Theory and practice in medical education at the University of Montpellier in the thirteenth and fourteenth centuries', *Journal of the History of Medicine*, 30 (1975), 103–23, and Agrimi and Crisciani, *Edocere medicos*, ch. 6.

[36] These versions are discussed by Peter Murray Jones, 'Four Middle English translations of John of Arderne', in Alastair Minnis (ed.), *Latin and Vernacular: studies in late-medieval texts and manuscripts* (Woodbridge, 1989), pp. 61–89.

operating, to the operation itself, the after-care of the patient, and then various related ailments which the surgeon may encounter. But, by comparison with the scholastic surgeries with their clear articulation and methodical approach, Arderne's *Practica* is lacking in structure.[37] It is difficult to imagine the text as the subject of a formal exposition to pupils, or as part of a curriculum which aspiring surgeons might follow.

Nor is the concentration on fistula-in-ano easy to reconcile with what we know of the teaching of surgery from the scholastic works. Commonly fistula-in-ano is dealt with in one chapter in the earlier surgeries, often with reference to the earlier discussion of fistula of the tear ducts. Sometimes it is not accorded a chapter to itself, but is discussed only within the wider handling of fistula in general. We would not expect to find such an extensive treatment of any surgical speciality in the scholastic authors, above all not for such an unglamorous subject as fistula-in-ano. In the scholastic surgeries disproportionate attention is devoted to surgery on the head in comparison with surgery on other parts of the body. The only operation discussed in anything like the detail found in Arderne is that for depressed fracture of the skull, which appears to have been the great set-piece operation for every Western surgeon from Roger of Parma onwards. But even for this operation the scholastic surgeons allocated only a few chapters within the larger section on surgery on the head, and there are no surviving *Practicae* dealing with this operation alone.

Arderne's procedure in the assembling of his text (*confeccio huius libelli*) on fistula-in-ano is not that commonly employed by the scholastic surgeons. Instead of a straightforward exposition of the *doctrina*, or a compilation based on extracts from the works of other authorities, Arderne interrupts his own exposition with at least one section which appears to have been taken verbatim from the extensive body of technical literature already in circulation in manuscript (there is no good English equivalent to the useful German term *Fachprosa* in reference to these short practical texts). The Latin texts of Arderne contain a section headed *Nota de cognitione signorum Lunae*, which consists of a short text explaining the method for finding the position of the moon on any given day by means of the calendar and a table of signs of the zodiac.[38] Following the table comes a passage which begins:

... thus argue the astrologers, viz Ptolemy, Pythagoras, Rhazes, Haly Abbas, etc., that the surgeon should not cut or burn in any member of the human body, nor let blood, while the moon is in the sign reigning over that member.[39]

[37] Compare, for instance, the Middle English surgery of 1392 edited by Grothé (note 8 above).

[38] Transcribed and translated in Power, *Treatises of the fistula in ano*, pp. 16–20.

[39] '... sicut volunt astrologi summi viz Ptolomaeus Pythagoras Rhasis Haly etc non debet cirurgus incidere vel urere in aliquo membro corporis humani nec facere phlebotomiam dum luna fuerit in signo regnante illud membrum' (Power, *Treatises of the fistula in ano*, p. 16).

This text is similar to several of the same kind that circulated independently of Arderne, and deals with the conditions under which surgery or blood-letting on any part of the body should be performed, or rather eschewed. It certainly has no special relevance to the operation for fistula-in-ano, and the style of this passage is not that of Arderne.[40] *Confeccio* seems to have involved the deliberate interpolation by Arderne of elements of technical literature originating elsewhere, a practice which has no parallel in the scholastic surgeries.

There are grammatical and lexical features of Arderne's writings which mark out Arderne not only as a weak Latinist, even by the standards of the scholastic surgeons, but as someone whose Latin seems not to have been put to the test of classroom exposure. It would hardly be an exaggeration to say that Arderne really provides a polyglot rather than a consistent Latin text. Parts of the *Liber medicinarum* are written in Anglo-Norman or Middle English, surrounded on either side by Latin.[41] Since Arderne does not seem to have had a university education, it is no surprise that the grammar of his Latin is like that of a man thinking in English but writing in Latin, as is often the case in the *experimenta* mentioned above.[42] Another feature of Arderne's Latin prose is the frequency with which he provides English or Anglo-Norman glosses to technical terms. The Latin lemma *vertile* (a peg) is glossed by Arderne *anglice a wraste*. Like the illustration of the peg provided in the margin, this gloss must have been meant to help identify the instrument. Of course we cannot be entirely sure that Arderne himself was the author of all the glosses. But the fact that these glosses are uniform in the Latin manuscripts seems to indicate at least an origin in some common ancestor rather than glossing by scribes. It is not possible to produce conclusive proof that these features of the Arderne text originated with the author himself, but, as with the illustrations, there is at least a strong supposition that they were integral to the first texts.[43]

Features like the glossing of Latin terms with vernacular are of course not exclusive to Arderne's text, but, taken together with the grammatical qualities discussed above, they add up to a text which is much less securely rooted in Latin scholastic culture than are the surgeries of Lanfranco, or

---

[40] Of course we cannot be certain that this passage was inserted by Arderne himself, rather than a later scribe, but the evidence of the manuscripts suggests that interpolation must have taken place at such an early stage as to preclude survival of any copies of the Latin text without it. The passage also fits well in the context of the discussion by Arderne of the preparations the surgeon should make before operating – it follows immediately on from a passage on the medicines and instruments the surgeon must make ready before the operation. The same procedure of interpolation of short *Fachprosa* texts is found elsewhere in the *Liber medicinarum* (Jones, 'Four Middle English translations', p. 67).

[41] Ibid., p. 68.

[42] See the cases of Adam of Everingham, Thomas Brone, and the chaplain of Colston, pp. 295, 298 above.

[43] See note 40 above. Glossing is found very frequently in Middle English translations of Latin texts. See Björn Wallner, 'On the .i. periphrasis in the NY Chauliac', *Neuphilologische Mitteilungen*, 88 (1987), 286–94.

Henri de Mondeville. Nevertheless it is striking that Arderne should have written in Latin, when it must appear that he thought and spoke in English. It is a measure of his respect for the tradition of the scholastic surgeries that he should have tried to emulate them despite the difficulties involved. Arderne also claims acquaintance with other Latin authors too, as he makes use of a number of tags from non-medical authors in the course of the *Practica*. Two examples where he can be shown to have quoted these authors occur in the deontological section near the beginning of the *Practica*. One is a quotation from the pseudo-Boethius, *De disciplina scolarium*: 'Since Boethius says in De disciplina scolarium "he is not worthy of the heights of sweetness who does not know what it is to taste the depths of bitterness".'[44] The quotation is accurate, and the work from which Arderne quotes was a very popular manual of education in the fourteenth and fifteenth centuries throughout Europe. Arderne may well have come across it if he attended a grammar school, but it was also used by some of the scholastic surgical authorities.[45] The second quotation run as follows:

But it cannot be doubted that if the aforesaid conditions are observed they will guarantee to the practitioner a gratifying degree of honour and wealth. Thus Cato says 'I think it a prime virtue to be able to bite on one's tongue'.[46]

Again the quotation is accurate, and the distichs attributed to a fourth-century Cato were very popular fodder for grammarians and moralists in Arderne's time. We can infer that Arderne's own Latin education was likely to have been of the conventional grammar school type, although his moral commonplaces may have been borrowed from earlier scholastic writers on surgery, rather than remembered from his own studies.[47]

Interestingly enough when Arderne makes use of a quotation from other surgical or medical authors in the *Practica* he does not acknowledge his

---

[44] 'Quia dicit boicius de disciplina scolarium / Non est dignus dulcoris acumine qui nescit amaritudinis inviscari gravamine' (Sloane MS 56, fol. 41r). Pseudo-Boethius, *De disciplina scolarium*, ed. Olga Weijers, Studien und Texte zur Geistesgeschichte des Mittelalters, 12 (Leiden, 1976), 4:22 (p. 115).

[45] Henri de Mondeville makes use of *De disciplina scolarium* to characterize the ideal *magister*, as is noted by Agrimi and Crisciani, *Edocere medicos*, p. 219.

[46] 'Sed non est dubitandum quod si premissa observantur qui ei excercenti ad culmen honoris & lucri prebibunt graciosum unde cato Virtutem primam esse puto compescere linguam (Sloane MS 56 fol.41v). Wayland Johnson Chase (ed.), *The distichs of Cato*, University of Wisconsin Studies in Social Science and History, 7 (Madison, 1922), Book 1, 3 (p. 16). Derek Pearsall, (ed.), *The Nun's Priest's tale* (A variorum edition of the works of Geoffrey Chaucer, vol. ii, *The Canterbury tales*, part 9 (Norman, Okla., 1983), p. 166, refers to the parody of banal pedagogic commonplace involved in Pertelote's citing Cato as an authority. See also Richard Hazelton, 'Chaucer and Cato', *Speculum*, 35 (1960), 357–80.

[47] For alternatives to Oxford and Cambridge as centres for higher education in England, see William J. Courtenay, *Schools and scholars in fourteenth century England* (Princeton, NJ, 1987), ch. 3. For English schooling of the period, see Jo-Ann Hoeppner Moran, *The growth of English schooling 1340–1548: learning, literacy, and laicization in pre-Reformation York diocese* (Princeton, NJ, 1985); and Nicholas Orme, *English schools in the Middle Ages* (London, 1973).

source in the same explicit way. Thus, for instance, a few words before the quotation from pseudo-Boethius mentioned above, Arderne makes direct, but silent, use of Lanfranco of Milan (who in turn was quoting Galen): 'Let the doctor therefore be ingenious enough in this operation to know more than is committed to writing, since everything that ought to be known about this operation cannot be expressed in words alone.'[48] This comes from the section on deontology in the *Chirurgia* of Lanfranco, and is repeated almost word for word by Arderne. But in the *Practica*, unlike the *Extracta emoroydarum*, Arderne seems to have been keen to give an impression that he had digested his surgical authorities, and was ready to incorporate them in his discussion without making it clear at all times when he was relying on authority. So, although at first sight the *Practica* gives the impression of floating free of surgical scholasticism, in a way that the *Extracta emoroydarum* definitely does not, this is misleading.

The contents of the Practica in relation to earlier surgeries

The real measure of the impact of the scholastic surgical tradition on Arderne must be the extent to which his *Practica* on fistula-in-ano embodies *doctrina* absorbed from his study of the masters. In order to make this indebtedness clear I will summarize the contents of the *Practica*, and then look at the scholastic tradition as it deals with the matters raised in Arderne's text.

As we have seen, Arderne's *Practica* begins with a list of cures of fistula-in-ano undertaken successfully by the surgeon. There follows a prologue which explains the circumstances of the *confeccio* of the text, corresponding in some ways to the traditional *accessus* to the literary or scholastic text.[49] This is succeeded by a section on deontology, the conduct of the surgeon towards his patient. Arderne would have been familiar with this device in Lanfranco, from whom he was quite happy to borrow, as we saw above. The *Practica* proper begins with a discussion of the instruments necessary for the operation of fistula-in-ano, by incision or by ligature, accompanied in most manuscripts by pictures of the instruments and a sequence showing the instruments in place. As we shall see, some of these instruments are clearly based on those described in earlier texts, though others are of Arderne's own devising.[50] He moves on to the nature of fistula, and how it develops from *apostemata*, and how the latter can be

---

[48] 'Sit igitur medicus ingeniosus in hac operacione ut plura quam in scriptis inveniat agere sciat quia omnia que circa tale opus fieri debent non possunt litteris exprimi' (Sloane MS 56, fol. 49r). The same words are used in Robert von Fleischhacker (ed.), *Lanfrank's 'Science of Cirurgie'*, Early English Text Society, original series 102 (London, 1894), p. 8, lines 11–12; and translated into English by Power, *Treatises of fistula in ano*, p. xxvi.

[49] See A. J. Minnis, *Medieval theory of authorship*, 2nd edn (Aldershot, 1988); R. K. French, 'A note on the anatomical accessus of the Middle Ages', *Medical History*, 23 (1979), 461–8; Danielle Jacquart, 'Aristotelian thought in Salerno', in Peter Dronke (ed.), *A history of twelfth century philosophy* (Cambridge, 1988), p. 414, n. 29.

[50] See below, pp. 315–16.

treated with medicaments in order to avoid fistulation. He then describes a number of different forms in which fistulae can present themselves to the surgeon, the number of holes and their position determining the difficulty of treatment. The surgeon is instructed how to ask his patient about his symptoms, in particular the discharge of *sanies*. The surgeon must then put his prognosis to the patient, and work out the best time for operation, making use of his astrological knowledge.

There follows the cure of fistula proper, beginning with a short definition of fistula in scholastic form. Arderne describes how, when the patient is strong and the fistula operable, to operate by cutting through the fistula to the walls of the rectum.[51] The procedure is described in great detail, and illustrated in most manuscripts on the basis of a pattern evidently suggested by the author. Directions are given for the staunching of blood after the operation. The after-care and bandaging of the wound are also specified minutely. If the patient is feeble, or there is a great distance between the fistulous hole and the anus, Arderne recommends a tight ligature through the fistula and rectum, to be left in place and tightened daily until the flesh between is cut away. Subsequently Arderne recommends a *diaflosmus* plaster, for which he gives exhaustive directions.

Next Arderne provides a number of case histories illustrating complications he has treated successfully. In cases where ulceration has occurred, Arderne tells how to treat it with *tapsimel* and *pulver sine pare*. Arderne also considers other specific related ailments like *bubo* of the rectum, a form of ulceration that gives rise to a hard swelling, and various kinds of sore on the flesh of the buttocks. Finally, Arderne provides a number of recipes and specifications for instruments used in the making of medicaments mentioned earlier in the *Practica*.

How far is this all based on the scholastic tradition of surgery?[52] There were of course no other works devoted specifically to this subject, and this goes not only for the scholastics but also for the authorities of late antiquity. But the subject did arise in the general surgical *Practicae*, albeit in a concise form, and discussion of fistula-in-ano goes back to the Hippocratic corpus.

---

[51] See below, pp. 317–18, for a comparison of Arderne's operation with that of the scholastics.

[52] For a brief but valuable modern survey of the development of surgery in the Middle Ages see Gundolf Keil, 'Mittelalterliche Chirurgie', *Acta Medicae Historiae Patavina*, 30 (1983–4), 45–64. The essays of Siraisi and Agrimi and Crisciani in this volume discuss scholasticism in Italian medieval surgery. Detailed analysis of the works of the surgeons may be found in E. J. Gurlt, *Geschichte der Chirurgie und ihrer Ausübung*, 3 vols. (Berlin, 1898); vol. III, pp. 744–8, deals explicitly with fistula-in-ano. Discussion of this operation up to the end of the eighteenth century and citation of sources is contained in Kurt Polycarp Joachim Sprengel, transl. A. J. L. Jourdan, *Histoire de la médecine* (Paris, 1815–32), Book 7, sect. 18, ch. 10, pp. 264–83. Karl Sudhoff, *Beiträge zur Geschichte der Chirurgie im Mittelalter*, vol. II (Leipzig, 1918), Studien zur Geschichte der Medizin, 11, 12, provides texts for a number of early surgeries. Salvatore de Renzi, *Collectio Salernitana*, 5 vols. (Naples, 1852–9) does the same service for Roger, Rolando, the Glosses of the Four Masters, and a number of other Salernitian *practicae* with surgical content.

The Latin translations of the Arab authors, particularly Haly Abbas al-Majusi, Rhazes and Albucasis, seem to have been the sources for most of what was written about fistula-in-ano in the West. These authors in turn depended chiefly on Paul of Aegina, who gave the longest and most circumstantial account of the operation in antiquity.[53] Arderne summarized the works of authors now known only through Paul's writings, particularly Meges of Sidon, who seems to have lived in the first century AD. There also survives a pseudo-Hippocratic treatise *De fistulis*, which deals principally with fistula-in-ano, but which could not have been widely known in the Latin West, though in some of its details – for instance, the use of horsehair in forming a ligature – its influence may have been felt indirectly.[54] But, for our purposes, Haly Abbas in the translation of Constantine, Rhazes and Albucasis are the direct sources for the operation or rather operations. The Latin scholastic authorities from the Salernitans onwards built on these foundations.

The description of the operative treatments for fistula-in-ano is given the fullest treatment by Albucasis.[55] He treats the subject at greater length than any of the subsequent surgical authors, excepting Arderne, and he is the most likely source for their ideas on the handling of this topic. Albucasis begins by describing how fistulae originate in knotting and thickening of the tissue near the anus, which becomes fistulous with time. These fistulae may perforate the rectum or bowel, or not. If they perforate the bowel the patient discharges faeces or foul matter, and often worms via the fistulae. Sometimes the fistulae may perforate the bladder and the urinary passages or reach the hip-joint or the coccyx. There is a test to establish whether the fistulae are penetrating or not, by passing the finger into the anus and a fine probe into the fistula. If finger and probe meet then the surgeon knows that the fistula has perforated the rectum. When the fistula has reached the bladder or urinary passages, it is signified by the passing of urine out through the fistula. In all cases of perforating fistulae, the absence of any medical cure makes surgery necessary.

In cases of non-perforating fistulae, the surgeon has the patient lie flat on his back, with his legs flexed back up to the stomach. Introducing a probe into the fistula, and the forefinger into the anus, the surgeon can decide

53 Paulus Aegineta, *Epitome medicae libri septem*, ed. I. L. Heiberg, Pars altera, Libri v–vii (Leipzig and Berlin, 1924), Corpus Medicorum Graecorum, ix.2, lib.6, sect 78, pp. 120–3; Francis Adams (transl.) *The Seven Books of Paulus Aegineta* (London, Sydenham Society, 1844), vol. ii, pp. 399–402.

54 'Des fistules', in Robert Joly (ed.), *Hippocrate*, Collection des Universités de France, 13 (Paris, 1978), pp. 131–45. Cf. Pearl Kibre, 'Hippocrates Latinus', *Traditio*, 34 (1978), 208, for one Latin MS, and the remarks of Vivian Nutton, 'Humanist surgery', in A. Wear, R. K. French, and I. M. Lonie (eds.), *The medical renaissance of the sixteenth century* (Cambridge, 1985), p. 77.

55 *Methodus medendi certa, clara et brevis ...* (Basle, 1541), lib. 2, cap. 80, pp. 132–4; M. S. Spinks and G. L. Lewis (eds.), *Albucasis on surgery and instruments* (London, 1973), pp. 502–11 (this English translation must be used with caution, as it supplies modern medical 'equivalents' for Arab terminology).

whether the fistula perforates or not. If it does perforate, Albucasis mentions a cure which may help in certain rare cases. The surgeon introduces a cautery iron into the fistula, burning away the little quills of superfluous flesh. Afterwards a dressing of healing ointments is applied.

If the probe does not come through to the finger in the anus, then there must be flesh intervening. If the fistula is close under the skin there, the surgeon can cut open the skin along the length of the fistula until the probe simply drops out of the wound. Then the superfluous quills of flesh are cleaned out as before. If the patient haemorrhages badly then the wound must be cauterized, which will help to stop the bleeding. Then the surgeon treats the wound with a dressing soaked in butter, or sulphur pounded with oil, until the area is putrefied and the burnt tissue falls away. Then he applies salves to encourage healing and the growth of new flesh.

If the fistula reaches deep into the anus, and is far from the surface of the body, then the surgeon must put in the finger and probe as described above. A barrier of flesh between probe and finger can only be treated in three hazardous ways. The first is to cauterize, as described above. Or the surgeon can cut open right to the end of the fistula, and insert a dressing. But he must be careful not to cut into the sphincter muscle controlling continence. Thirdly, the surgeon can perforate the barrier after incising to the area of the anus, either by using the probe or some other sharp-pointed instrument. Then he must clear away the bits of flesh, and treat as before. There is another way of cutting open the fistula. By using a probe with an eye like a shoemaker's needle, a thread can be introduced into the fistula and passed out through the anus with the help of the finger. The surgeon ties the thread at both ends and tightens at regular intervals until the flesh held by the thread (in fact five separate threads twisted together) is severed. Albucasis introduces illustrations both of the eyed probe and the curved scalpel used for incision. The major difference between his account and that of Paul is the recommendation of cautery, not found in Paul.

It is clear that the earliest Western surgeries of the twelfth century show no awareness of the Latin translation of Albucasis. Instead their main source was Haly Abbas in the translation of Constantine.[56] Haly Abbas follows Paul in his discussion of the difference between fistulae which perforate and those which do not, the test by probe and finger, and the laying open of the fistula surgically. But there is no mention of the use of a ligature, and in general his is a much simplified account. Roger Frugard of Parma, Rolando Cappelluti, and the glossators of these surgeries all discuss fistula-in-ano in a similar way, although Roger adds to Haly Abbas the suggestion that a ruptory ointment introduced into the depth of the fistula may do as well as laying open with the knife.[57]

[56] *Liber totius medicine* (Lyons, 1523), *Practica*, lib. 9, cap. 60, fol. 283.
[57] For Roger, see Renzi, *Collectio salernitana*, vol. II, pp. 485–6; Sudhoff, *Geschichte der Chirurgie*, pp. 225–6. For Rolando, lib. 3, cap. 37, see *Cyrurgia Guidonis de Cauliaco. Et*

It may well have been Ugo da Lucca who first introduced in the West material drawing on the more sophisticated surgery of Albucasis. At any rate it is not until the mid thirteenth century with Ugo's pupils Teodorico Borgognoni and Bruno Longoburgo, that we first meet the ideas of Albucasis applied to fistula-in-ano. Bruno Longoburgo acknowledges explicitly his debt to Albucasis. In fact his account follows Albucasis almost line for line in places, but without actually copying from his authority. He adds one refinement to the incision for fistulae – he suggests that the thread used for ligature can also be used to hold the flesh between fistula and rectum, so that the surgeon may cut with a *falx* or razor. In fact Bruno says incision after this method is better and safer than ligature, which is painful for longer and liable to give rise to complications. Bruno also quotes from Rhazes, *Liber Divisionum* on the reasons why penetrating fistulae cannot be cured except by surgery.[58] As on most other matters, Teodorico follows Bruno faithfully in everything to do with fistula-in-ano, even to Bruno's suggestion for use of the thread in incision and the reasons he gives for it.[59] Guglielmo da Saliceto is also a follower of Albucasis, but without the modifications suggested by Bruno and Teodorico.[60]

Lanfranco of Milan follows the procedures recommended by Albucasis, although he ranges rather wider than the earlier Western surgeons in his terminology and is less obviously dependent on an earlier authority. But we still find the causes of fistulation, the distinction between penetrating and non-penetrating fistulae, the test with finger and probe, and the alternatives of incision, ligature, and cautery for operating. The importance of avoiding damage to the sphincter muscle is stressed. Lanfranco follows Bruno in the use of the ligature to hold the flesh if the surgeon opts for incision. He devotes rather more space than Bruno and Teodorico to the option of cautery, and deals at some length with the possibility of using a ruptory ointment (like Roger) instead of the more radical (but in his opinion safer) cautery. Typically he makes this an occasion for an attack on those ignorant surgeons who try to use a *ruptorium* when there are counter-indications: 'those who do not have wine to drink, drink vinegar and scorn

---

Cyrurgia Bruni. Theodorici. Rogerii. Rolandi. Bertapalie. Lanfranci (Venice, 1498), fol. 159r. For the Glosses of the Four Masters, see Renzi, *Collectio Salernitana*, vol. II, pp. 656–7. In effect the later glossators and commentators added nothing to Roger in his discussion of fistula-in-ano.

58 Bruno Longoburgo, *Cyrurgia magna*, lib. 2, cap. 16, in *Cyrurgia Guidonis* (1498), fol. 101. Rhazes, *Liber divisionum*, cap. 97, in his *Opera parva* (Lyons, 1511), fol. xliii. See also *Ad Almansorem*, lib. 9, cap. 80, in the same volume (fol. clxxvii).

59 Theodorico, *Chirurgia*, lib. 3, cap. 42, in *Cyrurgia Guidonis* (1498), fol. 135v–6; Eldridge Campbell and James Colton (trans.), *The surgery of Theoderic ca. AD 1269*, vol. II (New York, 1960), pp. 114–18.

60 Paul Pifteau (ed.), *La chirurgie de Guillaume de Salicet achévée en 1275* (Toulouse, 1898), lib. I, cap. 46.

to seek another wine'. The wine of true *doctrina* is drunk by those who study their surgical authorities, as of course does Lanfranco himself.[61]

While Henri de Mondeville has nothing specific to recommend for fistula-in-ano (which he discusses in the context of fistulation in general), he does mention the perforating type of anal fistula and the danger of damage to the sphincter.[62] Guy de Chauliac summarizes the doctrine of his predecessors on the subject. In his account of the operative procedures he follows Albucasis and Lanfranco. He singles out Bruno and Teodorico for recommending the use of the actual rather than potential cautery in cases of non-penetrating fistula. He adds no comment then, but later censures them for recommending that after incision the surgeon should mortify the fistulous cavity and destroy all callosity therein instead of using incarnatives as Rhazes suggests.[63]

We know from the introduction to the *Extracta emoroydarum* that Arderne claimed acquaintance with a number of different surgical authors: Roger of Parma, Jamerius, Bruno, Lanfranco, and perhaps even Guy de Chauliac.[64] It is worth noting that none of the Arab surgical authors are on this list, although Arderne does refer to Rhazes and Haly Abbas in other sections of the *Liber medicinarum*. The *Practica*, however, does not name any of these surgical authorities though relying heavily on descriptions of the operation for fistula-in-ano derived from Albucasis and later authors. Despite the wealth of detail which Arderne supplies, which is not to be found in any of the early authorities, it is easy to pick out points in his *Practica* where he has clearly built on them.[65]

The passage on instruments which prefaces the cure of fistula introduces a number of instruments with which we are already familiar from the earlier authors. The *sequere me* of Arderne plays the same role in testing for perforation as does the probe in every authority from Haly Abbas onwards. The *acus rostrata* or billed needle (broader at one end with an eye at the other) is exactly the same instrument as that described by Albucasis as having an eye like that of the shoemaker's needle for passing the twisted thread through fistula and rectum. Arderne's *frenum cesaris*, made from *filum quadriplicatum*, fulfils the same function as the fivefold thread of Albucasis. Arderne has of course a razor for incision, and two other

---

[61] '... qui non habent vinum ad bibendum bibunt acetum & alium vinum petere dedignant' (Lanfranco, *Cyrurgia magna*, Tract. 3, doct. 3, cap. 12, in *Cyrurgia Guidonis* (1498), fol. 200v).

[62] J. L. Pagel (ed.), *Die Chirurgie des Heinrich von Mondeville* (Berlin, 1892), Tract 2, doct. 2, cap. 3, pp. 314–22.

[63] *Cyrurgia Guidonis* (1498), Tract. 3, doct. 2, cap. 7, fol. 43v; Björn Wallner (ed.), *The Middle English translation of Guy de Chauliac's treatise on ulcers*, part 1, Text, Acta Universitatis Lundensis, Sectio 1, Theologica Juridica Humaniora, 39 (Stockholm, 1982), pp. 124–6.

[64] Arderne's most quoted authority is Bernard de Gordon, who does deal with fistula-in-ano (see his *Lilium Medicinae* (Lyons, 1530), part 4, rubrica 9, p. 518), but not as a surgeon.

[65] The operation itself is found in Sloane MS 56, fols. 48r–51v, and Power, *Treatises of fistula in ano*, pp. 20–37.

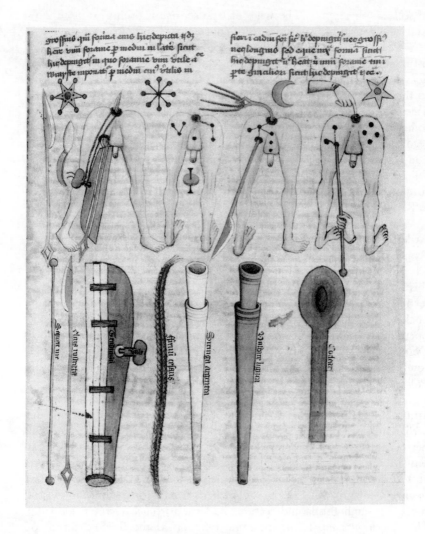

Figure 10   John of Arderne's operation for *fistula in ano*. Stages of the
operation are shown above the instruments to be used.

instruments of his own to add to the armamentarium, but these are for
refining well-established techniques rather than new operations.

Arderne makes the same basic distinction used by his sources between
those fistulae that perforate the rectum or bowel and those which do not.
Arderne describes the same test using a finger in the rectum and a probe
through the fistula:

... if there are a lot of holes, as is shown at this sign, he should probe thoroughly above the so-called index finger in the rectum. Then with his other hand he pushes in the instrument called *sequere me* to the hole of the fistula which is nearer to the anus.[66]

He also considers the difficulties raised by fistulae which penetrate to the bladder, urinary passages, or testicles (claiming to have cured an unidentified chaplain of Sir Geoffrey de Scrope of such an advanced case). He talks about the need to ask the patient whether any *egestiones* or *ventositates* escape via the fistula. These are of course all features of the received account of diagnosis in fistula-in-ano.

Following Rhazes, Arderne presents the surgeon with a stark alternative when confronted with a perforating fistula – he must either operate by incision or by ligature. In cases where the surgeon chooses incision, Arderne follows Bruno in making use of a ligature in order to hold the flesh tight as an aid to laying open the fistula. His refinement here is that he employs another instrument, the *tendiculum*, which is a wooden board with a hole for a peg, to tighten the ligature. By attaching both ends of the *frenum cesaris* to the peg, the surgeon can use the *tendiculum* to control the tightness of the ligature rather as a violinist tightens or loosens the strings of his instrument. The second new instrument also comes into play in incision, where Arderne directs that the surgeon's assistant holds the *coclear* or spoon so as to protect the wall of the rectum as the surgeon cuts down it. But the basic operation is that of Haly Abbas, Roger and the others. The use of the ligature is just as required by Albucasis. There is, however, no mention at all in Arderne's *Practica* of the use of cautery, and in this respect he seems to have followed Haly Abbas rather than Albucasis and the later Western surgeons.

Refinements must not blind us to the essential similarity between Arderne's operative techniques, and those described by the earlier scholastic surgeons who followed Haly Abbas, Albucasis and, ultimately, Paul of Aegina. This similarity led Puschmann to declare of Arderne: 'With the exception of a few modifications to the instruments, his method of operation shows no advance on that of Paul of Aegina or Celsus himself.'[67] Puschmann was too dismissive, since he overlooks the essential difference between Arderne and all the earlier writers on the subject, that Arderne sought to provide a comprehensive guide to the treatment of fistula-in-ano, of which the operations for incision and ligature form only a small

---

[66] '... si plura fuerint foramina sicut ad hoc signum depingitur & diligenter temptet super digitum in ano qui index dicitur quo facto cum altera manu impellat caput instrumenti quod dicitur sequere me in foramen fistule quod ano sit propinquius' (Sloane MS 56, fol. 48v).

[67] 'Mit Ausnahme einiger Modifikationen des instrumentariums zeigt jedoch die Beschreibung seiner Operationsmethode keinen Fortschritt gegenüber Paulus von Aegina und selbst Celsus' (Max Neuburger and Julius Pagel (eds.), *Handbuch der Geschichte der Medizin*, vol. 1 (Jena, 1902), p. 736).

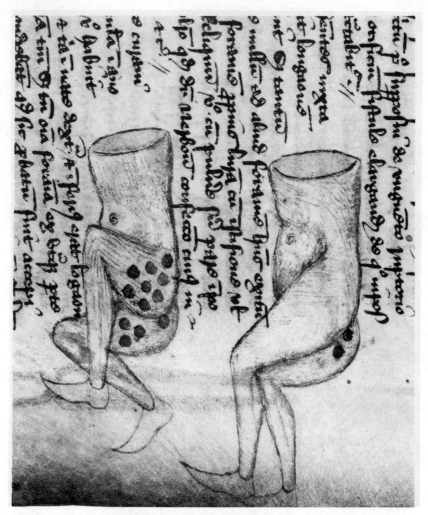

Figure 11 Two presentations of fistulae, as seen by the surgeon.

part.[68] Nor do any of the other authors describe these operations in the way that Arderne does, specifying each action in sequence and the construction of each instrument precisely. Characteristically he also supplies an element of personal observation and immediacy to his description of the different presentations of fistulae, missing from the scholastic authorities:

[68] The sections of the *Practica* dealing with the post-operative care of the patient – staunching of blood, treatment and bandaging of the wound – and with a variety of possible complications and related ailments are lengthy, and have no parallel in earlier discussions of fistula-in-ano.

Sometimes it happens that some have one hole appearing outside and running through the rectum below the anus for a distance of one or two fingers breadth, and next to that hole there is another which does not penetrate the rectum below, and I have seen some who have seven or nine holes on one part of the buttocks and five or six on the other, of which only one perforates the rectum as shown at this sign.[69]

He refers the reader to an illustration in the margin which shows the patient with numerous holes in both buttocks. But the basic distinction between penetrating and non-penetrating fistulae is still there. It brings home the extent to which Arderne's operative technique was founded on his close study of the earlier surgical tradition.

But the operative sections which are based on the scholastic authorities are relatively short in respect of the entire work. The length of Arderne's *Practica* and the amount of detail he includes in it raise larger questions about the audience to which it is addressed and the purposes Arderne intended it to serve. As we have seen, there are no other comparable treatises on a single branch of surgery surviving from the Middle Ages – the nearest parallel perhaps is the amount of space devoted in the longer surgeries to the operation for depressed fracture of the skull from Roger of Parma onwards. But even the descriptions of this operation lack the circumstantial detail found in Arderne.

Perhaps it is the brevity of the treatment of complex operations in the scholastic surgeries that needs to be explained, at least from a modern perspective. How could a prospective surgeon hope to master an operation on the basis of the skimpy detail provided in the scholastic surgeries? Presumably the answer is that the normal surgical *Practica* took for granted a context in which written instruction epitomized lengthier pedagogic expositions by the master-surgeons which may have included demonstration of the instruments and techniques used. The written text provided an epitome rather than an exhaustive treatise.

In Arderne's case this context could not be relied on. The amount of circumstantial detail he provides in his description of operative procedures, his precise directions for the preparation, preservation and use of medicaments, the designs he provides for instruments and bandages all suggest that he expected his readers to require step-by-step instruction in these things. No stage in the diagnosis, prognosis, or treatment could be left for the reader to supply from other sources of information, it would seem. What, then, can we infer about the intended audience for Arderne's

---

[69] 'Aliquando contingit quosdam habuere unum foramen tamen exterius apparens & per medium longaonis infra anum per spacium unius pollicis vel duorum illud perforans & iuxta illud foramen habeat aliud foramen exterius quod non penetrat longaonem inferius & aliquos vidi habuere vii vel ix foramina ex una parte natium .i. buttok & vi vel v ex altera quorum pullum eorum perforabat longaonem nisi unum tam sicut ad tale signum depingitur' (Sloane MS 56, fol. 45v).

treatise? His readers must have been expected to be able to follow a Latin text, but not to be able to rely on institutional teaching or a range of supplementary surgical texts. In one revealing passage in the *Liber medicin-arum*, Arderne prescribes a plaster for a case of *gutta*, and warns his readers: 'beware in case the patient or some other person sees, and keep it a great and precious secret, and reveal it only to your son or some chosen individual'.[70]

It is almost certain that he carried the same attitude over to the *Practica*, which contained many secrets of Arderne's specialist practice. At the end of his long life he was willing to communicate these secrets to his Latin-reading audience, who he supposed would preserve the *misterium* or *minis-terium* for themselves, their sons or daughters, or select apprentices. Perhaps he hoped that others would be able to reconstruct his techniques after his death. In any case the *Practica* was intended to divulge Arderne's secrets only to the master-surgeons, and those aspiring to be master-surgeons.

CONCLUSION

If scholastic surgery began as a movement away from the craft mystery towards the creation of a new *scientia* for a university environment, Arderne's *Practica* might seem almost an attempt to return that *scientia* to the craft surgeons.[71] After all, Arderne eschewed scholastic structure while silently borrowing much of the *doctrina* on fistula-in-ano he found through his reading of earlier writers. And he plainly hoped to instruct master-surgeons like himself with no university background, and to keep his knowledge out of the hands of the barber-surgeons. But this *Practica* can also be seen as an example of dissemination of learning, making scholastic *doctrina* available to a new audience. We know that it circulated com-paratively widely in England, and must have been one of the most frequently copied of prose instructional writings.[72] In the course of the fifteenth century it was translated into English in at least four separate versions, which meant that it was reaching a non-Latin-reading audience that Arderne may not have foreseen. Its popularity certainly surpassed that of the scholastic surgical authors, although Guy de Chauliac, Henri de Mondeville, Lanfranco, and Guglielmo da Saliceto achieved wide currency in fifteenth-century England.[73]

Yet John of Arderne seems to have had no imitators or successors in his adaptation of scholastic surgery to the English environment. The English

[70] ' . . . cave ne a paciente percipiatur nec ab aliquo alio sed magis secretum teneatur & carum & nisi filio vel tam dilecto reveletur' (Sloane MS 56, fol. 19v).

[71] See Agrimi and Crisciani, and Siraisi, this volume.

[72] As many as forty manuscripts of the *Practica* are known to survive from before 1532.

[73] See Linda Ehrsam Voigts, 'Editing Middle English medical texts: needs and issues', in Trevor H. Levere, (ed.), *Editing texts in the history of the science and medicine* (New York, 1982), pp. 47, 48, for remarks on the currency of these texts in England, and the numbers of surviving manuscripts.

surgery of 1392 studied by Richard Grothé is entirely scholastic in character, and is very closely related to the surgery of Henri de Mondeville.[74] It could just as easily have come from Paris or Montpellier, and does not attempt to adapt to English circumstances. Similarly, English surgical writings of the next century were excerpted from earlier and longer works – for instance, the compilation of Thomas Fayreford.[75] For surgeries with some resemblance to that of Arderne, we have to turn back to Italy. Lynn Thorndike drew attention to a pair of surgeries compiled in Italy, one by an anonymous surgeon at the end of the fourteenth century, and another by Leonardo Buffi da Bertipaglia, written in the 1420s. Thorndike talks of the wealth of personal and clinical detail included in the manuscript versions of the surgery of Leonardo Buffi (though not in the version printed in 1498 and subsequently), and of his 'quaint, garrulous, and rather breathless style'.[76] A more recent study by T. Pesenti Marangon has succeeded in placing Buffi in the context of his career as a teacher and surgeon at Padua. She sees him as in revolt against the abstractness of scholastic surgery (although leaning heavily on their *doctrina*) while a severe critic too of the irrational surgery of the empirics and barber-surgeons. With like-minded colleagues he sought to create a new surgical culture in Padua:

> Marginalized for the most part from academic science but sought after by patients, even from the richest social classes, these 'surgeon doctors' had ended up constructing a culture of their own, the expression of which is the anonymous manual of medicine and practical surgery written in Latin and the vernacular ...[77]

Yet Buffi, for all his use of personal and clinical detail, never reworked the conventions of scholastic surgery quite as drastically as did Arderne.

There is no evidence for Arderne having succeeded in creating the new surgical culture in England that has been claimed for Leonardo Buffi at Padua. But Arderne's works show how it was possible for a craft-trained surgeon with no university background to study the scholastic surgeries and to make their handling of a specific operation the basis of a *Practica* of his own. At the same time as this he changed the conventions of scholastic surgery to suit a new context in which his readers could not expect to have access to other sources of surgical information, and would need to have diagnosis, instruments and techniques spelt out for them.

---

[74] See note 8 above.
[75] See note 16 above.
[76] Lynn Thorndike, *Science and thought in the fifteenth century* (New York, 1929), chs. 3, 4 and p. 70.
[77] 'Emarginati per lo più dalla scienza accademica ma ricercati dai pazienti, anche dei ceti più ricchi, questi "medici ciroici" avevano finito con l'elaborare una propria cultura, di cui è espressione l'anonimo manuale di medicina e chirurgia pratica in latino e volgare ... ' (T. Pesenti Marangon, '"Professores chirurgie", "medici ciroici" e "barbitonsores" a Padova nell'età di Leonardo Buffi da Bertipaglia', *Quaderni per la Storia dell'Università di Padova*, 11–12 (1978), 1–38, at 20).

10

Documenting medieval women's medical practice

MONICA H. GREEN

It has been five decades since Muriel Joy Hughes published the first and, thus far, the only monograph devoted to medieval women medical practitioners.[1] In addition to the path-breaking computer-assisted analysis of French practitioners by Danielle Jacquart (who documented a total of 127 female practitioners),[2] some scattered new materials have come to light in recent years to supplement Hughes' still valuable synthesis.[3] None of them, however, overturn the general impression that women constituted no more than the tiniest percentage of medieval medical practitioners.[4] This paucity of documentation for women's medical practice is generally interpreted to be an accurate reflection of the insignificant role women played in medieval medicine, the few women that have been documented being aberrant exceptions who do not justify separate historiographical analysis. While not denying the persuasiveness of such arguments *ex silencio*, I would like to examine some reasons why the silence has been so profound.

In the intervening years since Hughes wrote in 1943, there has been an

---

[1] Muriel Joy Hughes, *Women healers in medieval life and literature* (New York, 1943; repr. Freeport, NY, 1968). Paul Diepgen's *Frau und Frauenheilkunde in der Kultur des Mittelalters* (Stuttgart, 1963) also discusses women's medical practice, though his principal concern is with gynaecology and obstetrics.

[2] Danielle Jacquart, *Le milieu médical en France du XIIe au XVe siècle: En annexe 2e supplément au 'Dictionnaire' d'Ernest Wickersheimer* (Geneva, 1981). In addition to the 121 analysed on pp. 47–55, there are six more listed in Jacquart's Appendix C.

[3] These are summarized in Monica Green, 'Women's medical practice and health care in medieval Europe', *Signs: Journal of Women in Culture and Society*, 14, no. 2 (1988–9), 434–73. One study that has come to my attention since the publication of that article is Francesco Pierro, 'Nuovi contributi alla conoscenza delle medichesse nel regno di Napoli negli ultimi tre secoli del medioevo', *Archivio Storico Pugliese*, 17, fasc. 1–4 (1964), 231–41, who adds the following to the Italian practitioners I noted: a Margherita practising surgery in the early fifteenth century during the reign of Ladislao of Durazzo; Virdimura of Catania, Jewess and wife of one Doctor Pasquale, who was licensed in 1276 to practise on paupers 'who cannot afford the immense fees of medics and physicians'; Donne Cusina di Filippo de Pastino and Bella di Paija, who are licensed to practise surgery in 1404 and 1414, respectively; and Tomasia da Castro Isae, another surgeon. (My thanks to Marta Petrusewicz for bringing this article to my attention.) See also n. 61 below.

[4] Even in Jacquart's comprehensive study, women constituted only 1.5 per cent of the total.

322

explosive development of the field of women's history in general.[5] While researchers of the medieval period have not yet accumulated data or analysed it as extensively as have scholars of the modern epoch, many important studies have appeared on such issues as women's relationship to the law and their participation in both household and market economies. These studies show not simply that women have a history, but that they have tilled fields, ruled kingdoms and feudal estates, engaged in a variety of occupations, committed crimes, and wielded economic power – in short, that they have been historical actors in most of the ways traditionally recognized for men. More importantly, these studies show that women have another, separate history created by the gendered divisions of medieval society, a history that will inevitably remain invisible until we set aside the androcentric perspective on the world which, by determining our manner of choosing data and asking questions, has caused most women of the past to fall through the methodological cracks of modern historiography.

Why should 'medieval women medical practitioners' constitute a category of historical analysis distinct from the men with whom they lived, practised, or competed? Thus far the question has gone largely unexamined. Never explicitly articulating their agendas, such earlier historians of medieval 'lady doctors' as Hughes, Charles Talbot and Ladislao Münster all seem to have been motivated by a modern concern to demonstrate that women's entrance into the upper echelons of the medical profession in the nineteenth and twentieth centuries was not without historical precedent or, in Münster's case, that Italy in particular had an early history of 'enlightened' attitudes towards women's medical practice.[6] Women's history has long since outgrown its original goal of simply chronicling 'women worthies' whose individual accomplishments could inspire modern women and confound their chauvinist critics. Historians of women are now as much concerned with the masses of middle- and lower-class women as with the few social elites, with the undistinguished but more common women and the parameters of their existence as women as with the atypical 'great' women, whose eminence was often due precisely to their individual opportunity to break free of the limitations encumbering most of womankind.[7]

Although obviously women must be placed squarely within the political

---

[5] This is not to say that the field is completely new, of course. For summaries of the historiographical traditions in several different countries, see Susan Mosher Stuard (ed.), *Women in medieval history and historiography* (Philadelphia, 1987).

[6] Hughes, *Women healers*; Charles Talbot, 'Dame Trot and her Progeny', *Essays and Studies* (The English Association), n.s. 25 (1972), 1–14; Ladislao Münster, 'Notizie di alcune "medichesse" veneziane della prima metà del Trecento', in *Scritti in onore del Prof. A. Pazzini* (Saluzzo, 1954), 180–7; and Münster, 'Women doctors in mediaeval Italy', *Ciba Symposium* (English edition), 10, no. 3 (1962), 136–40.

[7] See Natalie Zemon Davis, '"Women's history" in transition: the European case', *Feminist Studies*, 3 (1975–6), 83–103.

and socio-economic context they shared with men, the historical reality of medieval women's medical practice may have been different enough from that of their male counterparts to demand the use of special methodological techniques and analytical concepts that can take these different experiences into account. To demonstrate how the perspectives of women's history might fruitfully be employed in examining the experience of medieval women in medical practice, I would like to draw on some of the questions and conclusions proposed in a few recent studies of medieval women, especially those relating to women's work. In particular, I would like to explore two central issues: first, the intrinsic limitations for the study of women of the documents traditionally employed for gathering bio-graphical data on medical practitioners; and second, the different patterns in women's 'careers', which show greater fluctuation than men's, depending on their position in the life cycle or their marital status, as well as issues of occupational labelling. Finally, I offer two tentative local analyses of female medical practitioners based on data and documents that have recently been published. While I recognize that the geographical range I will be covering implies a European cultural uniformity which may have never existed, I think that at this early stage of investigation it is fully warranted, especially given the cross-national similarities in medieval women's work that have now been documented by recent research.[8] It should be noted that the bulk of the evidence I refer to relates more to urban situations than rural. This focus in itself undoubtedly obscures a vast amount of women's medical practice from view; however, I have not yet found sufficient material on medieval rural medical practice to attempt any kind of synthetic interpretation. The following comments in no way pretend to be definitive or methodologically prescriptive nor does my survey of the social-historical literature pretend to be exhaustive. Nevertheless, it is my hope that the observations offered here might provide some questions which social historians of medicine might ruminate on while in the archives.

THE INVISIBLE WOMAN

In recent years, historians of medicine have begun to reap amazing harvests from the wealth of archival material that social historians have been mining for years.[9] And there are still who knows how many resources that remain virtually unexplored. Stuart Jenks, for example, has shown how much

---

[8] Most of the social-historical materials I will be drawing on pertain to northern Europe rather than the Mediterranean. As research on women's labour patterns in southern Europe becomes more extensive, this northern bias will be corrected. See now *El trabajo de las mujeres en la edad media hispana*, ed. Angela Muñoz Fernández and Cristina Segura Graiño (Madrid, 1988).

[9] E.g., Luis García-Ballester, Michael R. McVaugh, and Agustín Rubio-Vela, *Medical licensing and learning in fourteenth-century Valencia*, *Transactions of the American Philosophical Society*, 79, part 6 (Philadelphia, 1989). For assessments of work in social history more

information on medical practitioners is yet to be retrieved even from such supposedly well-studied archives as the Public Record Office in London.[10] Such promises of yet-to-be discovered archival riches may make us optimistic of finding more female medical practitioners. But there will never be a radical change in the percentages of women we find if we cling solely to the sources and methodologies that have traditionally been employed to identify medieval healers.

Jenks' findings in fact reinforce a now familiar pattern: of the twenty-one practitioners he is able to document, none is a woman. Although women constituted 50 per cent (more or less) of the medieval European population,[11] were we to base our demographic understanding solely on the sources that are usually examined for evidence of medical practitioners we would form a very skewed impression of the medieval sex ratio. To take Jenks' data as an example, of the 145 people mentioned in the court cases relating to the practitioners he identified (i.e. plaintiffs, defendants, guarantors, witnesses and legal officials), only four are women. The resulting sex ratio (women:men) is a remarkable 100:3,525. This skewed representation of women forces us to acknowledge that simply because of women's different relationship to public life, there are intrinsic limitations to the documentation historians of medicine have been using. It is worth articulating what some of these limitations are.

Throughout most of the Middle Ages personal documents – autobiographies, diaries, private correspondence – were rare. With the exception of the learned elite classes (who left documentation of a different sort), most of the sources that we use to document medieval practitioners are those produced when an individual steps into 'public' life: when he or she makes a will, accuses someone or is accused of some offence in a court of law, buys or exchanges property, etc. Women's access to and participation in public life – their control over property, their accountability for their actions and debts – will therefore be directly influential in determining their presence in the documents.[12]

generally see, e.g., *Sources of social history: private acts in the late Middle Ages*, ed. Paolo Brezzi and Egmont Lee (Toronto, 1984); and the papers on the use of legal records for documenting English family history collected in *Journal of Medieval History*, 14, no. 1 (March 1988).

10 Jenks' search of ninety bundles of writs in the Public Record Office, London, produced evidence for twenty-one medical practitioners, only six of whom had been known to Talbot and Hammond when they compiled their register of English practitioners in 1965; see Stuart Jenks, 'Medizinische Fachkräfte in England zur Zeit Heinrichs VI (1428/9–1460/1)', *Sudhoffs Archiv*, 69, no. 2 (1985), 214–27.

11 There is considerable debate about this question. In relation to the questions addressed in this essay, it is worth noting that there is evidence to suggest that the sex ratio in late medieval towns was skewed in favour of females, with ratios ranging from 75 to 90 males per 100 females. See, for example, Maryanne Kowaleski, 'The history of urban families in medieval England', *Journal of Medieval History*, 14, no. 1 (March 1988), 47–63, esp. 55.

12 Cf. James Brundage's comments from the conference on English family history (*Journal of Medieval History*, 14, no. 1 (March 1988), 65–7) on the limitations of various forms of

A closer examination of Jenks' study will demonstrate how the legal incapacity of women removed them from visibility in the public sphere. All the ninety writs in the bundle Jenks examined are of the type *corpus cum causa*. This is a writ, as Jenks explains, by which the king orders the sheriff of a county (or any jailer of a district outside direct royal control) to bring a person held in the said sheriff's or jailer's gaol to the king's council and provide certification for the grounds on which the individual was being held. Persons mentioned in the writs are thus the plaintiffs, the defendants, the guarantors (in many cases between two and four men) who offered their own property as surety for the defendant, and the sheriffs charged to carry out the orders of the writ. Other individuals are on occasion mentioned as witnesses or as other parties connected to the affair. Women will appear in such documents only to the extent that they could serve in the office as sheriff, make accusations against their neighbours, be held accountable for their own alleged crimes, or serve as guarantors for their neighbours and kin.[13] Three of the four women who do in fact appear in the writs summarized by Jenks serve in only one of these roles, that of the accused; the other (already dead) is mentioned merely in passing as the author of a will whose executor is now suing for debt.[14] Before concluding from such documents as Jenks has used that there were no female medical practitioners, therefore, we need to recognize how limited the utility of such court records is for documenting *any* women, no matter what their occupation or status in society.[15]

Not all types of legal records present this same inherent bias against women. Women are not always entirely unrepresented nor are they even always drastically under-represented. In Provence between 1320 and 1400, for example, Jacques Chiffoleau has found that women's wills constituted between 35 and 40 per cent of the total, women often having made their testaments without the authorization of their fathers or husbands as was

---

documents for chronicling different sectors of medieval society. The studies of Lacey and Hutton on women's work in late medieval England are especially conscientious in articulating the special problems of documenting women. See Kay E. Lacey, 'Women and work in fourteenth and fifteenth century London', in *Women and work in pre-industrial England*, ed. Lindsey Charles and Lorna Duffin (London, 1985), pp. 24–82; and Diane Hutton, 'Women in fourteenth century Shrewsbury', in ibid., pp. 83–99.

[13] For an excellent summary of work on English women's legal history, see Janet Senderowitz Loengard, 'Legal history and the medieval Englishwoman: a fragmented view', *Law and History Review*, 4, no. 1 (Spring 1986), 161–78, and the revised version in *Women and the sources of medieval history*, ed. Joel Rosenthal (Athens, Ga. 1990), pp. 210–36. (My thanks to Professor Loengard for sharing her revisions with me in advance of publication.)

[14] Jenks, 'Medizinische Fachkräfte', pp. 220 (Agnes Mody), 220–1 (Angela Baste), 221–2 (Katerina Cave or Cove), and 227 (Margaret, wife of William Hurtby).

[15] For some studies of medieval women's legal status, see Loengard, 'Legal history'; *Recueils de la Société Jean Bodin pour l'histoire comparative des institutions*, vols. 11–12: *La femme* (Brussels, 1962); M. A. Duran (ed.), *Las mujeres medievales y su ámbito jurídico: Actas de las II Jornadas de Investigacion Interdisciplinaria* (Madrid, 1983).

theoretically required by law.[16] But, as Bernard Saint-Pierre points out in the same volume, representation in notarial archives is a function not only of sex, but also of personal wealth and social status.[17] If women medical practitioners ranked among the middling or lower artisinal classes (as they undoubtedly often did since higher social status seems to have rarely been attained by medical practitioners who were not university educated), they would be less likely to appear.

Class, of course, is an aspect of their social status that women share with men. What historians working on medieval women have increasingly been documenting, however, is that women's legal identity (and, correspondingly, their presence in legal documents) is dependent on their marital status to a degree completely unparalleled for men. That is, a married woman will have a different standing under the law than a woman who has never married or one who is widowed. Under English common law, for example, a married man could be held solely responsible not only for his own crimes or debts, but also for allegations or debts jointly incurred by himself and his wife, and even for those incurred by his wife alone.[18] Evidence is regularly found of men being accused and fined for their wives' activities in fields ranging from brewing ale to keeping brothels.[19] Widows and single women, however, having no husbands, were generally directly responsible for themselves under the law. The implications of this legal distinction will be obvious: although she may be performing the same activities as a single or widowed woman, not only will the married woman be invisible in the documents, but her husband may even appear to be engaged in activities that in reality she performed alone. Jeremy Goldberg, for example, notes that only widows and unmarried women are entered by name in the lists of those fined for illegal brewing activity in fifteenth-century Norwich and York. Although most brewing was carried out by women, if they were married only their husband's name was listed since he was legally liable to pay the fine.[20]

[16] Jacques Chiffoleau, 'Les testaments provençaux et comtadins à la fin du moyen âge: richesse documentaire et problèmes d'exploitation', in Brezzi and Lee, *Sources of social history*, pp. 131–52, esp. p. 134.

[17] Bernard Saint-Pierre, 'Le corpus notarial de Brignoles (XIVe–XVe siècles): critique et histoire sociale', in Brezzi and Lee, *Sources of social history*, pp. 23–48, esp. p. 42: 'La chance de figurer dans les archives notariales est donc directement fonction du sexe, du niveau de fortune et du statut social.'

[18] Married women did, however, have the possibility in some instances of pleading for the independent legal status of *femme sole*, thus granting them full responsibility for their economic actions. See Maryanne Kowaleski, 'Women's work in a market town: Exeter in the late fourteenth century', in *Women and work in pre-industrial Europe*, ed. Barbara A. Hanawalt (Bloomington, Ind., 1986), pp. 145–64, esp. p. 146.

[19] See, for example, Kowaleski, 'Women's work'; Lacey, 'Women and work'; and Ruth Mazo Karras, 'The regulation of brothels in later medieval England', *Signs: Journal of Women in Culture and Society*, 14 (1988–9), 399–433.

[20] P. J. P. Goldberg, 'Women in fifteenth-century town life', in *Towns and townspeople in the fifteenth century*, ed. John A. F. Thomson (Gloucester and Wolfboro, NH, 1988), pp. 107–28, esp. p. 115. See also Kowaleski, 'Women's work', p. 151.

Other aspects of women's legal position should also be assessed as we look for sources of historical documentation of female practitioners, such as whether or not women could join guilds,[21] or whether they could carry on a profession or trade in their own right when married, especially when they could not be held legally accountable for their debts or criminal actions.[22] Answers to all these questions must necessarily reflect the regional and more local variations (which may have been considerable) in formal and customary law and, of course, they must assess the gaps that may have existed between legal precept and actual practice. We must also be sensitive to change over time, since we cannot assume that levels of women's presence in notarial documents will not vary in different periods. Goldberg has noted a change in the English documentation within the fifteenth century itself, with women increasingly appearing in written records solely with reference to their husbands (whether they were still living or not) rather than in their own names as they had earlier in the century.[23]

Once we have acknowledged the ways in which women's legal status could affect their presence in the documentary record,[24] however, what do we do next? Everything I have said thus far could simply be turned into just another argument *ex silencio*, this one apologetic: there were thousands of female practitioners active in the Middle Ages who were simply never noted in contemporary documents. While we do have to acknowledge the intrinsic limitations of the historical record, sheer optimism provides no more solid a basis for historical understanding than does the pessimistic view I challenged at the beginning of this chapter. In fact, I do not believe the limitations of the historical record can fully explain the strikingly low percentage of women whom we have thus far identified as medical practitioners. Another, more profound limitation lies not in the data but in our methodology: the very criteria we use for identifying practitioners themselves preclude documentation of women's medical practice.

---

[21] Although women often enjoyed some of the religious, social, and charitable benefits of guilds through their husbands' membership, they were generally excluded from membership in their own right unless they were widowed, and even then their rights were severely circumscribed. For a recent summary of work on women in guilds in northern Europe, see Maryanne Kowaleski and Judith M. Bennett, 'Crafts, gilds, and women in the Middle Ages: fifty years after Marian K. Dale', *Signs: Journal of Women in Culture and Society*, 14 (1988–9), 474–501.

[22] It is interesting in this regard that in a case in Borja (Aragón) in 1330, *both* the husband and wife were charged for a failed cure that the wife alone had attempted. See Ioachim Miret y Sans, 'Les médecins juifs de Pierre roi d'Aragon', *Revue des Etudes Juives*, 57 (1909), 268–78, esp. 278.

[23] Goldberg, 'Women in fifteenth-century town life', p. 115.

[24] Interestingly, Ruth Karras suggests that ecclesiastical court records may present a bias *in favour* of women. Since many ecclesiastical cases involve moral offences and are less concerned solely with those fiscally responsible, there is no bias against women's presence; indeed, their greater moral accountability may make women more subject to accusation. See Karras, 'Regulation of brothels', p. 414.

WOMEN'S CAREERS (OR 'WHAT'S IN A NAME?')

When looking for medical practitioners in the historical record, most researchers have followed the quite reasonable principle of identifying individuals who are explicitly labelled practitioners in the sources. *Physicus, leche, chirurgicus, metgessa, apothecarius, obstetrix* – any of these labels will satisfactorily mark the individual as someone we can recognize as a medical practitioner.[25] Although he did not explicitly state his criteria for inclusion, Jenks seems to have used this same principle in identifying the twenty-one practitioners he found in the *corpus cum causa* writs. Yet here again, what's good for the gander is not always good for the goose. Of the 141 men mentioned in the cases Jenks cites, only eleven do not have an explicit label indicating (high) social status ('knight' or 'gentlemen') or, far more commonly, occupation (sheriff, physician, tanner, brewer, etc.). Of the four women, only one is identified by her occupation rather than 'wife of ...' The reason for the one exception is immediately clear: Katerina Cave, 'servaunt', is later referred to as Katerina Cove (*sic*), 'senglewoman'.[26]

The English example thus raises a question which needs to be asked of all our documents: to what extent are women, especially married women, ever identified by an occupational title? Kathryn Reyerson has found for late thirteenth- and early fourteenth-century Montpellier, for example, that women were identified by their husband's or father's name and occupation, sometimes by both. Some women (who may have been single) were simply designated *habitatrix*, 'inhabitant', of the town. Although geographic places of origin and residence were often given, only rarely were women identified by their own occupation.[27]

If identification by occupation was the exception rather than the rule for women, how many medical practitioners have thus automatically been obscured from our view? Did Agnes Mody, mentioned in Jenks' writs, practise as a surgeon alongside her first husband, the surgeon John Longe? We do not know. Did Margaret Hurtby assist her husband, William (with whom she was charged with trespass in 1455), in his practice as a physician? The documents don't tell us. Yet these are not idle questions. One of the patterns being noted in studies of medieval women's labour is that often (though by no means always) a woman upon marriage will join her husband in his craft, accepting responsibility for maintenance of the household (which was identical to the workshop in many cases), supervising apprentices and servants, and sometimes, in the event of her husband's

---

[25] There are, of course, many instances in Jacquart and other prosopographical studies of practitioners being identified contextually.

[26] Jenks, 'Medizinische Fachkräfte', p. 222.

[27] Kathryn L. Reyerson, 'Women in business in medieval Montpellier', in Hanawalt (ed.), *Women and work*, pp. 117–44, esp. p. 119.

death, taking over the family business.[28] The assumption that because married women are not identified by an occupational title they were 'merely' housewives (i.e. that the absence of an occupational label in fact proves that women did not engage in any economically significant labour) seems to owe more to modern nineteenth- and twentieth-century middle-class ideals of the leisured, idle wife than to anything we now know about medieval women's labour patterns.

But can we assume, at the other extreme, that beside every male that we can label surgeon, apothecary, or barber, we would find a wife who was aiding him in his craft, perhaps to the extent that she might practise it independently upon his death?[29] Since so little work has been done comparing medicine to other trades, it is not yet possible to say whether medicine generally conformed to the pattern of women functioning as part of the household craft, either as wives or as daughters assisting their husbands or fathers in the family trade. Husband and wife medical teams were, however, the ideal envisioned by Pierre Dubois when in 1309 he drafted a plan to recover the Holy Land, and his vision seems to have some correlation to medieval practice.[30] The Englishwoman Pernell was jointly arraigned with her physician husband, Thomas de Rasyn, in Sidmouth (Devon) in 1350 for their alleged ignorance and malpractice of medicine.[31] Though no mention is made of medical practice *per se*, a 1413 ordinance of the Archbishop of Canterbury decreed that 'no barber, his wife, son, daughter, apprentice, or servant work at haircutting or shaving on Sundays within the freedom of the city.'[32] Jacquart notes several French women who practised alongside their husbands.[33] Similar examples might also be found for daughters.[34]

Viewing medical practice in terms of household craft would help obviate the problem of explaining how widows, for whose practice there is no evidence during their marriage, 'suddenly' begin to practise medicine on the death of their husbands. Although we do not know what trade was practised by William of Lee, the late husband of the 'poor bedeswoman

---

[28] See, for example, Kowaleski, 'Women's work', and Goldberg, 'Women in fifteenth-century town life'.

[29] This formulation is perhaps applicable only to the medical crafts. Whether it would work equally well for university-educated physicians seems doubtful, though I currently know of no studies that have been done of women married to men of the professional classes. To the extent that such men were clerics, of course, they would (or should) have had no wives to assist them in any case.

[30] Pierre Dubois, *De recuperatione Terre Sante. Traité de politique générale*, ed. Ch.-V. Langlois (Paris, 1891), p. 62: 'Isti medici et cerurgi uxores habeant similiter instructas, cum quarum auxiliis egrotantibus plenius subveniant.'

[31] C. H. Talbot and E. A. Hammond, *The medical practitioners in medieval England: a biographical register* (London, 1965), p. 241.

[32] Hughes, *Women healers*, p. 85.

[33] Jacquart, *Milieu médical*, p. 52.

[34] Jacquart (ibid., p. 478) suggests that Sibille Lissiardi, *in predicta arte [sc. chirurgie] eruditissima*, may have been the daughter of the physician Lisuardus. See also n. 49 below.

Joan', who early in the fifteenth century sought permission from Henry IV of England to practice medicine 'without hindrance or disturbance from all folk' as she 'has nought whereby to live save by physic which she has learned',[35] among the seven Venetian women documented by Münster in the first half of the fourteenth century, Margarita, 'widow of master Menegellus, surgeon', Jacobina, 'widow of master Raynaldus, physician-surgeon', and *magistra* Beatrice, 'wife of the late physician from Crete', are practising medicine after their husbands' deaths, though only the latter two are accorded medical titles (*medica*) in their own right.[36]

Not all married women engaged in the same trade as their husbands, of course.[37] Jacquart mentions several women married to husbands who did not practise medicine – Asseline Alexandre who was married to a Parisian bourgeois, Guillemette Vyard to a tanner, Catherine Lemesre to a banker, Chandellier to a painter – yet all of these women practised as midwives, the only medical field in which (at this time period) men would hardly be expected to specialize.[38]

The case of midwifery and the sexual division of labour it implies brings up another aspect of medieval women's labour patterns that must modify – or at least make us seriously question – the model of near parity of male and female participation in medical practice that I have just suggested. As Judith Bennett has recently pointed out with sobering clarity, despite the rosy-eyed views presented by many historians, the medieval period was no 'golden age' for women where they enjoyed a 'rough and ready equality' with men, either in their access to various occupations or in the remuneration they received for their labours.[39] This is not the place, of course, to chronicle the whole history of women's economic oppression, but I would like to suggest that some recent key findings on women's labour patterns, particularly those relating to women's occupational identity, should urge us to reconsider the traditional male model of life-long work identity as an acceptable criterion for determining who is or is not a medical practitioner.

To take just a few examples, Maryanne Kowaleski, in analysing the full range of women's work in fourteenth-century Exeter, has found five basic

[35] Eileen Power, 'Some women practitioners of medicine in the Middle Ages', *Proceedings of the Royal Society of Medicine*, 15, no. 6 (April 1922), 20–3, esp. 23.

[36] Münster, 'Notizie', pp. 186–7. Lucia, wife of George of Santa Lucia, is considered legally responsible for herself even though (apparently) her husband is still alive. We should not be too quick to assume that widows would always be labelled as widows, however. Goldberg, 'Women in fifteenth-century town life', for example, notes that women are referred to as *uxores* even though it is clear from other sources that at the time of writing their husbands were already dead (p. 126, n. 98).

[37] Such occupational independence may in fact have been more the norm than the exception, in that many women worked in fields or tasks relegated to the separate, invariably lower status of 'women's work'.

[38] Jacquart, *Milieu médical*, p. 50.

[39] Judith Bennett, '"History that stands still": women's work in the European past', *Feminist Studies*, 14 (Summer 1988), 269–83. The phrase 'rough and ready equality' is Eileen Power's, as cited by Bennett, p. 270.

characteristics of female employment; (1) that women rarely benefited from formal training in the workplace, thus in effect segregating them into low- or unskilled jobs; (2) that, even when women did receive some skilled training, they still tended to be segregated into low-status, marginal positions within the trades; (3) that marital status and position within the household dictated the type and nature of women's involvement with work; (4) that female employment was often intermittent (perhaps due to varying demands of household and family), as opposed to the more typically male pattern of steady involvement in a single trade for years at a time; and (5) that women tended, far more than men, to engage simultaneously in more than one trade.

Though not dealing with the Middle Ages, a study by Natalie Davis on women in the crafts in Lyons has articulated most clearly a significant ramification of women's multiple involvements in the crafts and trades.[40] That is, that although engaging in many trades (either sequentially or simultaneously), women generally identified with none. This 'weak work identity' allowed women to change their trade upon marriage when they moved from the household of their father to that of their new husband. It had the added benefit (from the male point of view) of providing a semi-skilled labour force that could expand and contract as necessary, shifting as economic or family needs required. This expectation that women would never specialize might then have been used as a justification for not extending their training significantly in childhood. What Judith Brown, also working on the early modern period, has neatly termed 'occupational endogamy' (the marrying off of daughters to men in the same trade as the woman's father) seems to have been rare – which suggests that fathers did not invest heavily enough in their daughters' training to feel concerned that that training 'pay off' throughout their lives.[41]

A final commonality is women's general economic disability. Very few data on women's wages as compared to men's have yet been offered, though several indications suggest a pattern of significantly lower wages for women. G. d'Avenal finds that women's wages averaged only 68 per cent of men's for the same work in 1326–50, improving only slightly (up to 75 per cent) in 1376–1400 with the general inflation of wages following the Black Death.[42] A principal difficulty in directly comparing women's and

---

[40] Natalie Zemon Davis, 'Women in the crafts in sixteenth-century Lyon', in Hanawalt, *Women and work*, pp. 167–97; originally published in *Feminist Studies*, 8 (1982), 47–80.

[41] Judith C. Brown, 'A woman's place was in the home: women's work in Renaissance Tuscany', in *Rewriting the Renaissance: the discourses of sexual difference in early modern Europe*, ed. Margaret W. Ferguson, Maureen Quilligan and Nancy J. Vickers (Chicago and London, 1986), pp. 206–24 (notes, pp. 363–70), esp. p. 366.

[42] G. d'Avenal, as cited in Shulamith Shahar, *The fourth estate: a history of women in the Middle Ages*, trans. Chaya Galai (London and New York, 1983), pp. 198–9, 324. Simon A. C. Penn, however, finds more nearly equitable wages among women and men in agricultural labour in England after the Black Death; see 'Female wage-earners in late fourteenth-century England', *Agricultural History Review*, 35, part 1 (1987), 1–14.

men's wages, of course, is that men and women (often because of their different levels of skill) rarely did the same work, which probably only heightened the wage disparities. Judith Brown suggests that in Renaissance Tuscany a skilled male weaver could expect to earn three to four times more than an unskilled female.[43] Lower wages, access to only low-profit trades, limited control over property all meant that women had little wealth to invest. Kowaleski, for instance, notes that women's debts are on average significantly lower than men's, a reflection of how little capital they had at their disposal.[44] Karras, in turn, suggests that women were likely to enter trades that required little capital.[45]

How, then, assuming these general patterns of women's work will hold true for the field of medicine, might we imagine women's medical practice to have looked in the Middle Ages? Access to the highest-skilled level of the medical art – that acquired only in the university – was, of course, denied them. Likewise, they were generally denied full access to that other principal site of institutional privilege, the guild. But other than being denied the mastership, could women (either when married or as widows) join and reap the same benefits of guild membership as their male counterparts?[46] Did the daughters of apothecaries, surgeons and barbers only rarely receive extensive training in the technical skills of healing from their fathers? If not from their husbands or fathers, where did women get their training in medicine? Did women themselves ever act as teachers?[47] In studying sixteenth-century Morisco healers in Spain, Luis García-Ballester noted that Juan de Luna taught his daughter 'medical things', and she in turn taught her son Román Ramírez 'everything he knew about herbs and curing illness'.[48] Is there something peculiar about the medical art that encourages the formation of medical dynasties, like that of Juan de Luna, that include the female members of the family? Is there evidence of mother-daughter dynasties as well?[49]

. Once married, did daughters (whatever their early training) regularly

---

[43] Brown, 'A woman's place,' p. 218.
[44] Kowaleski, 'Women's work', pp. 149–50.
[45] See Karras, 'Regulation of brothels', p. 414.
[46] Jacquart, *Milieu médical*, pp. 51–2, notes that in the case of Montpellierain surgeons, at least, women could only join the guild as widows, and then only on the condition that they did not remarry.
[47] One well-known female instructor is the Jewess Sarah de Saint-Gilles, wife of Abraham, who in 1326 in Marseilles contracted to accept a boy, Salves de Burgonovo, as her apprentice. See Melina Lipinska, *Histoire des femmes médecins depuis l'antiquité jusqu'à nos jours* (Paris, 1900), pp. 116–17; and Ernest Wickersheimer, *Dictionnaire biographique des médecins en France au moyen âge*, 2 vols. (1936; repr. Geneva, 1979), vol. II. p. 732.
[48] Luis García-Ballester, 'Academicism versus empiricism in practical medicine in sixteenth-century Spain with regard to Morisco practitioners', in *The medical renaissance of the sixteenth century*, ed. A. Wear, R. K. French and I. M. Lonie (Cambridge, 1985), pp. 246–70, esp. pp. 264–5.
[49] Marina, one of the women documented by Münster, 'Notizie', is the daughter of the *medicatrix* Francesca.

take on the practice of their surgeon, barber, or apothecary husbands? And what did they do when they remarried? Did Agnes Mody, for example, change her area of work from surgery to stonemasonry when she remarried? Did she ever practice alongside either of her husbands or did she rather engage all along in such 'women's work' as spinning, retailing food or brewing ale?

Once trained (by whatever teacher and to whatever degree), did women regularly find themselves relegated, as Kowaleski suggests, to the low-status, marginal positions within the 'trade' of medicine? What, in fact, constituted 'low-status' or 'marginal' amid the array of medical practices? Does medicine in general require only a minimal capital investment, either for training or supplies? If so, this would seem to make medicine a very likely choice for women as it would involve considerably less financial investment than, say, the material and equipment investment involved in textile manufacture. Can the apparently common association of women practitioners with magic, charms and other religious types of healing also be associated with notions of status and an unstated hierarchy of medical practice?

Did women healers charge less than men, either because of the simple fact that they were women or because, being viewed as less skilled, more empirical in their knowledge, their services were seen to be worth less? (These two possibilities may not have been mutually exclusive; they may, in fact, have reinforced each other.) In either event, was male antagonism to women's practice thus economically motivated? Again, as mentioned above, there is little evidence available on wage differentials, though more work could certainly be done on assessing the relative value of the income of women we already know about. For example, among the English practitioners Marjory Cobbe, midwife to Elizabeth, wife of Edward IV, was granted an annual pension of £10 together with her husband. Matilda la Leche of Wallingford was assessed twenty pence in taxes in 1232, apparently more than any other woman of the town. Johanna, *Leche*, was paid 3s 6d for medicines in 1408–9 for a Brother Richard Merlaw and later 3s 3d, again for the same patient. The *medicus* (*sic*) Christiana was paid only in corn in 1313, while Elyot 'la middewyf' of Leicester, who attended the queen's birth in 1372, is only known to have been compensated by an annual gift of two carts of wood, granted her three years later by John of Gaunt.[50] In Birmingham, 'the commen midewyffe' was regularly allowed to occupy, rent-free, one of the houses owned by the guild of the Holy Cross, apparently in return for services to members of the guild.[51] How

[50] On Marjory, Matilda, Johanna and Christiana, respectively, see Talbot and Hammond, *Medical practitioners*, pp. 209–10, 211, 100 and 28. On Elyot, see *John of Gaunt's Register*, ed. Sydney Armitage-Smith, 2 vols. (Camden Society, 3rd ser., xx–xxi) (London, 1911), vol. ii, pp. 55 and 321.

[51] Joshua Toulmin Smith, *English gilds: the original ordinances of more than one hundred early English gilds*, Early English Text Society Publications, o.s. no. 40. (London, 1870), p. 249.

might Carole Rawcliffe's findings have been altered had she factored the 'profits of practice' of women into her impressive study of male practitioners?[52]

Obviously, to answer all these questions in terms consistent with other studies of women's work, we would need to have a better sense of how the medical crafts stood in relation to other artisanal fields. Perhaps the most consistent aspect of women's medical practice that we might find, I suspect, is that it is intermittent and 'part-time'. And it is precisely on this point that I think we most seriously need to question the criteria of what we are looking for when we attempt to identify medical practitioners, not only for the sake of studying women, but for any comprehensive study of the whole array of medical practice in the pre-modern world. As Margaret Pelling has recently stressed, nineteenth- and twentieth-century notions of 'professionalization' have seriously obscured and distorted many previous studies of medical practice in the early modern period.[53] Much the same tunnel vision has been operative in studies of the medieval period, I would argue, and with the same effects: obscuring from view the mass of unofficial, unlicensed, 'irregular' practitioners, both male and female, who practised medicine neither in the institutions nor under the limited specialist titles that have thus far been the primary foci of examination. Particularly for the countryside, Pelling suggests that in the early modern period healers, both men and women, practised along more or less the same lines as those I have sketched for the female model: they were more commonly unlicensed than licensed, they often used ritual, magic and prayer, they often practised medicine either simultaneously or alternately with other employments, and they may have had strong familial traditions in passing on medical knowledge (Pelling emphasizing especially the ties between mother and son). Indeed, Ronald Sawyer (as cited by Pelling) suggests that unofficial women practitioners constituted the most important stratum of care in Jacobean England.[54]

How might we apply Pelling's insights to the medieval period? First, I would suggest that we adopt Pelling and Webster's inclusive definition of a medical practitioner: 'any individual whose occupation is basically concerned with the care of the sick'.[55] Elsewhere, I modified that definition somewhat to make it more readily inclusive of female practitioners: 'Women who at some point in their lives would have either identified themselves in terms of their medical practice or been so identified by their

[52] Carole Rawcliffe, 'The profits of practice: the wealth and status of medical men in later medieval England', *Social History of Medicine*, 1 (1988), 61–78.

[53] Margaret Pelling, 'Medical practice in early modern England: trade or profession?', in *The professions in early modern England*, ed. Wilfrid Prest (London, 1987), pp. 90–128.

[54] Ibid., p. 109.

[55] Margaret Pelling and Charles Webster, 'Medical practitioners', in *Health, medicine and mortality in the sixteenth century*, ed. Charles Webster (Cambridge, 1979), pp. 165–235, esp. p. 166.

communities'.[56] Two points need to be stressed: first, that I emphasize 'at some point in their lives' since it is probably even more likely with women than with men that medicine will not be a life-long vocation; second, that in order to impose some limits on our work and not try to examine every act of healing, no matter how casual or inadvertent, I emphasize some level of identification with the medical art, either in that the woman actively 'sells' her craft to her community, or that the community itself makes that recognition and comes to her for healing. With this definition, an explicit label, though helpful in identification, is not necessary.

Even with explicit labels, however, there are some fuzzy areas that particularly complicate the question of what constitutes a 'medical practitioner' in the case of women. These involve three categories: *vetulae*, midwives, and nurses. We often find the term *vetula* used in connection with women who are healing, though literally the term means nothing more than 'old woman'. Jole Agrimi and Chiara Crisciani have studied the various representations of *vetulae* in religious and medical writings, finding that as the embodiment of all that was negative about femininity, old age, and *simplicitas*, the *vetula* came to stand equally for everything that was ignorant, illiterate, rustic, superstitious. To say that something was done *more* or *ad modum vetularum* was the ultimate disparagement. Indeed, a conflation of *vetulae* with other categories of practitioners was deliberately cultivated by physicians and learned surgeons, who attempted to denigrate those they saw as competitors and sources of all that their theoretical *doctrina* denied by lumping them together with the *vetula*. Henri de Mondeville, for example, speaks of *vetulae* in the same breath as barbers, fortune-tellers, *locatores*, *insidiatores*, tricksters, alchemists, prostitutes, midwives, converted Jews, and Muslims.[57]

Obviously, such polemics cannot be trusted to give us an accurate historical picture of the medical practices of 'old women'. Stereotyped and caricatured in the most ugly fashion, *vetulae* were spoken of by medical authors indiscriminately as a group (it seems to be exceedingly rare for any of them to be granted a personal name). What we can learn from such attacks, however, is that informal medical practice was widespread enough among women (though what proportion of women we cannot know) for physicians and literate surgeons to have wanted to take direct aim at these competitors. Documenting such women will surely be particularly haphazard: clearly not every *vetula* was a healer nor, as Agrimi and Crisciani brilliantly demonstrate, do religious writings – the most obvious alter-

---

[56] Green, 'Women's medical practice', p. 439.
[57] *Die Chirurgie von Heinrich von Mondeville*, ed. J. L. Pagel (Berlin, 1892), p. 65, as cited in Jole Agrimi and Chiara Crisciani, 'Immagini e ruoli della "vetula" tra sapere medico e antropologia religiosa (secoli XIII–XV)', paper presented at international congress, *Les pouvoirs informels dans l'église et la société du bas moyen âge* (Erice, 24–30 September 1989). I am most grateful to Professors Agrimi and Crisciani for sharing their paper with me in advance of publication.

native source of evidence – present any less biased or stereotypical representations of *vetulae*. (Indeed, the overlapping medical and religious conceptions of *vetulae* frequently led to alliances of *medici* and clergy in suppressing their activities.) Yet the medical practice of *vetulae* (or perhaps *mulieres* more generally, since they may not all have been old) will undoubtedly prove to be the largest area of women's involvement with healing, and it poses the greatest challenge to our ability to assess the religious, magical and physical modes of healing that were simultaneously operative in medical culture.

As for midwives, to a large extent we know so little simply because historians have done so little to learn about them. Virtually every study of the social context of practitioners of medieval medicine omits or marginalizes midwives. Indeed, few have ever queried why the documentation for midwives – the one field in which we would expect the *greatest* amount of evidence for female practitioners – is so minuscule. Irma Naso, for example, in an otherwise admirable study of the broad medical milieu of late medieval Piedmont, has nothing to say about *levatrices* other than to repeat the standard claim that they were associated with witchcraft. She does not even bother to document that any existed in her region.[58] One of the few exceptions to this neglect is Danielle Jacquart's supplement to Wickersheimer's biographical register of French practitioners, the original two volumes of which included no midwives at all. Most of Jacquart's additions to the roster of female practitioners, in fact, are *sages-femmes* and *matrones jurées*.[59]

Although historians' lack of interest is part of the problem, there are also several practical reasons why midwives seem so elusive. First is that they have no institutional identity comparable to the other, male-dominated medical fields. There are no guilds of midwives,[60] nor, apparently, are midwives being formally licensed before the early or mid fifteenth century. Second, is that alternative sources, in which midwives would be more likely to appear, have not yet been exploited by historians of medicine. Much evidence waits to be gleaned from parish and episcopal registers and other religious sources, the vast potential of which has been amply

---

[58] Irma Naso, *Medici e strutture sanitarie nella società medievale: il Piemonte dei secoli XIV e XV* (Milan, 1982), pp. 130–5. The insightful observations of David Harley on the highly uncritical (and largely undocumented) association of midwives with witchcraft will, one hopes, put this myth to rest and force a more probing evaluation of the primary sources. See David Harley, 'Historians as demonologists: the myth of the midwife-witch', *Social History of Medicine*, 3, no. 1 (April 1990), 1–26.

[59] Jacquart, *Supplément* to Ernest Wickersheimer, *Dictionnaire biographique des médecins en France au Moyen Age* (Geneva, 1979).

[60] David Herlihy, '*Opera muliebria*': *women and work in medieval Europe* (New York, 1990), seems to have over-interpreted Jacquart's references to *sages-femmes jurées* (*Milieu médical*, p. 49) in claiming that 'guilds of midwives existed at Paris, Rheims, Orleans, Dijon and Lille' (p. 173). No evidence has yet been produced that midwives themselves banded together to form formal guilds.

demonstrated by the recent studies of Annie Saunier and Pierre André Sigal.[61] By analysing the visitation records of the archdeacon Jean Mouchard – one of whose tasks was to oversee the appointment of midwives in his parishes – Saunier is able to document the existence of no less than 113 midwives in the area to the south and west of Paris in the thirteen-year period from 1458–1470. Sigal, on the other hand, uses the accounts of miracles from various canonization procedures and collections of miracle stories from France and Italy from the mid thirteenth through fifteenth centuries. From these sources he culls surprisingly rich information about the realities and attitudes towards sterility, pregnancy, birth, concern for the infant's soul, etc. Although, as Sigal notes, these sources cannot be taken at face value as evidence for daily practice, they do offer interesting clues about the role, even the number of midwives present at births.

Considerable attention has been paid by historians of medieval medicine to the development of the terms *medicus, physicus, surgicus,* and *apothecarius* and to how the varying use of the terms reflects new concepts of professional identity and specialization. No similar study has been done of the evolution of the term *obstetrix* (or its vernacular equivalents), although it has been noted that few identifiable women seem to have been called *obstetrices* before the late thirteenth century, even though the Latin term had always existed in medical literature.[62] Michel Salvat has suggested a gradual development from a situation where a body of knowledge (midwifery) was commonly shared among many women to the creation of a specialist field with certain individuals now acknowledged as having greater knowledge than other women. Annie Saunier suggests that even in the brief period of her study of the later fifteenth century a gradual spread of ecclesiastical appointments of midwives – and so the creation of a specialist identity – can be discerned.

In order to chronicle the history of this increasing specialization of midwifery, there will be need for greater care than is usually the case in the identification of certain women as midwives. As I have argued elsewhere, other categories of women (including *vetulae*) are simply assumed to be midwives whether or not they are specifically designated as such in the sources, thus obscuring how impoverished the documentation for specialist midwives really is.[63] This is especially true of descriptions of certain legal

---

61   Annie Saunier, 'Le visiteur, les femmes et les "obstetrices" des paroisses de l'archidiaconé de Josas de 1458 à 1470', in *Santé, médecine et assistance au moyen âge,* Actes du 110ᵉ Congrès National des Sociétés Savantes, Montpellier, 1985 (Paris, 1987), pp. 43–62; and Pierre André Sigal, 'La grossesse, l'accouchement et l'attitude envers l'enfant mort-né à la fin du moyen âge d'après les récits de miracles', in ibid., pp. 23–41.

62   Michel Salvat, 'L'accouchement dans la littérature scientifique médiévale', *Senefiance,* 9 (1980), 87–106, esp. 92; Jacquart, *Milieu médical,* p. 48. F. Vercauteren has found the word *obstetrix* used to describe a woman in the early twelfth-century *Life of Saint Arnulf;* see 'Les médecins dans les principautés de la Belgique et du nord de la France, du VIIIᵉ au XIIIᵉ siècle', *Le Moyen Âge,* ser. 4, vol. 6 (1951), 61–92, esp. 66.

63   Cf. Green, 'Women's medical practice', pp. 438–9 and 453–6.

proceedings that, unlike most, do regularly document women: determinations of virginity or pregnancy which, so it is often claimed, were always made by midwives. James Brundage, for example, claims that 'midwives' were consulted by Ivo, Bishop of Chartres (1091–116), regarding the normal length of gestation, even though the text of Ivo's letter refers only to 'upright and mature women' ('honestae mulieres et veteranae').[64] Likewise, Erwin Ackerknecht asserts that 'midwives' gave legal testimony in court throughout the Middle Ages. He claims, for example, that in 1220 (*sic*) Pope Gregory IX (1227–41) ordered that women should be examined by midwives in annulment proceedings involving the husband's impotence. (The husband was deemed to be impotent if the wife was found to still be a virgin.)[65] Yet what Gregory's *Decretals* actually established as canon law was that the woman should be examined by a group of women, variously described as 'discerning and upright matrons' or 'matrons of good reputation, trustworthy and expert in marital affairs', one text specifying that there should be seven of them.[66] True, *obstetrices* are mentioned in an earlier collection of canonical laws, the *Decretum* of Gratian (fl. 1130–60), but Gratian was simply quoting a letter of Cyprian (d. AD 258) who was reflecting the very different medical environment of late antiquity.[67] Gregory's immediate predecessor, Pope Honorius III (1216–27), in fact asserted that an assembly of matrons provided more reliable testimony than midwives:

And because, as the canon says, the hand and the eye of midwives are often deceived, we wish and command that in this matter you take care to depute upright, discerning and prudent matrons to inquire whether the said girl is still a virgin.[68]

It seems that no particular medical expertise was expected of such women other than that which they would have acquired in the course of their own pregnancies and their attendance at the lyings-in of their neighbours. Thomas Forbes has documented this for determinations of pregnancy and

---

[64] James A. Brundage, *Law, sex, and Christian society in medieval Europe* (Chicago, 1987), p. 224; Ivo of Chartres, *Epistula*, CCV, in *Patrologia cursus completus ... series Latina*, ed. J.-P. Migne, 221 vols. (Paris, 1844–64), vol. CLXII, col. 210.

[65] Erwin H. Ackerknecht, 'Midwives as experts in court', *Bulletin of the New York Academy of Medicine*, 52, no. 10 (December 1976), 1224–8.

[66] *Decretales Gregorii P. IX* in *Corpus iuris canonici*, 2nd edn, 2 vols. (Graz, 1955), vol. II, lib. IV, tit. xv, c. 6: 'quasdam matronas suae parochiae providas et honestas ad tuam praesentiam evocasti ... ut mulierem ipsam prudenter inspicerent, et perquirerent diligenter, utrum idonea esset ad viriles amplexus'; ibid., c. 7: 'a matronis bonae opinionis, fide dignis ac expertis in opere nuptiali, dictam fecistis inspici mulierem'; lib. II, tit. xix, c. 4: 'quam testimonio septem mulierum probavit, quae per aspectum corporis eam esse virginem asseverant'.

[67] *Decretum magistri Gratiani* in *Corpus iuris canonici*, vol. I, caus. XXVII, q. I, cc. 4–5.

[68] *Decretales*, lib. II, tit. xix, c. 14; 'Et quia, ut dicit canon, saepe manus fallitur et oculus obstetricum, volumus et mandamus, ut adhuc honestas matronas providas et prudentes deputare curetis ad inquirendum, utrum dicta puella virginitatis privilegio sit munita ... ' The fallibility of the midwife had already been asserted by Cyprian.

virginity in England,[69] while Alberto Chiappelli has found a case in Pistoia where three 'discreet and honest women', together with two male physicians, were called in to determine an alleged pregnancy in 1375.[70] (See also the discussion of the Manosquin practitioners below.) It seems likely that the later use of official midwives for legal testimony is the result of the Church's institution of its own system of appointing midwives, chosen (as has been noted by several commentators) as often for their moral probity as for their medical skill.[71]

Admittedly, chronicling the creation of a legal and medical category of midwife over the course of the later Middle Ages will not constitute a history of midwifery *per se* since assistance at birth is obviously being provided whether or not a specialist label is used. Indeed, the image we get will be all the more incomplete and undoubtedly distorted since we are dependent on sources primarily written by men – themselves excluded from the birthing room – which document the male-controlled legal, political, religious and educational systems. Nevertheless, the variation in terminology applied to women functioning as birth attendants does suggest a real change in perceptions of the role and it encourages us to consider whether 'midwife' is really the transhistorical (and hence ahistorical) category that it has been assumed to be.[72]

---

[69] Thomas R. Forbes, 'A jury of matrons', *Medical History*, 32, no. 1 (January 1988), 23–33. It is notable that often knights were asked to supervise the women in their determinations in order to establish the credibility of their testimony.

[70] Alberto Chiappelli, 'Di un singolare procedimento medico-legale tenuto in Pistoia nell'anno 1375 per supposizione d'infante', *Rivista di Storia delle Scienze Mediche e Naturali*, 10, nos. 5, 6 (1919), 129–35, esp. 130–1. The men, Maestro Vincenzo di Salvi and Maestro Francesco di Feo di Arezzo, were paid six gold florins between them; the women, who (typically) are not named, were paid 10 soldi each. Chiappelli implies (p. 130, n. 5) that the women were obstetrical specialists, though he cites nothing to that effect from his document.

[71] See the literature cited in Green, 'Women's medical practice', pp. 449–50.

[72] Andrew Cunningham has suggested to me that another question that could be broached is whether midwives can be considered medical specialists at all. Is childbirth a medical 'condition' and does the work that the birth attendant performs constitute an act of healing? This question has been widely discussed in modern feminist critiques of the 'medicalization' of childbirth, i.e. the view that birth is a pathological condition that demands constant physician intervention within the antiseptic, rigidly controlled environment of a hospital, with the woman becoming a helpless patient, not an active party to her delivery. In this context, the debate whether childbirth is medical or not is more of an issue of patriarchal control and choice than medicine *per se*. Such criticisms are irrelevant to the medieval experience, when (male) physicians were rarely involved with birth and hospitals were the last place most women would deliver. Nevertheless, I think the question is valuable as it forces us to consider how medieval people (especially women themselves) would have categorized the *obstetrix*. Certainly, many male physicians claimed to turn to the *obstetrix* as their helper – as their eyes and hands – when they needed to do intimate examinations of female patients or when certain therapies needed to be administered. That many of these physicians did not consider midwives *learned* in medicine probably reflects something other than a belief that what they did was not medical. (See Agrimi and Crisciani, 'Immagini e ruoli'.) Midwifery's lack of integration into the medieval medical establishment, I would guess, is due to issues of gender stratification rather than

The category of 'nurse' is problematic mostly because some modern commentators cannot rid themselves of the medical connotations of the term fixed by the development of professional nursing in the nineteenth century. Hughes is perhaps most culpable here, for she included in her chapter on 'nurses' all the women involved in any kind of healing or charitable care that she could not fit under her other, more specialized headings. Thus we find here virtually all religious women, whether in orders or not, and any woman who worked in a hospital. In her appendix listing female practitioners individually, however, Hughes included under the heading 'nurses' only the twelve women identified as 'nourrices' in French sources. Herlihy follows Hughes in likewise identifying these 'nourrices' as medical practitioners. Neither raises the possibility that these women may have been wet-nurses or nannies, which would certainly seem conceivable in that most of them are identified as servants in the households of individual employers.[73] Such conceptual carelessness would hardly be worth comment except that through random confusion of religious healers, hospital attendants, nuns, wet-nurses and nannies, the healing activities of large numbers of medieval women become hopelessly obscured behind other forms of care that have little or nothing to do with medicine.[74] The modern, quite specific professional medical connotations of 'nurse' have no place in the Middle Ages, and it would seem best to restrict the term to those women (usually wet- or dry-nurses of children) who were so designated in medieval documents.[75]

Even with less ambiguous categories of practitioners there is need for greater attention to medieval usage. When a woman was called a *chirurgica* as opposed to a *medica*, did the speaker have in mind the same distinctions that differentiated a *chirurgicus* from a *medicus*? Does the context of the citation make a difference? Are these practitioner labels terms that women used to describe themselves or were they imposed by their contemporary society, the scribe who wrote the document, or (possibly) by modern editors? I am not by any means suggesting that we dismiss these labels as insignificant. Rather, I think we need to challenge our comfortable

a belief that childbirth has nothing to do with medicine. But these comments are impressionistic only; more research is obviously needed.

[73] Hughes, *Women healers*, pp. 114–34 and 147; and Herlihy, '*Opera muliebria*', p. 147. Hughes did demonstrate a passing awareness of these other possibilities on p. 86, but she carried it no further.

[74] While I agree with Peregrine Horden that the 'care or cure' dichotomy of studies of medieval hospitals obscures more than it clarifies their function, surely a focus on the provision of health care (and not charity more generally, as is Horden's concern) merits greater care in analysis. See Peregrine Horden, 'A discipline of relevance: the historiography of the later medieval hospital', *Social History of Medicine*, 1 (1988), 359–74.

[75] See Christiane Klapisch-Zuber, 'Blood parents and milk parents: wet nursing in Florence, 1300–1530', in Klapisch-Zuber, *Women, family, and ritual in Renaissance Italy*, trans. Lydia Cochrane (Chicago and London, 1985), pp. 132–64; and Leah L. Otis, 'Municipal Wet Nurses in Fifteenth-Century Montpellier', in Hanawalt (n. 18 above), pp. 83–93. Neither makes any claim for medical responsibilities on the part of wet-nurses.

assumption that we know what these terms meant and look instead at precisely what significance medieval people themselves attached to them and what kind of medical practice they implied. We might also explore the possibility that they may say something about hierarchies that existed within the community of female practitioners, paralleling those that existed among men.

TOWARDS A HISTORY OF WOMEN'S MEDICAL PRACTICE IN THE MIDDLE AGES

I have attempted here to suggest some possible ways in which research on medical practitioners might become more comprehensive of women when our questions and methodologies are informed by an understanding of the different legal and economic conditions of the female half of the medieval population. All of these questions and speculations need to be tested against both the evidence we already have and that which, one hopes, will come to light in the near future.[76] The proper realization of that task must, of course, be left to historians with hands-on experience in the archives and familiarity with the salient details of local social, legal and economic history. These are, I must stress, speculations and I will be more than happy to see them challenged by future research.

Once we have assembled a broader body of documentation on women who practised medicine, our next task will be to determine how we can move from the disconnected anecdotes about isolated women that have characterized previous studies toward a synthetic historical analysis that can tell us not only about the commonalities of medieval women's medical practices, but also about the range of medieval medical practice as a whole. Since the historian's vision of what kinds of interpretations are possible will inevitably affect how she or he sifts through the original documents, it is worthwhile to sketch out here some ways in which a broader interpretative study might be framed.

As Ladislao Münster demonstrated in his study of six women practising in Venice in the first half of the fourteenth century,[77] paucity of documentation, although obviously rendering our work difficult, need not deter us altogether. Setting his analysis into a broader context of medical regulation in late medieval Venice, Münster concluded: (1) that in the Republic of Venice women, although not officially licensed, were allowed to practise under the official status 'per grazia', thus rendering their practice in no way

---

[76] Kowaleski, 'Women's work', p. 162, feels that documenting women's work in medicine is inherently more difficult than other fields that were more regulated than medicine and so produced more documentation. While this is undoubtedly the case for England, it is not necessarily true for the continent (especially Italy) due to the earlier introduction there of licensing and the incorporation of medical testimony in judicial proceedings.

[77] Münster, 'Notizie'. Although the documents pertain to only six women directly, a seventh, Francesca, *medicatrix*, is mentioned as the mother of Marina.

different from men's; (2) that their practice was not limited to women and children but included men as well (in this regard, therefore, also paralleling the practice of men); (3) that they not only practised general medicine but also cultivated certain specialities, particularly in surgery; (4) that those who were called *medichesse* learned their art not from special courses, but from their husbands, who were, like them, physicians or surgeons; (5) that those not called *magistra* or *medica* practised the art only occasionally and, to some extent, secretly, often simply preparing medicaments (hence their name, *medicatrices*); (6) that the professional position of those who practised by consent of the government differed not at all from their male colleagues', as the College of Physicians and Surgeons never found anything to say against their activity; and (7) that the city of Venice, although not the seat of a university, was excelled by no other Italian region (except Sicily and the Republic of Florence) in having so many female practitioners. Münster leaves many of the implications of his assertions unexplored (e.g. the possibility that it was precisely *because* Venice did not yet have a university that women practitioners could thrive), nor can he explain why, at least as indicated by the extant documents, it is only in the first half of the fourteenth century that women seem to be appearing.[78] Particularly limiting is his bias against unlicensed practitioners: interested in neither midwives nor religious healers, Münster even finds it necessary to call the *medicatrices* 'the female representatives of charlatanry'.[79] Nevertheless, precisely because Münster takes such care to set his women into the medico-legal context of their city and to explore questions of their training and range of practice, his locally focused study offers a model of how we might analyse information about medieval women's medical practice so that it can be used for broader comparative work.

An analysis of the data provided by recent studies on two very different French cities, Paris and Manosque (in Provence), may illustrate this further. A glimpse of female medical practitioners in Paris at the turn of the fourteenth century can be gleaned from the statistical analyses of David Herlihy and Béatrice Coury.[80] Both studies draw on the *livres de la taille*, the tax rolls for the city of Paris in 1292, 1297 and 1313.[81] Herlihy's focus is on women's labour in general as reflected in the *tailles*, while Coury's is on medical practitioners. Neither has much to say about female medical

---

[78] Compare the findings of Katherine Park, who found women matriculated in the Florentine Guild of Doctors, Apothecaries and Grocers only in the *second* half of the fourteenth century, i.e. after the Black Death had opened up the profession somewhat. See *Doctors and medicine in early Renaissance Florence* (Princeton, 1985).

[79] Münster, 'Notizie', p. 186.

[80] Herlihy, '*Opera muliebria*'; Béatrice Coury, 'Contribution à l'histoire sociale des praticiens parisiens à la fin du moyen âge: aspects méthodologiques', *Sources: Travaux Historiques*, 5, (1986), 13–28.

[81] Coury omits the *taille* of 1296 (which has also been published) from her analysis as it is incomplete and differs little from that of 1297. Herlihy draws mostly on those of 1292 and 1313.

practitioners, yet a synthesis of their findings produces an intriguing profile.

The *taille* of 1292 was the most inclusive, with a total of 14,516 hearths (foca) being assessed. Groups exempt from the *taille* included clergy and students (which would account for the absence of physicians from the list). Three groups – 'Lombards' (i.e. Italians), *menus genz* (poorer but none the less taxable individuals) and, for the most part, Jews – were assessed separately and so likewise are not always represented in the *tailles*. In the 1292 *taille*, 2,238 women appear as heads of hearths (15 per cent), while 735 women (11 per cent) head hearths in the *taille* of 1313, which drew on a smaller but apparently richer section of the populace.[82]

In the survey of 1292, 39 per cent of the women are entered with a designation of occupation; in that of 1313, 47 per cent of the women are shown with an occupational title. They engage in 172 different areas of work in 1292, 130 in 1313. Medical practice is by no means the most prominent of these. Herlihy includes 'nurses' (whom he assumes to be medical practitioners) among the fifteen most common occupations for women in 1292; no medical field falls into the top fifteen in 1313.[83]

No practitioners explicitly labelled as surgeons, male or female, are included in any of the *tailles*.[84] As for barbers, in the 1292 *taille*, Coury counts 146, thirteen of whom are women. In 1297, there are 101, including five women. In 1313 (perhaps because of the restricted nature of the survey, noted above) the overall number has dropped to 68. Only one female barber (not noted by Coury) is found for this last year.[85] Of the *miresses*, Coury counts eight in 1292 (out of a total of 36 *mires*), five in 1297 (out of 20), and one in 1313 (out of five).[86] Two midwives (*ventrières*) are included in the *taille* of 1292,[87] two in 1297, and none in 1313.[88]

Most unfortunately, although Coury has noted the number of women in her total figures, she does not sustain a separate analysis by sex in her otherwise useful examination of the assessed taxes (and hence the wealth) or the geographic distribution of these practitioners within the city of Paris. Still, her enumeration is helpful in drawing a few simple observations. The percentage of female barbers dropped from 8.9 per cent in 1292, to 4.9

[82] Herlihy, '*Opera muliebria*', pp. 132–4.

[83] Ibid., pp. 143 and 146.

[84] Coury, ('Contribution à l'histoire', pp. 15, 20) is puzzled by this omission, though she suggests that the term *mire/miresse* may have comprehended surgeons. Cf. Jacquart, *Milieu médical*, p. 54.

[85] See *Le livre de la taille de Paris*, ed. Karl Michaëlsson, Acta Universitatis Gotoburgensis, 1951 (Göteborg, 1951), p. 88, for Aveline la barbière. Herlihy, ('*Opera muliebria*', p. 147) is in error in claiming there are thirteen female barbers in this *taille*.

[86] Herlihy suggests ('*Opera muliebria*', p. 146) that the three women referred to as *mestresses* in 1292 may have been doctors, too.

[87] Coury mentions only one, but see Hughes, *Women healers*, p. 146. Hughes (p. 110) suggests that Jehanne, called 'la sage' in the *taille* of 1292, may also have been a midwife.

[88] Coury, 'Contribution à l'histoire', p. 14–15.

per cent in 1297, to 1.5 per cent in 1313. This seems a sharper decline in female representation that one would expect from the overall drop of taxable female heads of hearths from 15 per cent to 11 per cent in the same twenty-one-year period. Does this reflect increased restriction of women's practice as barbers? Or merely a drop in their income? The *miresses*, on the other hand, remain at a fairly steady percentage of 22.2 per cent (1292), 25 per cent (1297), and 20 per cent (1313). The small total numbers make percentages distorting, of course. Nevertheless, since the *tailles* in general under-represent women to a far greater degree than men of their same economic level, these figures may suggest something near parity in the numbers of men and women practising under the nebulous title *mire/ miresse*. The minuscule evidence for midwives in what was perhaps the largest city in Europe at the time suggests the very low economic status of midwives and/or the fact that 'midwife' was only then becoming a recognized specialist function.

These are obviously very meagre data indeed, especially in comparison to Manosque, a town perhaps one-fiftieth the size of Paris. Joseph Shatzmiller, drawing on a rich series of notarial registers and the registers of judicial inquests, has gathered more than eighty documents relating to healers involved in judicial and legal matters in Manosque for the years 1262–1348.[89] Although this does not pretend to be a fully comprehensive social history of Manosquin practitioners (most of the documentation that relates solely to the identified practitioners' non-medical affairs, for example, is omitted), over the course of the ninety some years of his study Shatzmiller is able to identify forty-one medical practitioners (excluding apothecaries, midwives and 'charlatans') in this moderate-sized town of about 3,000 to 4,000 inhabitants. Three of the forty-one (7.3 per cent) are women. One of these, the Jewess Mayrona, is a member of a medical family; her father, Benedictus, is a physician, as is (possibly) her husband Leo Frances.[90] With a dowry of 100 livres (the same as that of the daughter of another male practitioner), she clearly came from a wealthy family. Mayrona, *fisica*, is in fact never documented in the act of healing. Rather, in most of the forty-five documents known to mention her (which are not included in Shatzmiller's collection) she appears instead in her other occupation of money-lender. In this respect, however, she resembles at least a few of her fellow male practitioners, who are also seen carrying on other occupations besides healing.[91]

The *surgica* Fava is likewise Jewish and likewise a member of a medical family, in her case of surgeons. She is married to the 'patriarch' of the

[89] Joseph Shatzmiller, *Médecine et justice en Provence médiévale: documents de Manosque, 1262–1348* (Aix-en-Provence, 1989). There is a lacuna for the years 1265–85 due to the poor state of the documents.

[90] Precisely why Shatzmiller suggests that Leo is a physician is unclear.

[91] Ibid., p. 6–7 and 242–3. Professor Shatzmiller informs me (personal communication, 8 February 1990) that his reference to Mayrona on p. 11 of his book as 'sirurgica' is in error.

family, Astrugus, and has a son and two grandsons who also practise the family trade. Fava appears in a case in 1321–2 recounting an attack on Ponçon, the crier of the hospital. Wounded by a kick to his testicles, Ponçon sought out Fava to treat him and she complied with plasters 'and other necessary things'. Asked by the court if she had actually palpated his wound, she replied no. That task had been left for her son, Bonafos, also a surgeon, who examined Ponçon and was later asked to give the formal medical testimony in court as to whether the wound was old or new.[92]

The third woman, Laura, appears in a case of 1292 in which a man is being ordered to pay several physicians and surgeons for determining the extent of the wounds suffered by his son. The surgeon Elias and 'master' Finus are to be paid ten *livres* each, while another six 'surgeons and physicians', among whom is Laura, *habitatrix Manuasca*, are each to be paid ten *sous*, an amount that seems standard for surgical care for wounds.[93] No other information is given about Laura, however; we do not know whether she is a 'surgica' or a 'fisica' nor what her exact role in the examination was.

What can we conclude from these few individuals about women's medical practice in Manosque from the mid thirteenth to the mid fourteenth century? Schatzmiller, tentatively extrapolating from the fragmentary data that remain, hypothesizes that in any given year throughout the period of his study there were on average eight or nine physicians and surgeons practising, producing a practitioner:patient ratio of 1:450–500.[94] For the single years in which Laura, Fava and Mayrona are documented (1292, 1321 and 1343), they constitute, respectively, 1 of 8, 1 of 8, and 1 of 2 physicians or surgeons known to be practising that year. It is also notable that this general ratio of male: female practitioners holds within the Jewish community as well (which, as only about 5 per cent of the total Manosquin population, was itself over-represented among medical practitioners), where women are two of the eleven documented practitioners. It would be rash, however, to assume at this point that this male-to-female ratio was in any respect 'typical'. While it is admissible to posit a basic supply-and-demand argument for estimating the number of practitioners as a ratio to total population (Shatzmiller cites estimates similar to his own for many other cities), since these three women seem to have provided no services not duplicated by their male counterparts, the only reason to assume that this male-to-female ratio was normal is if women in medical families were regularly participating in the family trade. (A supply-and-demand argument would, however, seem admissible in estimating the number of midwives, who perform a regularly needed and unique function.)

Although the limited documentation does not allow us to say much

[92] Ibid., pp. 150–1.
[93] Ibid., pp. 74–6. Cf. pp. 78 and 113.
[94] Ibid., pp. 17–18.

about the scope of their practice, the Manosquin *fisicae* and *sirurgicae* were clearly not restricted to the treatment of women, which (except for obstetrics) seems to have been a field open to everyone. In 1263, Guilhem Fouques called in master Stephanus of Montpellier to cure his daughter for the promised sum of 25 *livres*. In 1310, Raimon Sauneri contracted the physician Isaac to care for himself, his wife and his children for the following four years. In 1319 the surgeon Bonafos (Fava's son) testified to having determined, by direct palpation of her right side, that the wound of one Astruga was not serious. In 1334, Bonafos is also promised 20 *sous* for the cure of the daughter of Langerius Langerii and his wife Gallia. In 1341, a Christian woman, Alaxia Collarda, asked Crescas de Nîmes, a Jewish physician, to come to her house, first to cure her daughter, and then again several weeks later when she herself fell ill. (Crescas responded by asking for payment in the form of sexual services.)[95] In the two cases where men are involved in matters pertaining to female reproduction, the outrage is that they have allegedly provoked an abortion or used 'diabolical' methods to effect cures of infertility and impotence that do not materialize, not that, as men, they have no business involving themselves in 'women's affairs'.[96]

If we can judge from Ponçon's decision to seek out Fava first for aid to his wound, or the judgement that Laura should be paid the same as her male counterparts, it would seem that women practitioners were respected by their communities and deemed equally competent with men. Nevertheless, their visibility within the medical community was not particularly great. True, seventeen of the thirty-eight men are, like Fava and Laura, known from only one document, so the women are not unusual in their minimal documentation. But Fava's husband, Astrugus (who was also a goldsmith and so can not be considered a 'full-time' medical practitioner), is called in at least six times to give medical testimony; her son, Bonafos, appears in a medical capacity thirty-four times. Perhaps Fava did not normally attend to the more drastic wounds that demanded legal inquiry and that would consequently bring her into the judicial documents studied by Shatzmiller. Still, it is striking that as a member of perhaps the most prominent medical family in Manosque (no other individual comes close to Bonafos' popularity) there is not more evidence of her working either in concert with her relatives or on her own.

Nothing is known about the training of these women practitioners (though in the case of Mayrona and Fava, it would be reasonable to expect that it came from their male relatives), nor whether any of them were licensed. It is interesting to note, however, that the one practitioner who was prosecuted for having practised medicine despite being illiterate (in

---

[95] Ibid., pp. 61–2, 123–4, 140, 194, 229–30.
[96] Ibid., pp. 80–5 and 176–83.

Latin?) and inexperienced was a male.[97] With regard to non-physical methods of healing, the one instance of use of charms, etc., that Shatzmiller documents is likewise of a male practitioner (the infertility expert). Whether women also practised a kind of informal, magical medicine cannot be determined from these documents.

In addition to Mayrona, Fava and Laura, specialist birth attendants also practised in Manosque. A case from 1289 shows that there were perhaps three practising *c.* 1265. In an attempt to determine whether one Raimon Gaus has reached majority, testimony is provided by several women, who recount the circumstances of Raimon's birth and those of one Guillaume and one Romeu who are, in conflicting reports, said to have been born at the same time as Raimon.[98] Even though other women were clearly present at these births, it seems that the key question in authenticating the birth, is 'que bajula levavit eum'. Not as technically specific as *obstetrix*, *bajula* (French *baille*) seems to have taken on the meaning of 'midwife' by this point in time, although it is also used to refer to wet-nurses, suggesting a continuing vagueness of professional identity.[99]

As far as the court was concerned, *bajulae* had no monopoly as forensic experts. Shatzmiller, in discussing cases of expert testimony given by people other than medical practitioners, notes that the court depends on 'femmes "vieilles et expertes en affaires matrimoniales"' to establish the virginity of a woman, thus conforming to the dictates of canon law discussed above. It then later calls in a midwife, *obstetrix*, to confirm the women's conclusions, which seems to be the only documented instance in which the technical term *obstetrix* is used.[100] Beyond this one case, there seems to be no privileging of the midwife's expertise over the experience which most women might have gained in the course of an ordinary lifetime. Two women, Ayglentina and Peyrona, are asked in 1314 to

---

[97] Ibid., pp. 113–14. Why the accused's mother, Emenrarda, is implicated in the case is not clear.

[98] The two witnesses who were present at Romeu's birth agreed that Asalgarda was the *bajula* who delivered him. There was disagreement, however, on who delivered Raimon: one witness (who was present at the birth) said it was Alacia Vegreria, another (who was not) said she had heard it was Guillelma Vexaria. No *bajula* is mentioned in connection with Guillaume's birth.

[99] See Shatzmiller, *Médecine et justice*, p. 67, where *bajula* is also used to refer to the woman who *nursed* (lactavit) the infant Raimon. It is unclear what function Elisabet, *bajula liberorum* (p. 82) performed. Jacquart, *Supplément*, notes a Marie 'la Bayle' (fl. 1485 in Apt) and Perrote de Pouy, 'dite "la Baille"' (b. c. 1268 and practising in Troyes), both of whom are apparently 'sages-femmes' (pp. 205 and 222). See also Frédéric Godefroy, *Dictionnaire de l'ancienne langue française et de tous ses dialectes du IXe au XVe siècle* (Paris, 1880; repr. Vaduz, 1965), vol. I, p. 555, s.v. *baille*. Interestingly, Professor Shatzmiller has suggested to me that *bajula* may have also been used to refer to the matrons of brothels (personal communication, 8 February 1990).

[100] Shatzmiller, *Médecine et justice*, p. 32, citing from the unpublished master's thesis of Andrée Courtemanche, 'Regard sur la femme médiévale: la délinquence féminine à Manosque au tournant du XIVe siècle' (Université Laval, Quebec, 1981). Shatzmiller does not reproduce these documents.

examine a woman who has been beaten and to determine if she is pregnant and whether the beating will cause her to lose the child. Yet the two women are simply called *mulieres* and *matronae*.[101] In the case of Raimon and Romeu, when asked how she knew how long women were accustomed to lie in childbed, a witness, Alasacia Maurella, replied that this was what is seen and heard: that she herself had had five children, and she had also seen very many women in childbed. She makes no claim to 'expert' (let alone 'learned') authority nor does she imply that anyone else has it.[102] Apparently, no *bajula* was called in to testify on this issue.

How representative are these legal and notarial documents for women's medical practice in Manosque? Of the approximately 620 individuals named in Shatzmiller's texts, some 80 (12.9 per cent) are women. Women do serve as witnesses and are held financially accountable for the payment of some debts and fines (even for those of male family members). Interestingly, aside from a few servants, the *fisicae*, *sirurgicae*, and *bajulae* are the only women referred to by any kind of functional title. All the rest are identified as daughters, wives, widows, sisters, nieces, or mothers of men. Shatzmiller, however, has presented only a small slice of the extant materials. A truly comprehensive study of female Manosquin practitioners would obviously have to draw on *all* the extant documents in order to situate these women more firmly within the legal, social and economic framework of the town.

The work of Andrée Courtemanche on women in Manosque around the turn of the fourteenth century lays the foundation for such a broadly based analysis.[103] She finds that the range of occupations for women in Manosque overall was quite narrow, certainly in no way comparable to the diversity found in Paris (see above). The two principal areas of employment for Christian women are seasonal agricultural labour and domestic work, while others are employed in the production and sale of bread and clothes, the sale of wine and other foodstuffs, medical care, wet-nursing, and

---

[101] Shatzmiller, *Médecine et justice*, p. 131. Because the document is fragmentary, it is not clear to whom the phrase *matronis presentibus* applies. Shatzmiller interprets it as applying to the two examining women, whom he refers to in his summary of the document as 'sages-femmes'. Jacquart (*Milieu médical*, p. 48) identifies the fourteenth- and fifteenth-century French *matrones jurées* as midwives, yet the use of the term seems fluid enough in medieval documents to caution us against a too easy equation of all *matronae* with specialist *obstetrices*. For example, a Latin gynaecological text from the thirteenth century is intended for *matronae*, though it seems that the author means women in general (*matronae* being a polite address), not medical specialists *per se*. See *Collectio salernitana*, ed. Salvatore De Renzi, 5 vols. (Naples, 1852–9), vol. IV, p. 1. I have found no evidence in dictionaries of medieval Latin that *matrona* was used to mean anything other than 'wife', 'lady', or 'godmother', or as an honorific title for religious women. To my knowledge, its use in a particular legal or medical sense has not yet been studied.

[102] Shatzmiller, *Médecine et justice*, p. 68.

[103] Andrée Courtemanche, 'Les femmes juives et le crédit à Manosque au tournant du XIVe siècle', *Provence Historique*, fasc. 150 (1987), 545–58. I have not seen her thèse de doctorat, 'La condition des femmes dans la société manosquine (1290–1369)' (Université Laval, Quebec, 1907 (*sic*, for 1987?)).

money- and grain-lending. Jewish women engage in none of these except the sale of wine and grain, medical care, wet-nursing and, above all, lending, a field in which some thirty Jewish women were involved during the three decades of Courtemanche's study. Although not a principal area of women's employment, medical care was nevertheless as important an area of labour as several other occupations, especially in the case of Jewish women, who had fewer alternatives for generating income.

As these sketches of Parisian and Manosquin practitioners show, far more information about women's medical practice can be squeezed out of the extant documents than might at first seem possible. Even more could be obtained if historians were willing to devote special attention to female practitioners, taking into consideration the representativeness of the documents being used and any local legal factors that might be relevant.

If we had a solid foundation of such closely focused studies, it would be possible to answer some broader questions about women's medical practice in the high and later Middle Ages. Are there, for example, differences in women's medical activity between small towns and large? Between large towns with a university and those without? Is the gradually increasing restriction of women's practice (which thus far has only been sporadically documented) moving at an equal pace throughout Europe? Jacquart, for example, has noted that, with but one exception, every known *femme médecin* who practised in Paris was in some way harassed by the medical faculty.[104] No such universal (or at least effective) repression has yet been documented elsewhere, even though laws restricting women's practice are being promulgated.[105]

Particularly interesting in this regard are the implications of recent suggestions that the increasing professionalization of medicine from the thirteenth century on was spurred directly by the growth in medical knowledge that came with the adoption of ancient and Arabic medical learning into the core of the university curricula and the dissemination of that learning even among practitioners far removed from the Latinate culture of the *studia*.[106] As theoretical learning came to be increasingly valued in the legal assessment of the curative merits of healers, would it not be inevitable that women's capabilities be increasingly devalued since they had so little access to that learning? The common belief in women's feeble intellectual abilities could only have enhanced prejudices against them further.

A final issue worth exploration is what is termed 'the construction of gender' – that is, how what constitutes 'masculine' and 'feminine' is

---

[104] Jacquart, *Milieu médical*, p. 54.
[105] E.g., in Valencia. See García-Ballester et al. (n. 9 above), pp. 29–32.
[106] García-Ballester, McVaugh and Rubio-Vela, *Medical licensing*; and Nancy G. Siraisi, *Medieval and early Renaissance medicine: an introduction to knowledge and practice* (Chicago, 1990), esp. ch. 2.

actually defined and elaborated by a given culture.[107] Although at some point or another one can find women working in almost every kind of craft and manual labour in the Middle Ages, at particular points in time and in particular localities there were in fact very defined notions of the proper division of labour by sex. How and to what extent was medical practice 'gendered' – i.e. to what degree was medical practice associated with one or the other sex, either horizontally, by field, or vertically, by position on the ladder of prestige and social or economic power? I have argued elsewhere that, with the exception of normal childbirth, which seems to have been almost exclusively relegated to women, there was no simple and universal sexual division of medical labour on the basis of the sex of the patient: female practitioners do not seem to have always restricted their practice to women, nor males to men.[108] There may, however, have been more subtle divisions that have not yet been explored. Aside from the obvious division of labour (or at least of prestige) created by university education, were there any other lines along which tasks could be apportioned by gender – paralleling, say, the ways in which different aspects of textile production (carding, spinning, weaving) were segregated by sex? At what point did the practice of medicine as a whole (except for midwifery) become a task not to be entrusted to women? Questions such as these might serve to remind us that formal legal prohibition is not the only way such gender-based restrictions are effected. The force of custom and cultural expectations must also be assessed before we blithely conclude (with today's mythical 'liberated woman' in mind) that, in the absence of laws explicitly forbidding their practice, women had complete freedom of opportunity and merely 'chose' not to practise medicine.

Documenting the historical experience of women practitioners must be the concern of all social historians of medicine, not simply those who specialize in women's history. There are no 'women's archives' where documents on women's experiences are kept separate from those of men, nor, with the possible exception of midwifery, is there a separate occupational category with a documentary foundation pertaining to female practitioners exclusively. More important than the nature of the historical materials, however, is the question of historiographical integrity. While licensed or university-educated physicians and surgeons may make more interesting subjects for prosopographical studies precisely because their

---

[107] For a general consideration of the notion of gender, see Joan W. Scott, 'Gender: a useful category of historical analysis', *American Historical Review*, 91 (1986), 1053–75.

[108] Green, 'Women's medical practice'. Such extreme sexual segregation may have been operative on a local level, however. Many of the licences for women surgeons in the Kingdom of Naples cited by Calvanico quite explicitly state that modesty demands that female practitioners care for other women; see Raffaele Calvanico, *Fonti per la storia della medicina e della chirurgia per il regno di Napoli nel periodo angioino (a. 1273–1410)* (Naples, 1962), e.g. item nos. 1872, 3571, 3572 and 3643. The problem, of course, is penetrating through the formulaic legalese of these documents and determining how much their rhetoric reflected everyday practice.

practice is better documented, the fact remains that the medieval populace drew on a variety of resources for medical care, of which the learned medical elite (from which women were largely excluded) constituted only a portion. Women's involvement in the provision of health care took a variety of forms, not all of which can be neatly classified under the distinct practitioner labels that imply 'professional' identities.[109] If we agree with Roy Porter and others that the historian of medicine's task is to document both the practitioners' and the patients' experience in past times,[110] then documenting medieval women's medical practice becomes doubly incumbent upon us, since if we choose to ignore women's medical practice we simultaneously choose to ignore the health care received by a significant portion of the medieval population, male and female.

ACKNOWLEDGEMENTS

My thanks to the participants in the Barcelona Conference and to Judith Bennett, James Bono, Maryanne Kowaleski and Miriam Shadis for their suggestions.

[109] In addition to those discussed above, some further possibilities of women's involvement in medicine are suggested by Gundolf Keil, 'Die Frau als Ärztin und Patientin in der medizinischen Fachprosa des deutschen Mittelalters', in *Frau und spätmittelalterlicher Alltag: Internationaler Kongress, Krems an der Donau, 2. bis 5. Oktober 1984* (Vienna, 1986), pp. 157–211, esp. pp. 200–10.

[110] *Patients and practitioners: lay perceptions of medicine in pre-industrial society*, ed. Roy Porter (Cambridge, 1985).

11

A marginal learned medical world: Jewish, Muslim and Christian medical practitioners, and the use of Arabic medical sources in late medieval Spain

LUIS GARCÍA-BALLESTER

The Christian conquest of Muslim-ruled areas in that part of the Iberian peninsula within the confines of present-day Spain did not mean that the Arabic language disappeared from those areas. From the late eleventh century onwards the frontiers of Castile included such important cities as Toledo (from 1085 onwards); during the course of the thirteenth century the Guadalquivir valley was incorporated (with the conquest of Cordoba, 1236, and Seville, 1248), as was the Kingdom of Murcia (1243 onwards); the Muslim Kingdom of Granada was not conquered until 1492. For their part, the Christians of the Crown of Aragon, in the eastern coastal area of the Iberian peninsula, conquered the Kingdom of Valencia, as far as the frontier with Murcia, in 1237–40. All these cities and regions contained a population whose everyday language of communication was Arabic, and who, to a great extent, remained settled in the area after the conquest. Furthermore, Arabic maintained its role as a language of scholarly communication and as the vehicle which allowed continued access to medical sources of unquestionable theoretical and practical value.[1]

---

[1] On the small number of medical works written in or translated into Arabic, which were translated into Latin, see Danielle Jacquart and Françoise Micheau, *La médecine arabe et l'occident médiéval* (Paris, 1990), pp. 230–43. On the role played by knowledge of the Arabic language in the medical training of the Jewish and Muslim physicians practising in medieval Spanish kingdoms, see L. García-Ballester, 'Medical science in thirteenth-century Castile: problems and prospects', *Bulletin of the History of Medicine*, 61 (1987), 183–202, and L. García-Ballester, Lola Ferre, and Eduard Feliu, 'Jewish appreciation of fourteenth-century scholastic medicine in the Western Mediterranean', in McVaugh and Siraisi (eds.), *Renaissance medical learning* (*Osiris*, 2nd series, 6 (1990), 85–117). The conclusion reached by L. P. Harvey after the analysis of two medical consultations, the one in 1492 and the other in 1501, between Christian patients and Muslim practitioners, one of them, a woman, about the situation of Arabic medicine among Muslim practitioners living under the new

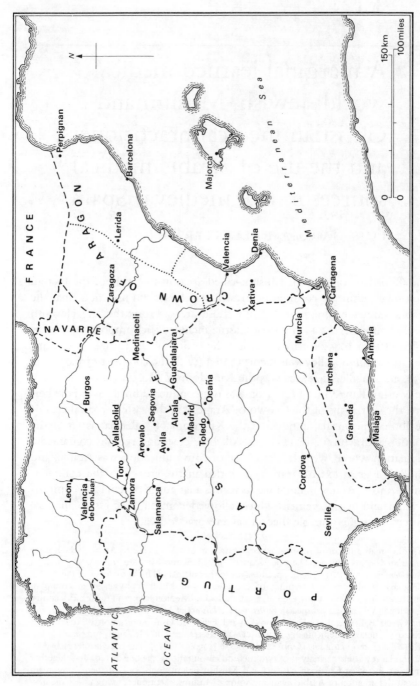

The Iberian peninsula in the thirteenth, fourteenth and fifteenth centuries.

During the last few years, various experts on Arabic culture in medieval and Renaissance Spain have discovered, described and studied surviving manuscripts of all kinds written in Arabic that were used by members of the three religious groups (Christians, Muslims and Jews) that lived alongside each other in the Christian kingdoms of Spain between the eleventh and sixteenth centuries. The most recent and most complete of all these works is that produced by P. S. van Koningsveld.[2] He describes 105 manuscript codices. Twenty-four of them contain a total of sixty-five medical works with various texts by Hippocrates, Galen, Dioscorides, Avicenna, Rhazes, Maimonides, Averroes and other lesser authors. All the manuscripts with medical contents were copied between c. 1150 and 1480. This is fundamentally the material upon which this chapter, which continues and brings up to date other earlier contributions on the same subject,[3] is based.

The present chapter is divided into three parts. In the first we shall describe the uses these manuscripts were put to by physicians of the three religious groups (Christians, Muslims and Jews) that lived alongside one another in the peninsular Kingdoms of Castile and the Crown of Aragon from the twelfth to the fifteenth centuries and who are recorded as having made use of the Arabic language to establish the foundations of their medical knowledge. In the second part, we shall offer a general panorama, based on an analysis of the evidence of reading and transmission present in the manuscripts themselves. This analysis demonstrates the continued use of (Greek and Arabic) medical sources written in Arabic, which contributed to the development of the medieval Galenism of these physicians (who were most commonly of Jewish origin, although the other two groups should not be forgotten). If our analysis is basically restricted to Castile, this is due to the fact that all the *surviving* Arabic medical manuscripts which circulated in Spanish Christian lands come from this Kingdom, with the exception of two (one from Barcelona, the other from Valencia, both of which were cities of the Crown of Aragon). The close relationship existing between the population of the lands of Castile and the

Christian conquerors is highly illustrative of the situation: 'Granada [we could say also Valencia or Murcia] was a place where the culture of the conqueror was for a time challenged by the continuing reality of the culture of the conquered': see 'In Granada under the Catholic monarchs: a call from a doctor and another from a *curandera*', in *The age of the Catholic monarchs, 1474–1516, Literary studies in memory of Keith Whinnom* (Liverpool, 1989), pp. 71–5.

[2] P. S. van Koningsveld, 'Andalusian-Arabic manuscripts from Christian Spain: a comparative, intercultural, approach', *Israel Oriental Studies*, 12 (1992), 75–110; van Koningsveld, 'Andalusian-Arabic manuscripts from medieval Christian Spain: some supplementary notes', in *Festgabe für H.-R. Singer* (Frankfurt a. M., 1991), pp. 811–23. I have used the typescript version of both papers by courtesy of the author.

[3] The first attempt to use this approach on the medieval medical manuscripts written in Arabic and preserved in Western libraries, especially El Escorial and Biblioteca Nacional of Madrid, was made by L. García-Ballester, *Historia social de la medicina en la España de los siglos XIII al XVI* (Madrid, 1976), pp. 31–42.

people of the Crown of Aragon has meant that it is advisable to make reference to events that took place in the Crown of Aragon, when it is relevant. The third part will be dedicated to the analysis of the intellectual characteristics of the only medical work written in Arabic in the first third of fourteenth-century Castile to survive to the present day. This is the *Kitab al-tibb al-qastali al-maluki* (Book of regal Castilian medicine), an important systematic medical treatise, written by an anonymous Jew from Toledo (*fl.* 1295–1312).[4] It will enable us to consider in great depth the role played by the rationalist Jewish minority in the maintenance and growth of the medical literature that circulated among the Jewish minority in Castile. In addition, as will be seen, this medical literature acted as a support for a particular approach to professional practice. Thus, the medical activity of certain physicians – to be more precise Jewish practitioners – was not limited to mere empiricism, nor to the blind application of prescriptions repeated from generation to generation; it was, in fact, the manifestation in practice of theoretical knowledge, transmitted and developed in accordance with an 'open' system, distinct from that of the Latin scholastic university world.[5]

I

Three population groups continued to use Arabic as a language of communication in Christian Spain: Muslims, Jews and Christians, both those of Arabic culture (Mozarabs) and those formed in Latin culture. The survival of the Arabic language among these different groups was not uniform; the time and other circumstances of a social and intellectual nature influenced the survival of Arabic among them to a greater or lesser extent.

Christians

One of the most interesting peculiarities of the new area conquered by Christians from the north – especially in the case of Toledo, but also of other cities – was the presence in them of communities of Christians of Arabic culture, who had lived as a minority in what had hitherto been Muslim territories, and who, after the conquest, remained alongside their brothers-in-religion of Latin culture. They received the name *Mozarabs*.[6]

---

[4] L. García-Ballester, and Concepción Vázquez de Benito, 'Los médicos judíos del siglo XIV y el galenismo árabe: el *Kitab al-tibb al-qastali al-maluki* (Libro de medicina castellana regia), *c.* 1312', *Asclepio*, 42 (1990), 119–47.

[5] On the relationship between both systems of medical training in western Mediterranean countries, see García-Ballester, Ferre and Feliu, 'Jewish appreciation'.

[6] On *Mozarabs* and medicine, see F. Girón-Irueste, 'Los médicos mozárabes y el proceso de constitución de la medicina árabe en Al-andalus, siglos VIII–X', *Asclepio*, 30–1 (1978–9), 209–22, which, in my opinion, over-emphasizes the role of *Mozarabs* in this process. See also Jacquart and Micheau, *La médecine arabe*, pp. 134–53, and P. S. van Koningsveld, *The*

The strength of Latin culture and the continuing uneasiness of the Church at the presence of Christians of Arabic culture, whether they were Christians of long standing or recent converts, meant that Mozarabic culture underwent a rapid process of decline, already apparent in the early thirteenth century.[7] Even though it is possible to identify documents composed in Arabic by members of this Christian minority in the early fourteenth century, all available indications point to this language rarely being used from the second half of the thirteenth century onwards by those individuals among them who practised medicine. None of the surviving medical manuscripts in Arabic that have come down to us, and which are known to have circulated in Christian lands, were copied by or belonged to a member of the Mozarabic community.[8]

Christian physicians trained in Latin culture were not averse to using Arabic medical manuscripts. Throughout the thirteenth century, and even at the beginning of the fourteenth century, nobody among the Christian intellectual minority of Europe doubted that an effective way to gain access to medical learning was still through a knowledge of Arabic.[9] Moreover, Christian scholars were aware that there existed valuable medical works unknown to scholastic medical circles because they had not been translated into Latin. Very few Christian university physicians were capable of handling these Arabic sources directly. Moreover, Arabic medical manuscripts do not seem to have been particularly abundant in the late thirteenth century and the first decades of the fourteenth century, to judge from the available information. However, the Arabic medical manuscripts that were in existence in Christian lands were highly regarded, and were used habitually by Christian physicians and scholars, either in Latin translation, or, by those few with sufficient knowledge of Arabic, in the original.

One of the few Christian physicians of this period who is known to have had a knowledge of Arabic was Arnau de Vilanova (*c.* 1240–1311), who spent part of his life in those areas of the Crown of Aragon where the majority of the population – for example in the Kingdom of Valencia –

Latin Arabic glossary of the Leiden University Library. A contribution to the study of Mozarabic manuscripts and literature (Leiden, 1977).

[7] This mistrust of the Spanish Catholic Church, and the relationship of this phenomenon with the medicine practised by the appropriate minority, have been studied within the context of the so-called 'Moriscos' or new Christians compulsorily converted from the Muslim religion at the beginning of sixteenth-century Spain: see L. García-Ballester, *Los moriscos y la medicina. Un capítulo de la medicina y la ciencia marginadas en la España del siglo XVI* (Barcelona, 1984).

[8] Van Koningsveld, 'Andalusian-Arabic manuscripts from Christian Spain', pp. 29–30 of his typescript, and 'Andalusian-Arabic manuscripts from medieval Christian Spain', number xiv of the Appendix.

[9] Roger Bacon's (d. 1294) opinion with regard to this is very well known. See J. S. Brewer (ed.), *Fr. Rogeri Bacon opera quaedam hactenus inedita* (London, 1859), vol. I, *Compendium studii*, cap. 8, pp. 467–8, and 471–2.

spoke Arabic.[10] He is known to have translated at least three works of medicine from Arabic into Latin: *De tremore, iectigatione et spasmo* by Galen; *De viribus cordis* by Avicenna and *De simplicibus medicinis* by Abu Salt (1067–1134), a physician from Denia, Valencia.[11] He appears to have undertaken his translations in Barcelona, during the time of his first period in the service of the King of Aragon (1280s).[12] From his own writings we know that he also frequently used medical works in Arabic to discuss unclear passages in the Latin versions.[13] On his death, in the inventory of his library, which was located in the city of Valencia, there figure eight works 'in arabica lingua', two of which we know were certainly of medical content.[14] Evidence of Arabic texts similarly being either translated or used to check accuracy can be seen in the request that Guillelmus de Biterris directed (1302), via the king, to the Jews of Catalonia for the loan of 'certain books of medicine written in Arabic, which were necessary for him'. In this way he intended to increase the number of Latin medical manuscripts at, and to improve the quality of those already in the possession of, the recently created University of Lerida, where on the orders of the king, he was establishing a faculty of medicine.[15]

The Christian university doctors who did not know Arabic turned to those of their Christian pupils who came from lands where Arabic was a living language to translate for them the medical writings in which they were interested. Such was the case of Bernard de Gordon (fl. 1283–1308), a colleague of Arnau at the faculty of medicine in Montpellier, who asked Berenguer Eymerich of Valencia to translate the work entitled *De cibariis infirmorum*.[16]

---

[10] J. A. Paniagua, 'L'arabisme à Montpellier dans l'œuvre d'Arnau de Vilanova', *Comptes-rendus du XVIe Congrès International d'Histoire de la Médecine.* (Montpellier, 1958), pp. 163–9; L. García-Ballester, 'Arnau de Vilanova (*c.* 1240–1311) y la reforma de los estudios médicos en Montpellier (1309): el Hipócrates latino y la introducción del nuevo Galeno', *Dynamis,* 2 (1982), 97–158, at 141–5.

[11] The three translations are being published in *Arnaldi de Villanova opera medica omnia* (AVOMO hereafter) (Barcelona, 1975–), see M. R. McVaugh (ed.), *Translatio libri Galieni de rigore et tremore et iectigatione et spasmo* (Barcelona, 1981), AVOMO, vol. XVI.

[12] McVaugh, *Translatio,* pp. 30–7.

[13] '... nec est imputandum errori transferentis, quia in omnibus libris arabum, quos invenire potuimus, sic invenimus contineri; nec similiter imputandum est defectui vocabulorum in illa lingua, quod ad notificandum dolorem secundo modo acceptum scimus in ea copiosos esse sermones', *Commentum supra tractatum Galieni de malicia complexionis diverse,* ed. by L. García-Ballester and E. Sánchez Salor (Barcelona, 1985), AVOMO, vol. XV, p. 192, lines 15–20.

[14] R. Chabas, 'Inventario de los libros, ropas y demás efectos de Arnaldo de Vilanova', *Boletín de la Real Academia de la Historia,* 9 (1903), 189–203, nos. 48, 65, 76, 93, 115, 150, 173 and 183; at least nos. 76 and 173 are medical works.

[15] Archive of the Crown of Aragon (hereafter ACA) in Barcelona, C., reg. 299, fol. 52v, 2 September 1352, published in A. Rubió y Lluch, *Documents per l'història de la cultura catalana mig-eval* (Barcelona, 1921), pp. 13–14, doc. 16.

[16] Probably a part of the 28th book of Albucasis' (az-Zaharawi) *Tasrif,* which circulated in Latin with the title of *Liber servitoris,* and where the author shows how to prepare medical prescriptions. Berenguer Eymerich's translation has never been edited: see

Another place where Christian scholars used Arabic manuscripts was in the recently conquered territory of Murcia, which became part of the Kingdom of Castile. There, the context was different from that which has been seen in the Crown of Aragon. In Murcia the active scholars were members of the mendicant orders (Dominicans and Franciscans) and Italian scholars, who showed enough intellectual curiosity about natural and medical sciences contained in Arabic manuscripts to maintain a limited programme of translation and study. These regions were unique in bordering territories of Arabic culture (the Muslim Kingdom of Granada, North Africa), as well as the Mediterranean Sea, which meant that after the Christian conquest an intense commercial and cultural interchange was quickly established with meridional regions of Europe (Italy, among others) and with the nearest Arabic countries.[17]

The first translations from Arabic to Latin in these territories were made by the Franciscan Pedro Gallego (*c.* 1200–67), who was named first Bishop of Cartagena (Murcia) in 1250. During the seventeen years of his bishopric he completed translations of four works of natural philosophy with implications for medicine: an abridgement (with personal touches) of the *Liber de animalibus* (from *Historia animalium*, Books 1–9) of Aristotle; an abridgement of Averroes' compendium to the *De partibus animalium* (from *Historia animalium*, Books 1–2, chapter 2) of Aristotle; and a text on *Oeconomia* (*in regitiva domus*), probably based on the pseudo-Galenic work. He also wrote a *Summa astronomica*, in which he appears to summarize the treatise of Al-Fargani, *Elementa astronomica*.[18]

The second place in Murcia where medical works were translated was the school of Arabic and Hebrew languages ('Studium Arabicum et Hebraicum') founded by the Dominicans in 1266 for missionary and apologetic purposes. This school was similar to others created in the thirteenth century in territories on the frontiers of Christendom ('Germania', 'Hungaria', 'Hispania'). For reasons unknown to us, Rufinus Alexandrinus (from Alessandria in Italy, to the north of Genoa) arrived in Murcia to learn Arabic. He was taught the language there by a Dominican, Dominicus Marrochinus.[19] With the latter's help he translated at least two works: the first was an ophthalmic work, which he finished in 1271;[20] the second was a group of works collected in a manual like those used in teaching medicine, and entitled in Latin *Liber questionum medicinalium discentibus in medicina*, attributed to 'Huneyn filius Ysaac medici qui latine dicitur

---

L. García-Ballester, *La medicina a la València medieval* (Valencia, 1988), p. 92, n. 163. These kinds of work were much appreciated by medical practitioners: see Jacquart and Micheau, *La médecine arabe*, p. 210.

[17] See, García-Ballester, 'Medical science in thirteenth-century Castile', p. 199.

[18] Ibid., pp. 199–200.

[19] Ibid., p. 200.

[20] Berne, Bürgerbibliothek, MS 216, fols. 1ra–43vb. This copy dates from 1279 (fol. 43vb).

Johannicius'.[21] This second item is an authentic student textbook. That this Arabic-language students' manual should have been current in Murcia between the years of 1270 and 1280 is of great interest, and tells us of the presence and circulation among the Muslim population of a medical literature elaborated and prepared for didactic purposes.[22]

After the treaty of Alcaraz (1243), the Muslim Kingdom of Murcia was subjected to Castile, although it maintained a certain degree of autonomy (language, religion, land ownership, even the Muslim monarch himself remained until the early 1260s). Around 1257 the Christians started seriously to contravene the terms of the settlement, and an increasing exodus of Muslim inhabitants in the direction of the neighbouring Kingdom of Granada can be detected; in 1264 a rebellion broke out among the Muslim inhabitants of Murcia.[23] From that moment onwards, the situation of tolerance that had previously existed disappeared. It is known from Arabic sources that the Muslim scholar and physician, Abu Bakr M. ibn Ahmad al-Riquti, remained in Murcia after the advent of the Christians, at least until 1272. During these years he resisted pressure from King Alfonso X of Castile to convert to Christianity, unlike other Muslim scholars of Murcia such as Bernard the Arab. Bernard translated a treatise on a kind of astrolabe (*azafea*) by Al-Zarqali (Azarquiel) from Arabic to Castilian with the collaboration of the Jew don Abraham in Burgos in 1278. Until recently, the presence of al-Riquti has been associated, although without any documentary support, with the translating activity of Pedro Gallego, and also with the existence of a possible *Madrasa* or school of Islamic studies, which may have functioned in Murcia during those years in which this Muslim scholar remained in this land. This last point springs from the well-known evidence of Ibn al-Khatib, in which he affirms that 'the tyrant-king of the Christians knew [his scholarship], and built for him, after he had conquered Murcia, a *Madrasa* in which he could teach Muslims, Christians and Jews and [where] he continued to be held in esteem by him [i.e. the king]'.[24] Nevertheless, there is no documentary

---

[21] Erfurt, Staatsbibliothek Amploniana MS, F 271, fols. 11ra–25rb. In the copy (fol. 18vb) there is a mention of 'Huneyn filius Ysaac medici qui latine dicitur Johannicius'. See also M. Steinschneider, *Die hebräischen Übersetzungen des Mittelalters, und die Juden als Dolmetscher* (Berlin, 1893), pp. 710–11. It could be the variant *Kitab al-masa 'il fi t-tibb* of Hunain ibn Ishaq's introduction to medicine: see Jacquart and Micheau, *La médecine arabe*, pp. 46–7.

[22] Another problem is why this translation did not become diffused through Latin Europe. The Murcia translation has been preserved only in the above-mentioned manuscript.

[23] J. Torres Fontes, 'El obispado de Cartagena en el siglo XIII', *Hispania*, 13 (1953), 339–580.

[24] Ibn Al-Khatib, *Al-Ihata fi akjbar Gharnata*, ed. by M. A. 'Inan, 4 vols. (Cairo, c. 1975–7), vol. III, pp. 67–8. Van Koningsveld gives an English translation of the passage from al-Khatib: see his 'Andalusian-Arabic manuscripts from Christian Spain', pp. 9–10 of his typescript. The Muslim King of Granada, Yusuf surnamed 'Al-Faqih' (1272–1302) of the Banu Nasr family, took in al-Riquti and gave him facilities for teaching and practising medicine. On the Banu Nasr of Granada, see R. Arié, *L'Espagne musulmane au temps des Nasrides, 1232–1492* (Paris, 1973).

evidence to prove that this institution ever functioned. Van Koningsveld has recently brought to light new evidence, also from Arabic sources, unknown until now. It comes from Abu 'Ali al-Husain ibn Rashiq (*fl* 1275), who lived in Murcia after the Christian conquest. It is of great significance, firstly because it confirms the existence of scientific manuscripts in Arabic among the Muslim population that remained after the conquest. Secondly it provides information about the attraction exerted by the knowledge of natural and medical things contained in these manuscripts upon Christians. In addition, it enables us to appreciate how members of the enlightened Muslim minority perceived this situation. It thus complements what is known about Pedro Gallego and the *studium* founded by the Dominicans.

I was in the city of Murcia – may God restore it! – during the days when its inhabitants were afflicted by the *dain* [i.e. by subjection to a non-Muslim ruler] . . . At that time a group of their priests and monks had come to that city on behalf of the Tyrant-King of the Christians, in order to dedicate themselves – as they thought – to devotion and scientific study, eagerly stretching out their necks to look into the sciences of the Muslims and to translate them into their own language, for the sake of criticism – may God thwart their effort! They were especially fond of disputing with the Muslims and had a blameworthy intention in attracting weak minds.[25]

We have evidence about the existence in Murcia of Arabic manuscripts on natural philosophy a few years later, around 1325. But this evidence is no longer associated with the Muslim minority or with Christian scholars. Now the information comes from Jewish sources and the users were likewise Jews. We refer to Samuel ben Judah of Marseilles, who, on being expelled by the King of France, sought refuge, like so many other Jews, in the Christian Kingdoms of the Crown of Aragon and Castile. He went to Murcia (1324) where he traced the Arabic version of Alexander of Aphrodisias' *De anima*, which he translated into Hebrew.[26] In the fifteenth century – when Arabic had been abandoned by the scholars in favour of Latin, Greek or Romance languages – there appear two further Christian physicians from Valencia who knew Arabic and who handled scientific manuscripts in circulation there; they were Martín Villarroya (*fl.* 1414–21) and Juan de Bosnia (*fl.* 1456–84).[27] After that date we have to wait until 1540 to find Christian physicians in Valencia in possession of medical

---

[25] Muhammad Hajji (ed.), *Abu' l-'Abbas Ahmad ibn Yahya, Al-Mi'yar al-mu'rib wa-al-jami' al-mughrib 'an fatawa 'ulama Ifriqiyah wa-al-Andalus wa-al-Maghrib*, 13 vols. (Rabat, 1981), vol. XI, p. 155. Quoted and translated into English by van Koningsveld, 'Andalusian-Arabic manuscripts from Christian Spain', p. 11 of his typescript.

[26] L. V. Berman, 'Greek into Hebrew: Samuel ben Judah of Marseilles, fourteenth century philosopher and translator', in A. Altmann (ed.), *Jewish medieval and Renaissance studies* (Cambridge, Mass., 1967), pp. 289–320, on pp. 317–18.

[27] See, García-Ballester, *Historia social de la medicina*, pp. 72–3.

manuscripts in Arabic (Avicenna's *Qanun*) and with sufficient knowledge of this language to enable them to read such works.[28]

The Muslim minority

As regards the Muslims that remained in Christian lands after the conquest, the educated minority emigrated southwards, to those areas of the peninsula still in the hands of Muslims, or alternatively, to the areas occupied by present-day Morocco. In spite of this, attitudes towards the Arabic language and medical writings were not the same in the various parts of Spain in the later Middle Ages. The Muslim inhabitants of Castile soon lost all knowledge of Arabic, to the point that by the fifteenth century even the Koran had to be read to them in a Romance language, since Arabic was unintelligible to them.[29] After 1265, there is no evidence that any of the surviving medical manuscripts among those that circulated in Christian zones of Castile were copied by Muslim scribes. In the case of those surviving from before that date (between 1166 and 1265), which were copied by Muslims in either Castile or Catalonia, all the scribes were prisoners of war, who carried out their work for Jewish masters.[30] In spite of this we know that still in 1346 there were Muslims in Toledo with enough knowledge of Arabic to translate notarial documents written in Arabic into Castilian to be used by the king.[31] However, the only surviving manuscript with medical contents belonging to Castilian Muslims is of the fifteenth century and is partly in 'aljamiado' (Castilian in Arabic letters) and partly in Arabic. Empirical and magical elements are predominant in this work.[32]

The same did not occur in the lands of the Crown of Aragon, where there was a substantial Muslim population with a certain level of literacy, which we can establish with documentary evidence. As an example, it is possible to find in the notarial archive of Zaragoza (Aragon) many documents from the second part of the fourteenth century, related to business between Muslim people and Christians or Jews, which are signed in Arabic with the name of the Muslim participants.[33] There is fifteenth-century evidence

---

[28] See, García-Ballester, *Los moriscos y la medicina*, pp. 24–8.

[29] *Tratados de legislación musulmana* (Madrid, Real Academia de la Historia, 1853), pp. 7 and 248, quoted by A. Castro, *Sobre el nombre y el quién de los españoles* (Madrid, 1973), p. 276.

[30] See, van Koningsveld, 'Andalusian-Arabic manuscripts from Christian Spain', p. 21 of his typescript.

[31] See, F. Fita, 'Marjadraque, según el fuero de Toledo', *Boletin de la Real Academia de la Historia*, 7 (1885), 360–94, document no. 5, pp. 371–6, where are given the names of two 'mudéjares' (Muslims) – don Mahomad Xaraffi and his son don Hamete – who translated into Spanish for the king some documents written in Arabic, which were stored in the archive of Toledo Cathedral.

[32] J. Albarracín Navarro and J. Martíinez Ruiz, *Medicina, farmacopea y magia en el 'Misceláneo de Salomón'. Texto árabe, traducción y glosas aljamiadas, estudio y glosario* (Granada, 1987).

[33] Notarial Archive of Zaragoza (ANZ hereafter), Pedro López de Anso, 22 February 1361, fol. 27; the document is signed by Abrayim Avenjucez, mayor of the Muslim community of Azuara, a little town near Zaragoza; a witness of the document is Muça de Jamez, a

from both Aragon and Valencia that members of the Muslim minority
maintained contact with the medical sources of their own culture expressed
in Arabic. We are referring to – as far as Aragon is concerned – the
existence of regular medical studies in the *Madrasa* of Zaragoza, where in
1447 and 1495 it can be demonstrated that medicine was being taught
together with its foundations in natural philosophy; Avicenna's *Qanun* and
the same author's *Uryuza fi-l-tibb*, among others, were being used as the
standard texts for this purpose.

These significant pieces of information are derived from the contents of
both a colophon of an Arabic manuscript copied in 1447 (19 June 851) 'in
the Madrasa built by the Muslims of the city of Zaragoza', and a letter
written by a Muslim student of medicine to his master, Abu 'Abd Allah M.
al-Gazi, *alfaquí* of Belchite (Aragon) from Zaragoza in 1494. The documents were published in Arabic by Ribera.[34] The fact that the letter had
not been translated into a western language was probably the reason why it
was not taken into consideration until 1975, the year in which it was
translated into Spanish and its contents analysed.[35] The letter has two parts,
both of which are important for our purposes. In the first, the student,
whose name was Muhammad al-Qurasi, promised his master, among other
things, that he would not forget to send him a copy of some commentaries
on writings of Al-Yasiti (d. 1189), in all probability the well-known
Malikite theologian who was so influential among Spanish Muslims.[36] In
the second part, he informs his master about his medical studies:

As regards your request that I should send you the commentaries on the writings of
al-Yaziri ... I do not have the copies of the commentaries with me, except a few
insignificant fragments ... However ... when Muhammad b. Yusuf comes, I shall
ask him for these commentaries so as to make a copy of them and to be able to send
them to you ... And if I have other business to attend to, I shall abandon it in order
to be at your immediate service ...

Concerning your kind enquiries about my situation and the way of teaching for
the goal that I am pursuing [i.e. to be a physician], I inform you that I am in perfect
health, thanks to God, and that I have just read the commentary on Avicenna's
Uryuza, and that, with the will of God, I shall start to read the first book of the
Canon. I shall have to work day and night to achieve my goal, because the
above-mentioned work deals with the general aspects of medicine, which are:
knowledge of the limits of medical science; the mixture of the humours; the
elements; the nature of bodies; the science of the necessary things, such as meals,

---

Muslim barber from Zaragoza. ANZ, Rodrigo López Castillón, 23 February 1363, *s.f.*;
the document is signed both by Moçat de Marquna and Ali de Marquna, boilermakers
from Huesca, who were contracted to repair the bathtub of the king.

[34] J. Ribera, 'La enseñanza entre los musulmanes españoles', in *Disertaciones y opúsculos*
(Madrid, 1928), vol. I, pp. 229–359; colophon and letter are on pp. 351–4.

[35] See the Spanish translation in García-Ballester, *Historia social de la medicina*, pp. 68–9
(letter) and p. 71, n. 171 (colophon).

[36] See, W. Hoenerbach, *Spanisch-islamische Urkunden aus der Zeit der Nasriden und Moriscos*
(Bonn, 1965), p. xxxiii.

drink, sleep, wakefulness, movement and rest; knowledge of illness and its causes; and many other things which I shall not detail. All this forms but some of the subtleties of this science, which also takes into account logic and philosophy. And all this can only be accomplished by means of effort and application.[37]

We have to emphasize the significance of the presence of the Malikite theological tradition within the context of the only surviving document in fifteenth-century Spain in order to understand medical teaching among the Muslim minority in Aragon.[38] Van Koningsveld, after analysing the manuscripts that are known to have belonged to members of the Muslim or Morisco minority, emphasizes the leading social and intellectual role of religious institutions (mosques) and leaders (*alfaquies*) among the Muslim minority living in Spanish Christian lands.[39]

In this context, we believe it to be acceptable to connect what has just been mentioned on the subject of the teaching of medicine among the Muslim minority in Aragon with recently discovered evidence. This has been provided by van Koningsveld and relates to the copying, in Valencia in 1480, and subsequent circulation of a medical work by ibn Rushd, the *Mansuma fi-l-tibb*, a medical poem (like the *Uryuza*) used in teaching.[40] Together with these points we should also mention the presence, also in the Kingdom of Valencia, of an *alfaquí* (fl. 1450–6) from Paterna, a small town with a largely Muslim population near the city of Valencia. This *alfaquí* brought from Cairo a manuscript describing the *Sexagenarium*, the Latin name for the instrument used by Egyptian astronomers, which, by means of the graphic application of trigonometrical formulae, in accordance with Ptolemaic science, provides equations for the centre of the earth and the theory of the planets.[41]

These data from Aragon (1447 and 1495) and Valencia (1450 and 1480), all concentrated in the central and final years of the fifteenth century, have a further common feature in that all of them can be found in Spanish Muslim sources. The plentiful Christian documentation preserved in the archives says nothing of these matters, yet, in contrast, it provides numerous examples that point to the lack of cultural (and medical) integration which Muslim communities experienced in Christian lands. Unfortunately, it is impossible to go beyond what has already been said, in view of the paucity of sources we are faced with. Moreover, we lack similar data for the thirteenth and fourteenth centuries. Nevertheless, by the sixteenth century, scarcely two generations after 1495, two significant developments should provide food for thought. In the first place, the Muslim tradition of

---

[37] Arabic text in Ribera, 'La enseñanza', vol. I, pp. 352–4.
[38] See García-Ballester, *Historia social de la medicina*, pp. 50–3 and 69.
[39] Van Koningsveld, 'Andalusian-Arabic manuscripts from Christian Spain'.
[40] Ibid., Appendix I, no. 70; see P. K. Hitti, *Descriptive catalog of the Garrett Collection in the Princeton University Library* (Princeton, 1938), p. 343.
[41] E. Poulle, 'Théorie des planètes et trigonométrie au XVè siècle, d'après un équatoire inédit, le sexagenarium', *Journal des Savants*, 3 (1966), 129–61.

medical teaching had been completely forgotten by the old Christian society of Aragon when they thought of creating a new faculty of medicine in Zaragoza (1584); and, secondly, the descendants of Muhammad al-Qurasi, who proclaimed that 'medical science ... can only be achieved by means of effort and application', were only able to write their medical works, fundamentally based on magic, in 'aljamiado' (the text of Spanish written in Arabic characters).[42]

Everything seems to indicate that in the period between the thirteenth and fifteenth centuries, and at a faster rate in Castile than in the Crown of Aragon, a series of factors led the Muslim minority in Christian lands towards a state of progressive cultural disintegration, with consequent repercussions on the form of medicine which they practised, which drifted towards empirical and magical forms as the dominant style of medical activity. Among these factors we might mention: (1) The social and economic conditions in which they were obliged to live (in effect as serfs to Christian lords). (2) The possible influence of their own religious leaders, around whom the cultural and political life of Muslim communities revolved. These leaders were heavily influenced by Malikism, the dominant spiritual movement among the Spanish Muslim population, both in Castile and the Crown of Aragon, and this was not at all well disposed towards intellectual activity, such as natural philosophy. (3) The fact that it was impossible for them to enter centres of medical teaching (faculties of medicine and schools of surgery) which were accessible to Christians (we only have the exception of Zaragoza in the fifteenth century and in this particular case our reference is to a specifically Islamic institution). (4) The flight of the intellectual minority to nearby Muslim territories (Granada and Morocco), where members of the medical profession could practise freely. Although there is little definite evidence on this last point, we can cite two examples, first the already mentioned intellectual and physician Abu Bakr M. ibn Ahmad al-Riquti (fl. 1264–78) from Murcia, who went on to practise and teach medicine in courtly circles of the Muslim monarch of Granada, 'Al Muhammad b.M.b. Yusuf (1272–1302);[43] and second, that of Muhammad al-Safra (c. 1280–c. 1350), a surgeon from Crevillente (Valencia) who left for Granada (probably in 1318) and later Fez (1344),

---

[42] Nevertheless, I am in agreement with Harvey and with van Koningsveld about the fact that in Christian Spain there was a survival of Arabic culture (and a fortiori of Arabic medicine) from the thirteenth through to the sixteenth century, embodied first in the Muslim minority and finally in the Morisco minority: L. P. Harvey, 'The literary culture of the Moriscos, 1492–1609. A study based on the extant manuscripts in Arabic and Aljamia, 2 vols., Ph.D. thesis (University of Oxford, 1958); Harvey, 'The survival of Arabic culture in Spain after 1492', Actes du 8me Congrès de l'Union Européenne des Arabisants et Islamisants, Aix-en-Provence, Septembre 1976 (Aix-en-Provence, 1978), pp. 85–8; van Koningsveld, 'Andalusian-Arabic manuscripts from Christian Spain', p. 20 of his typescript; see also García-Ballester, Los moriscos y la medicina, passim.

[43] See note 24 above.

where he died shortly afterwards.[44] All these four factors, at least, were present simultaneously and help to explain the progressive disintegration of the minority's intellectual and cultural life, which also affected the medicine they practised, in so far as the medicine practised by a social group is an integral part of its cultural identity.

Paradoxically, a factor that tended to assist this disintegration of medical culture was the pressure applied by Christian authorities via control of medical practitioners of non-university origins. This control was exerted through an examination which reproduced at a lower level the procedures of the Christian schools of medicine. It was in fact an indirect method of acculturing the scholastic medical model among those Muslim or Jewish practitioners who wished to open the circle of their medical practice wider to the Christian population. It is noteworthy that in the Kingdom of Valencia – whose Muslim population in many areas was not just the dominant, but also the only community – we have been able to find only four requests from Muslims for a medical licence in the whole of the fourteenth and fifteenth centuries (Hamet Hatequia in 1338, Maymó Abdochaxis in 1388, Cahat Azeit in 1434, and Abdalla Gasí in 1445).[45] Obviously, this number of licences bears no relation to the actual number of practitioners in the Muslim community. It is extremely difficult, of course, to know what kind of health care was available to the large numbers of Muslims in the Kingdom of Valencia, or who attended them; yet, in spite of a lack of documentation providing concrete details, everything seems to indicate that they were treated by healers from their own community who, with rare exceptions, did not practise among Christians or Jews. For instance, in the two hundred and fifty years between 1250 and 1500, we have not been able to trace a single document in which there appears a Muslim physician or surgeon contracted by a municipal council, either of a large or a small town, to exercise medicine or surgery among its inhabitants. Quite the opposite occurred in the case of Jewish physicians and surgeons, whose presence among the practitioners hired by Christian municipal councils was frequent. Muslim healers appear in Catalan or Valencian records only when a member of the Muslim community accepted the professional model of the Christian society and requested an examination; or, more often, when he was prosecuted for illegal medical practice. In these latter instances, our little data reveal in effect 'sub-profess-

---

[44] H.-P.-J. Renaud, 'Un chirurgien musulma du royaume de Grenade: Muhammad al-Safra', *Hesperis*, 20 (1935), 1–20; Arié, *L'Espagne musulmane*, p. 430; García-Ballester *Historia social de la medicina*, pp. 21–2.

[45] ACA, C., reg. 863, fol. 161r (Hamet Hatequia); Archive of the Kingdom of Valencia (ARV hereafter), Justicia Civil, 550, fols. 30r–31r (Maymó Abdochaxis); ARV, Real, 264, fol. 133 (Cahat Azeit), and ARV, Real, 51, fols. 111v–112 (Abdalla Gasi). On the first two, see L. García-Ballester, M. R. McVaugh, and A. Rubio-Vela, *Medical licensing and learning in fourteenth-century Valencia*, Transactions of the American Philosophical Society, 79, part 6, (Philadelphia, 1989), pp. 17, 25–6 and 98–101.

ionals' (quacks, both men and women), and show us how deeply medicine was affected by the broad cultural disintegration that afflicted the Valencian Muslims living under Christian rule.[46]

In connection with this last point, we should also mention the prestige that scholastic medicine, and its Christian professionals, acquired from the thirteenth century onwards among the members of the non-Christian religious groups. We have been able to demonstrate this point among the 'rationalist' minority of the Jewish community,[47] but, despite the scarcity of information, it is also known to have taken place among the scholarly members of the Muslim minority who, before they emigrated to Muslim-ruled areas, lived in lands conquered by the Christians. Such was the case of the above-mentioned surgeon Muhammad al-Safra. After his arrival in Fez (1344), he wrote his *K. al-Istiqsa wa al-ibram fi-cilay al-yiraha wa al-awram* (*On the treatment of wounds and tumours*), a surgical treatise in which he denounced the poor position of surgery among the Muslims, and emphasized his training in Valencia with the Christian surgeon 'magister Bernard'.[48] We can also confirm the view that Christian medicine was prestigious among the Muslims from evidence that has been gathered about the wish of the Muslim monarch of the Kingdom of Granada to be attended in his illness by Christian physicians (13 August 1378), in particular by the famous Majorcan surgeon, Pere ça Flor, surgeon to the King of the Crown of Aragon.[49] What can be confirmed in connection with the Muslim minority remaining in Christian areas is that during the period under consideration (the thirteenth to fifteenth centuries), there is no indication that any of its members wrote a medical work of any description.

The Jewish minority

Nothing seems to indicate, on the other hand, that the Jewish population followed the steps of the cultivated Muslim minority. On the contrary, some of them achieved a high level of penetration and influence even among the Christian ruling circles themselves.[50] Their medical practitioners (both physicians – *phisici* – and surgeons – *cirurgici*) can be traced in any Christian community during the fourteenth and fifteenth centuries, both in Castile and the Crown of Aragon. They were hired by the Christian municipal authorities for the medical attention of the community

---

[46] This is the hypothesis proposed by García-Ballester, McVaugh and Rubio-Vela, *Medical licensing and learning*, pp. 25–9.

[47] See García-Ballester, Ferre and Feliu, 'Jewish appreciation'.

[48] See note 44 above. I have not been able to identify this Christian master of surgeons.

[49] Archive of the Kingdom of Majorca (ARM hereafter), Gobernación, LR-30, fol. 187r, 19 July 1378. We give particular thanks to Manuel Becerra, who called our attention to this document.

[50] For a general view of the Jewish minority in medieval Spain, see Y. Baer, *A history of the Jews in Christian Spain*, 2 vols. (Philadelphia, 1978).

and shared this activity with Christian medical practitioners, in spite of ecclesiastical prohibitions to the contrary.[51]

Thus, Jewish physicians were held in high esteem by the members of Christian society. On the other hand, during the fourteenth century, part of the learned Jewish minorities was intellectually drawn towards Christian scholastic medicine. These physicians belonged to the so-called 'rationalists'. We may summarize intellectual activity in the heart of Jewish communities under three headings. Firstly, there were the rabbis, whose principal interests were oriented towards problems of the faith and Talmudic exegesis; secondly, the Cabalists, whose concern was with what we might call theosophic speculation; finally came the rationalists, who were interested in natural philosophy, and whose intellectual sphere was centred upon knowledge of nature.[52] The latter made the practice of their Jewish faith compatible with the rational study of nature (natural philosophy). Physicians who were members of this group made an effort not to reduce medicine to a mere application of remedies and routine practice but to make it an activity based on natural philosophy. As a result, this minority was also drawn by the intellectual attraction of natural philosophy and the medicine based on it, that is, of Latin scholasticism, which, from the late thirteenth century onwards, was able to offer practical and intellectually worthwhile responses to the specific medical problems (both of a theoretical and a practical nature) that contemporary Europe posed. For the first time there appeared in Europe new medical works in Latin, together with Latin translations (on natural philosophy and medicine) of classical writers (Aristotle, Galen), which were able to compete in quality with those works hitherto only available in Arabic. Jewish physicians belonging to rationalist groups tried to incorporate into their own culture, by means of translations into Hebrew, the new written intellectual product of the Latin medical scholasticism elaborated in the university circles of Montpellier throughout the fourteenth century. They considered it to be useful, both as a tool in medical practice and as an intellectual model to follow.[53]

As for the question that concerns us here – the survival of Arabic as a vehicle for scientific communication – it would seem that the behaviour of the Jewish minorities was not identical in Castile and in the Crown of Aragon. The Jewish communities of this second area (like those of Provence and other territories of the south of present-day France), or at least the rationalist minority, gradually forgot Arabic as the fourteenth century

---

[51] L. García-Ballester and M. R. McVaugh are preparing a book on medicine and Jewish practitioners in the fourteenth-century Crown of Aragon.

[52] Berman, 'Greek into Hebrew', pp. 289–90 and 293. On the division of Jewish medieval society into three rival social groups, see also the Hebrew grammar by Profiat Duran (Perpignan, 1340/5–1414), *Ma'ase Efod* (Vienna, 1865). We are grateful to Eduard Feliu (Barcelona) for this piece of information.

[53] García-Ballester, Ferre and Feliu, 'Jewish appreciation'.

progressed, and as a result lost the ability to read medical manuscripts in Arabic, using instead Hebrew, Romance languages or Latin itself.[54]

In the case of Castile, the first clear evidence for the intellectual fascination that Latin scholastic natural philosophy exercised over the Jewish minority belongs to the last third of the fourteenth century.[55] This, however, did not mean that the Jewish minority abandoned contact with medical sources written in Arabic, and they continued to produce them in this language almost until their expulsion. We have proof of this in the Castilian communities of Toledo and Guadalajara. Even after their conversion to Christianity, some *conversos*, such as García de la Estrella b. Juan Gozalbez b. Gato (*fl.* 1420) of Toledo, continued to make use of Arabic to copy medical manuscripts written in that language.[56] This does not mean that they lived without any contact with the Christian medical works that were being produced. As we shall have occasion to see, there is evidence that in the early fourteenth century scholastic medical writings of the last third of the thirteenth century (in all probability Teodorico Borgognoni of Lucca's *Cirurgia*) were known to Castilian Jewish physicians, who argued about these works from a position of full intellectual equality.

The Jews were the only non-Christian socio-religious group in Castile that could count on a minority within their number who were interested in natural philosophy and in a form of medicine related to it, and who at the same time were actively practising medicine. This medical practice was not limited to members of their own communities, but also included the Christian population.[57] As will be seen below, their activity (as that of Christian practitioners) was basically itinerant, which provided them with detailed knowledge of Christian people and places. This knowledge was by no means irrelevant for their knowledge of medicine. In fact, as will also be seen at a later stage, some of them were able to integrate these new aspects derived from their itinerant practice of medicine into the doctrinal *corpus* of a demanding form of Galenism, written in Arabic, that was nourished by a wide range of medical sources by Greek and Arab authors.[58] Their interest in a medicine based on natural philosophy was rooted in their own

---

54 Although they have not been conserved, it is known that medical manuscripts in Arabic circulated among the Jewish communities of Catalonia in the first decade of the fourteenth century: ibid.

55 Steinschneider, *Die hebräischen Übersetzungen*, p. 210 (don Meir Alguadez ben Salomo, physician of Enrique III, King of Castile, 1390–1406).

56 F. Guillén Robles, *Catálogo de los manuscritos árabes existentes en la Biblioteca Nacional de Madrid* (Madrid, 1889), no. 101–10, p. 248. See R. Kuhne, 'El Sirr Sina'at al-Tibb de Abu Bahr Muhammad b. Zakariyya' Al-Razi', *Al-Qantara*, 3 (1982), 347–414, at 352; P. Leon Tello, *Judíos de Toledo*, 2 vols. (Madrid, 1979), under Abengato.

57 See note 51 above. Even the community of canons of Avila Cathedral (Castile) hired two Jewish physicians (R. Meyr and R. Yuçé Cohen), Spanish National Archive (AHN hereafter), Clero, lib. 816, fols. 37r, 50r, 167r, 179v and 218v (2 July 1460 to 19 February 1468); AHN, cod. 411–B, fols. 5v and 85v. I am grateful to Carlos Carrete (University of Salamanca) for these pieces of information.

58 See the third part of this chapter.

intellectual rationalist tradition. In Castile, these rationalist Jewish physicians were able to preserve sufficient knowledge of the Arabic language to enable them not only to read these Arabic medical sources, but also to use Arabic as a means of written communication as late as the first third of the fourteenth century and even later. This demonstrates at least the following: in the first place that the circulation of medical manuscripts in Arabic was normal among members of Castilian Jewish communities; secondly, that there existed a public that was by no means indifferent to medical matters as part of natural learning; thirdly, that part of this public was made up by those who wished to learn the physician's craft and to take the first steps in medical learning; fourthly, that medical manuscripts were indeed copied and transmitted. We shall have occasion to see that some Castilian Jewish physicians, at least until the first half of the fourteenth century, maintained a degree of contact with medical science and did not limit themselves to being mere readers, copiers and/or transmitters of other authors' medical works: they also participated in the process of intellectual creation. We have direct evidence of this through a fascinating medical work written by a Jewish physician, probably of Toledo, in the first third of the fourteenth century.[59] However, as we shall have the opportunity to see, we can demonstrate the presence of medical manuscripts in Arabic at the heart of Castilian Jewish communities until the fifteenth century, almost until the same year as their expulsion from Spain (1492). Unfortunately we do not have evidence in the fourteenth-century Crown of Aragon of such medical intellectual creativity by a member of the Jewish community. This does not imply its total absence. We have evidence, for example, of the presence in the Jewish quarter of Xàtiva (Valencia) in 1347, prior to the Black Death, of either a school where medicine was taught, or a prestigious master in medical teaching.[60] Were any medical works produced by such masters? It remains unknown to us.

II

The socio-religious norms according to which the Jewish and Muslim minorities had to live in the later Middle Ages became increasingly strict in the course of the fifteenth century. One of the results of these conditions was the conversion of members of the Jewish and Muslim communities to Christianity, a process which did not at all aid the survival of manuscripts composed in Arabic. We should not forget that conversion to Christianity also meant encouraging a change in cultural model. As has already been noted, the Christians' cultural model was dominated by the Latin scholastic model. The same pressure from Latin culture (both direct and indirect) that

---

[59] See García-Ballester and Vázquez de Benito, 'Los médicos judíos castellanos del siglo XIV y el galenismo árabe'.
[60] I am very grateful to Michael McVaugh for this piece of information.

was felt by Christians of Arabic culture (*Mozarabs*) was also exerted on converts. Furthermore, Latin scholastic scientific and medical culture could rely on the strength of its own prestige. After the expulsion of the Jews and the conquest of the Kingdom of Granada (the last part of the Iberian peninsula with inhabitants of Arabic language and culture, who continued to live in their land after the conquest), both of which occurred in 1492, a political tendency to seek uniformity in language, religion and culture gained strength among Christian rulers. After the enforced conversions to Christianity of the early sixteenth century, the use of Arabic became identified with the old Muslim faith. The use of Arabic was soon to become an activity that might arouse political or religious suspicion. The Christian political and religious authorities, both within and outside the Inquisition, made the use of Arabic a political matter. The possession of texts in Arabic (let alone speaking it) became something rather suspicious and even dangerous.[61] These were all rather unfavourable circumstances for the conservation of manuscripts written in Arabic, even though they might contain medical and/or scientific material, both of which were subjects that Christian scholars and rulers were trying to preserve. In spite of all this, a considerable number of medical manuscripts in Arabic that were copied or circulated among these minorities of Christian Spain both in the Crown of Aragon and in Castile have been preserved, spread amongst various libraries. This must mean that many more have been lost, as has happened in the case of almost all those that are known for sure to have circulated in the Crown of Aragon until the first third, at least, of the fourteenth century.[62] Those that have been preserved allow us to analyse the phenomenon – unique in European Christian lands – of the actual use of medical manuscripts in Arabic in Christian areas by members of the three cultures then co-existing in Europe between the mid twelfth century and the last decade of the fifteenth century (see table on p. 372).

The medical manuscripts in Arabic that were copied or circulated in the kingdoms of the Iberian peninsula (Portugal has not been considered here) under Christian rule can be divided into three groups on the grounds of their origins:[63] (1) Those that were composed in the Muslim period and that survived after the Christian conquest. (2) Those that went from the Muslim areas of the peninsula (whether old or new copies) to the Christian

---

61 The Belgian humanist Nicolas Clénard found great difficulties in Seville (1539) in learning Arabic because Muslim people recently converted to Christianity refused to talk in Arabic in order not to show any signs of their old faith: see A. Roersch (ed.), *Correspondance de Nicolas Clénard*, 3 vols. (Brussels, 1940–1), vol. I, pp. 151–2, nos. 34–49. For an analysis of the medical contents of this correspondence and its relationship with the role played by Arabic language for recovering Greek medical sources in the European Renaissance, see L. García-Ballester, 'The circulation and use of manuscripts in Arabic in sixteenth-century Spain', *Journal for the History of Arabic Science*, 3 (1979), 183–99.

62 See note 54 above.

63 Van Koningsveld, 'Andalusian-Arabic manuscripts from Christian Spain', pp. 1–2 of his typescript.

Places and years in which medical manuscripts in Arabic were written, corrected or used in medieval Spanish kingdoms. *The figures indicate the number of medical works*

	Twelfth century								Thirteenth century													Fourteenth century														Fifteenth century										Total
	13	18	26	45	64	65	82	90	13	26	27	29	30	32	37	48	65	66	80	94	96	23	33	41	44	46	56	61	75	76	79	85	87	88	89	13	24	25	28	32	66	80	83	94	undated	Total
Alcala																				1	1																									5
Almeria					1																													2	1											1
Barcelona				4																																										5
Cordoba																																					1									5
Granada	1																								1	4																				4
Guadalajara															1													1										1	3	1					1	8
Malaga																																	1								1					1
Murcia																			3																											3
Ocaña																	1	1																												2
Purchena							1																																			1				2
Seville			1																																											3
Toledo				1	1	1	1	1			1	2	2	1								4	1				12		1	1														3		43
Valencia									1	1	2																		1																	
Zaragoza																																													2	2

Sources: Catalogues from the libraries of El Escorial, BN Madrid, BN Paris, and Princeton (Garret Collection). The two MSS from Zaragoza (1494) have not survived. Indirect description by J. Ribera, 'La enseñanza entre los musulmanes españoles' (see note 34 above).

areas of the north. There even seems to have existed a real market of copyists in the Muslim south (Kingdom of Granada) that accepted orders from people living in Christian regions. All the orders that are known are from Jews living in thirteenth–fourteenth-century Castile, a group which played an important part in scientific communication between Muslim and Christian Spain. We have to remember for instance the travels to Granada of the Jewish physician Yusuf ibn Waqqar of Toledo (*fl.* 1312–40), and his friendship with Ibn al-Khatib (1313–75), a Muslim medical writer at the royal court of Granada.[64] (3) Those copied in Christian lands. These make up the largest group. As has already been mentioned, some were copied by Muslim scribes who were prisoners of war. The majority, however, were copied by Jewish scribes and physicians for their own personal use, and they remained in the hands of Jewish families for several generations between the twelfth and the fourteenth centuries (for example, the Banu Susan family, Toledo), or fourteenth–fifteenth centuries (the Banu Waqqar family, Guadalajara–Toledo). All except two of the surviving medical manuscripts belonged to members of Jewish communities. These circumstances led van Koningsveld to state that 'the Jews ... [were] the main heirs of the specifically secular, purely scientifical elements of the Arabic civilization in medieval Christian Spain'.[65] However, we must not forget the survival of Arabic medical culture amongst the practitioners and the people of the numerous Muslim minority of Christian Spain.

If we arrange the surviving medical manuscripts chronologically (see table), it can be observed that they range from 1113 until 1494. With the exception of information from Valencia, Zaragoza and Ocaña (all of fifteenth-century date), the rest of the evidence is concentrated in towns with large Jewish communities. The most active centres were Toledo and Guadalajara (fourteenth and fifteenth centuries). Of particular significance was the Jewish community of Toledo, where a substantial number of medieval manuscripts in Arabic were composed, copied or transmitted. The fact that Toledo was the leading western centre for the translation of medical and scientific works from Arabic to Latin between 1150 and 1300 was, I believe, not unrelated to this state of affairs. Moreover, members of the Jewish community had a decisive role in this process.[66]

It can also be seen from the table that from the 1390s onwards there appears to be an interruption in the copyists' activity and, therefore, clearly

---

[64] See M. M. Antuña, 'Una versión árabe compendiada de la "Historia de España" de Alfonso el Sabio', *Al-Andalus*, I (1933), 105–54, at 116 (Arabic text) and 129 (Spanish translation), where the *A'mal al'a'lam* by Ibn al-Khatib is edited. On the Waqqar family, see *Encyclopaedia Judaica* (Jerusalem, 1972), vol. VIII (1205–7), and Steinschneider, *Die hebräischen Übersetzungen*, pp. 598–9, and 921–2; on Ibn al-Khatib, see *Encyclopédie de l'Islam* (Leiden and Paris, 1971), vol. III, pp. 859–60.

[65] Van Koningsveld, 'Andalusian-Arabic manuscripts from Christian Spain', p. 28 of his typescript.

[66] On this process see Jacquart and Micheau, *La médecine arabe*, pp. 131ff.

in the case of Toledo a slowing down in the rhythm of transmission and circulation of medical literature in Arabic. In the first half of the fifteenth century this was restricted to the activity of the Banu Waqqar family. In the last part of the century we have only the Valencia manuscript and information from Zaragoza, both cases involving Muslim communities. This situation must have been a consequence of the clear crisis of co-existence between the dominant Christian group and the other two minorities in the late fourteenth century; this crisis was expressed in social terms in many cities, both in the Crown of Aragon and Castile, by a series of pogroms, which were repeated in the fifteenth century and culminated in the expulsion of those members of the Jewish minority who did not convert to Christianity.[67] Another factor which must have been influential in the almost total cessation of the copyists' activity was the gradual loss of knowledge of Arabic on the part of Jewish rationalist physicians, and its replacement by Hebrew, Latin or a Romance language.[68] Both factors – one of a social nature (the crisis of co-existence), the other of intellectual scope (the gradual disappearance of Arabic from the intellectual horizon) – might well explain the void observable between the fourteenth and fifteenth centuries.

If, instead of arranging the surviving medical manuscripts on a chronological basis, their contents are analysed, we find that the Hippocratic corpus is represented, but only by the *Aphorisms* and books from the *Epidemics* and *On prognostics*; that is to say, it is represented by books that were eminently didactic and clinical in character. On the other hand, the available material includes the most interesting of Galen's extensive medical output, ranging from his treatises on anatomy and physiology (*De usu partium*, and *De facultatibus naturalibus*) to his semiological writings (*De symptomatum differentiis*, *De differentiis febrium*), writings on pathology (*De locis affectis*, *De crisibus*, *De diebus criticis*, *De differentiis morborum*), on therapeutics and dietetics (*De compositione medicamentorum*, *De alimentorum facultatibus*), and on hygiene (*De sanitate tuenda*). One of the manuscripts contains, grouped together, the collection of Galen's most important medical (pathological and clinical) works, which in Latin scholastic medicine was to be known by the title of *De morbo et accidenti*, and was to be the nucleus of the important commentaries on general pathology in the freshest and most attractive scholastic writing during the transition from the thirteenth to the fourteenth century, especially in Montpellier.[69] Another manuscript contains Dioscorides' *Materia medica*, the most important source of Galenic therapeutics. Together with this impressive sample from

[67] Baer, *History of the Jews in Christian Spain*.
[68] See García-Ballester, Ferre and Feliu, 'Jewish appreciation'.
[69] See Fernando Salmón, 'La couleur dans les théories visuelles des cercles médicaux universitaires à la fin du XIIIè siècle', Colloque 'Maladies, médecines et sociétés' (Paris, May 1990, in press).

the Galenic corpus, works of the great masters of Jewish and Arabic medicine were also in circulation; the writings of Rhazes, Avicenna, Haly Abbas, Avenzoar and Maimonides were copied frequently and assiduously. It is interesting to note that the text used most often was the *Continens* (*al-Hawi*) of Rhazes, followed by the *Canon* of Avicenna.[70] While the *Canon* was not well received in Al-Andalus,[71] it was however popular among the Jewish minorities living in Christian Castile at least from the beginning of the fourteenth century;[72] in the Latin West;[73] and among the Jewish minorities of Provence and Catalonia.[74] Many of these writings had not been translated from Arabic into Latin in late twelfth-century Toledo, and some of them, by both Greeks (Galen) and Arabs (Rhazes, Avenzoar), would not appear in Latin until the 1270s or 1280s, when they contributed in a decisive way to the renovation of scholastic medicine in European university circles.[75] The presence and circulation of these works among Jewish communities in thirteenth-, fourteenth- and fifteenth-century Castile tells us of the vitality of medical practice among this minority, whose knowledge of Arabic guaranteed them access to the most authentic sources of a form of medicine based on natural philosophy.

Another example of the intellectual vitality of these Jewish physicians was the way they put this medical literature to use. Although the amount of evidence available is very restricted, the contents themselves of some of the surviving manuscripts demonstrate that these works were used for the teaching of medicine, for the production of medical works of a systematic nature, and in order to provide an intellectual and doctrinal basis for medical practice, at least for the most learned physicians. In the following section, we shall analyse the only surviving work, which can serve to illustrate the last two points mentioned.

Some of the extant manuscripts do not reproduce a medical work by a classical author, but tend to be of the nature of medical *florilegia*. These were Arabic manuscripts copied at Toledo in 1379 and at Guadalajara in

---

[70] For a critical description of these manuscripts in van Koningsveld's papers on Andalusian-Arabic manuscripts, see note 2 above. For a detailed description of the contents of manuscripts, see H. Derenbourg, 'Notes critiques sur les manuscrits arabes de la Bibliothèque Nationale de Madrid', in *Homenaje a don Francisco Codera* (Zaragoza, 1904), pp. 571–618; H. Derenbourg and H.-P.-J. Renaud, *Les manuscrits arabes de l'Escurial*, vol. II, fasc. 2: 'Médecine et histoire naturelle' (Paris, 1941).

[71] R. Arnaldez and A. Z. Iskandar, 'Ibn Rushd (Averroes)', in *Dictionary of Scientific Biography* (*DSB* hereafter), ed. C. C. Gillispie (New York, 1981), vol. XII, pp. 7b–8. The popularity of the *Hawi* of Rhazes is testified to by the great number of manuscript copies transmitted and written by Castilian Jewish physicians: see Derenbourg and Renaud, *Les manuscrits arabes*, nos. 806–18, *passim*.

[72] See the third part of this chapter.

[73] Nancy Siraisi, *Avicenna in Renaissance Italy. The 'Canon' and medical teaching in Italian universities after 1500* (Princeton, NJ, 1987), pp. 43–76; Jacquart and Micheau, *La médecine arabe*, pp. 79–85 and 167ff.

[74] García-Ballester, Ferre and Feliu, 'Jewish appreciation'.

[75] García-Ballester, 'Arnau de Vilanova y la reforma de los estudios médicos', pp. 119–45; Jacquart and Micheau, *La médecine arabe*, p. 176.

1387 and 1425 using clinical and dietetic texts by Hippocrates, Galen, Paul Aegineta, Rhazes, Maimonides, Mesue, Avenzoar and others. Their educational nature is obvious since they adopt the question-and-answer format.[76] Another of the manuscripts copied in Guadalajara in 1432 by a member of the Banu Waqqar family for his son appears to have a similar educational purpose; it contains extracts from Avicenna's *Canon*.[77] As will be seen shortly, the one surviving work of a systematic nature, written in the first third of the fourteenth century and copied in 1376, was also composed with a clear didactic intention. Some fragments of the late manuscripts have an astrological character, such as tables to establish the astrological profile of a patient.[78]

In this context, it is interesting to remember what has been noted concerning the existence of regular medical teaching in the Islamic *Madrasa* of Zaragoza in the fifteenth century. We do not know whether it was being undertaken in previous centuries. Neither do we know anything after the year 1494. Teaching activity is likely to have given rise to some form of medical writing. But we do not have any evidence for this either. However, the only medical manuscript that has come down to us from the Muslim minority of Valencia, a medical poem by Averroes, copied in 1480, was for didactic purposes.[79]

III

As has already been pointed out, the Jewish physicians of Castile – probably those belonging to the rationalist group – did not limit themselves to reading and handing down classical works, however important these may have been, but were also involved in a second and parallel task, the creation of new medical works. Only one has been preserved: the *Kitab al-tibb al-qastali al-maluki* (*Book of regal Castilian medicine*).[80] Its author, whose name has not been preserved, was a Jew, as he himself informs us (fol. 21r). The work was probably written at some time in the first two decades of the fourteenth century and in any case before 1348, for there is no mention whatsoever of the plague of that year in the analysis that the author makes in his ninth chapter of the unusual illnesses that affected Castile in a particularly virulent fashion during the period of his medical practice. From the evidence of the author we know him to have been physician to

---

[76] Derenbourg and Renaud, *Les manuscrits arabes*, no. 873,8 (Toledo, 1379), no. 873,11 (Guadalajara, 1387), and no. 870,1 (Guadalajara, 1425), pp. 83–4.

[77] Ibid., no. 870,4, pp. 77–8.

[78] Ibid., no. 873,1, p. 81. The astrological fragments are being studied by Margarita Castells (University of Barcelona).

[79] *Manzuma fi'l-tibb*, with glosses in Latin and Spanish: see note 40 above.

[80] On the description of the two surviving manuscripts, see García-Ballester and Vázquez de Benito, 'Los médicos judíos castellanos del siglo XIV y el galenismo árabe'. Our references are to the oldest copy, Madrid, Biblioteca Nacional, Arabic MS, no. 601, fols. 1r–38v.

Ferdinand IV, King of Castile (1295–1312) (fol. 19v). The constant advice about how the physician should behave in the presence of members of the nobility and royalty, abundant throughout the work, together with the recommendations he makes concerning the *regimina sanitatis* dedicated to such persons, is indicative of how familiar this physician was with courtly circles in Castile. We also know by the author's own admission that he wrote this work when he had reached a considerable age. In fact, throughout the work there appear references to how beneficial 'experience' can be in medical practice, as well as other remarks to the effect that the arguments adduced were 'what has been obtained during my lengthy experience' (fol. 26r). From the manner in which he constantly alludes to Toledo, he must have retired to that city after having practised for the greater part of his life in the lands of Castile. The constant references to Burgos, and to specific patients in that city, also lead one to consider that he may have been a physician there under contract to the town council.[81] Also apparent from his work is the itinerant nature of his medical practice, a particular characteristic of these Jewish physicians, who were hired by Christian town councils for periods of rarely more than five years, or, alternatively, who used to follow the court, or who went to wherever the king or nobles called for their services. His professional activity enabled him to get to know an extensive part of the Kingdoms of Leon and Castile. To be more precise, the cities of Leon, Valencia de Don Juan, Toro, Valladolid, Burgos, Segovia, Arevalo, Avila and Medinaceli, as well as Toledo and Seville to the south, are mentioned in the work (see map).

A description of the contents and structure of the work is the best way to penetrate the intellectual background and purposes of the author. The work consists of two clearly differentiated parts. The first is an introduction of the natural philosophical foundations of medicine and the activity of the physician, all of which tends to justify the purpose and suitability of the work (fols. 1–7v). It is divided into five brief sections: in the first, the concept of illness is expounded and the task of the physician within society is justified, everything connected with health and illness being claimed as the latter's rightful field of activity. The second section presents the conceptual foundation of the work as a whole. It is none other than the Aristotelian scheme of the four causes (material, formal, final and efficient). The author adapted to this what was known in the Latin West by the name of *res naturales* and *res non-naturales* (the naturals and the non-naturals). He makes obvious use of medical sources other than Johannitius' *Isagoge*, the translation of which into Latin and the subsequent diffusion of which was,

---

[81] We know the name of at least one of these Jewish physicians contracted by the municipality of Burgos in 1388 and in 1411, 'don Salomon el Leví': see Municipal Archive of Burgos, Libros de Actas, 30 April 1388 and 6 April 1411. See J. A. Bonachia Hernando, *El concejo de Burgos en la Baja Edad Media, 1345–1426* (Valladolid, 1978), pp. 118 and 188. I am very grateful to Carlos Carrete for this piece of information.

as is well known, the starting point for the medieval scheme of Latin Galenism (together with the res praeter naturam) from the twelfth century onwards.[82] The work in question does not devote a specific section to the group of things against nature formed by illness, its causes and its manifestations or signs (res praeter naturam), although they are present in the book. On the basis of Avicenna's Canon, with slight modifications,[83] this Castilian Jew distributed what he called 'natural causes' in the following way: material causes (elements, humours, spirits and limbs or organs), formal causes (complexion, qualities and virtues, including the natural, the vital and the animal), final cause (essential operations) and efficient causes. The last, denominated 'natural causes of health and illness' by the author, were grouped in the following six sections, according to their order of importance: air, food and drink, evacuation and repletion, motion and rest, sleep and wakefulness, and accidents of the soul.[84] If the physician is to use procedures consonant with nature, his intervention in health and illness has to be carried out through these six 'efficient causes'. However, the physician's activity is not limited to them; he may intervene in the processes of illness and health by means of procedures that are not at all natural, such as 'medication and manual operation [surgery]' (fol. 2v). In the third section, the author explains the reasons for focusing his work on the 'six natural [efficient] causes', without nevertheless thereby renouncing the use of medicines. On the other hand, he rejects surgery. He takes special care to emphasize that his work aims to be 'useful' (intafa'); it is for this reason that he decides not to develop at length the components that make up the other three causes (elements, humours, spirits, etc.), all of which are subjects more appropriate in a work of natural philosophy. The author made a particular effort to stress the physician's capacity to manipulate these six components, both for the preservation of health (what in the Latin West was to be known by the name of regimina sanitatis), and for the cure of illness, by means of the therapeutic use of diet. This last point was something on which the author placed great importance, preferring this technique to treatment involving medicines, whether simple or compound; however, he did not renounce medicinal treatment out of hand. From this point onwards, the author repeatedly insists on the importance of the air. The complex Galenic concept of 'climate' was in effect to be one of the principal axes around which the whole work revolved; on this the author based the comparative analysis that he carried out throughout the work, distin-

---

[82] D. Jacquart, 'A l'aube de la renaissance médicale des XIe–XIIe siècles: L'Isagoge Johannitii et son traducteur', Bibliothèque de l'École des Chartes, 144 (1986), 209–40.

[83] The work I describe here is a very interesting testimony to the diffusion and popularity of Avicenna's Canon amongst learned Jewish physicians of this time.

[84] We have to remember the importance given by Rhazes to these 'non natural things', following the path opened up by Hunain ibn Ishaq: see Rhazes' Introduction to medicine, edited with Arabic text and Spanish translation by C. Vázquez de Benito, Libro de la introducción al arte de la medicina o 'Isagoge' (Salamanca, 1979).

guishing between different cities and regions of Castile (Burgos, Leon, Valladolid, Toro, Segovia, Avila among others), on the one hand, and what he calls Al-Andalus centred upon Toledo, on the other. The fourth, very brief, section is devoted to pointing out the importance of the curative action of nature through the 'natural causes', without there being any need for action on the part of the physician. In the fifth and final part the greater or lesser significance of the 'six natural [efficient] causes' is considered once again, the 'necessity' that man has of each one of them in order to maintain life being used as a comparative factor. The result of these deliberations is a hierarchy of these six groups, at the top of which is situated the air, followed by food and drink. Both – but more especially the first one – acted as a support for the four remaining ones. The author does not hide his interest in writings on food, a subject constantly present throughout the work.[85]

The second part is the longer (fols. 7v–38v). It consists of ten chapters, of very variable length, preceded by a section in which the different chapters are listed and a brief summary of each of them is presented. The work concludes with an appendix containing a collection of prescriptions (*agrabadin*) with compound medicines suitable for the people of Castile. This appendix has been lost. The contents of the different chapters are as follows: in the first (fols. 7v–13v) 'the illnesses in which the patient should abstain from consuming any sort of meat, and also the circumstances in which [the physician] allows the patients of the region [Castile] to eat it' are mentioned (fol. 7v). The second (fols. 13v–17v) 'deals with the illnesses in which patients in this region should refrain from consuming wine, and in which they need not; and also the various classes of wine and their characteristics, according to the different places' (fol. 13v). All the third chapter (fols. 17v–23r) is dedicated to 'the rules which should be observed when blood-letting, the [appropriate] quantity of blood to extract, and a list of the illnesses of this region in which it can or cannot be undertaken' (fols. 17v). The fourth chapter (fols. 23r–24r) 'deals with the application of cupping-glasses, scarification and leeches in Castile' (fol. 23r), special attention being devoted to the technique of scarification as applied to children and adolescents. The fifth chapter (fols. 24r–27r) is totally devoted to 'the prescription of purgatives in this region [Castile]' (fol. 24r). Chapter six (fols. 27r–v) deals with 'the norms concerning vomiting (that the physician should observe) in this region' (fol. 27r). Chapter seven (fol. 27v–31r) deals with baths. After a reminder of Galen's bio-energetic scheme (the three digestions that take place in the human body), with the consequent

[85] This kind of medical literature became highly prestigious among Jewish physicians according to manuscripts listing books of foodstuffs, which have been preserved in El Escorial's Library: see Derenbourg and Renaud, *Les manuscrits arabes*, nos. 833,4 (1265), 871,2 (1336) and 873,2 (n.d.), pp. 42, 79 and 81.

problem of the elimination of waste matter, the author makes a more detailed analysis of the problem of baths in Castile, showing his preference for the 'dry bath' (sauna), the technique of which is described in detail. According to the author, this type of bath – one not without risks – was frequently used in Castile, and Christian physicians also demonstrated their preference for it. The eighth chapter (fols. 31r–34r) is devoted to the use of cold water 'both in a state of health and in illness', bearing in mind the complexional characteristics of the people of Castile, the climate of the region and its particular illnesses. For obvious reasons, this chapter is closely related to the second one, the one that deals with wine. The ninth chapter (fols. 34r–38r) has two clearly differentiated parts: the first is devoted to the conceptual foundations of such terms as 'putrefaction' (*al-'afuna*), 'pestilential air' (*al-hawa al-wubai*), 'celestial causes' (*al-sabab samawi*) among others, as well as the suitable means of treatment for certain unusual illnesses of sudden widespread appearance, in particular 'smallpox' (*yudari*); the author was witness to one outbreak of an especially virulent nature – 'that not even old people of sixty knew' (fol. 35r) – during his career. The author insists that all these illnesses are produced by natural causes (*al-amr al-tabi'i*). The second part is dedicated to explaining the mechanism of production of 'the specific illnesses of this region', that is to say, what we might call the standard pathology of Castile during the author's lifetime (*c.* 1270–*c.* 1340). The most frequent illnesses were 'nasal and chest catarrhs, consumption, lung ulcers, those illnesses that affect the tendons [painful and particularly common owing to the cold climate of the region], back pains [kidney stones and colics located in the intestinal zone] and the illnesses proper to each season' (fol. 35r). He ends the chapter with a digression on the therapeutic use of cauterization, especially indicated in chronic illnesses that exhibit pain (pains in joints, gout, tendon conditions). A technique of cauterization not described by the most frequently used authors, nor employed in Al-Andalus, is detailed – 'in my opinion it is a treatment characteristic of this region [Castile]' (38r). It consisted of provoking a wound by means of cauterization in one of the lower limbs, between the knee and the heel, which takes in both sides of the leg where the veins run; to keep the wound purulent use was made of a shackle of the same size as the wound provided with a hole through which the 'superfluous humour accumulated at the point of the chronic illness' is eliminated (fol. 37v). The tenth chapter (38r–v), the last in the work, is very brief. In it the author endeavoured to answer the problem of what therapeutic and preventive attitude the physician should adopt when faced with people who were born in regions other than Castile, but who had gone to live there. The book finishes with the following epilogue:

This is the end of our book. May God help us. Praise be to Him. Those who believe in Him will be saved. This book was finished in Toledo – may God protect it. Praise be – on the tenth day of February in the year 1414 of the Christian Era

[= A.D.1376], by the hand of Musa b. Sasun [*sic*]. May God protect him! (fol. 38v).[86]

As has already been stated, the manuscript does not preserve the appendix containing compound medicines. We do not know whether the author never managed to draw it up, or if the exemplar for the surviving copy did not include it, or whether the copyist had no interest in it.

This is a work written in Arabic as a response to the particular intellectual, clinical and therapeutic problems of his times. It demonstrates that at the time when it was composed (*c.* 1312–40) and copied (Toledo, 1376) there existed a certain level of debate concerning medical problems within the Jewish community of Toledo, to which the author probably belonged. According to the evidence of the author, the atmosphere of intellectual discussion on medical and natural questions had also spread to other cities, both to the north (e.g. Burgos) and to the south (Seville); indeed, he indulged in a polemic with a physician among his contemporaries from the latter city – the Jew Abu Harun b. al-Lawi (fols. 20v–21r). Furthermore, the fact that reference is frequently made to specific works by Galen, Rhazes, Isaac Israeli and Avicenna as a matter of course, together with the polemic which he sustained on certain of the doctrinal points of Avicenna, indicates a personal knowledge of all these works; in addition, it indicates that they were accessible and familiar to those of his kind for whom the author wrote. The process of creating a new medical work, with explicitly clinical and therapeutic purposes – and thus aimed at informing others of the author's own medical experience – clearly shows the existence of points of common understanding between the author and his audience. These intellectual points were in the form of easily accessible references, a shared technical vocabulary and scientific methodology, in addition to a whole complex, elaborate common intellectual background which allowed the author and his readers to communicate with each other in an intelligible fashion. We should not forget that in order to achieve a reasonable degree of understanding, a thorough appreciation of all the methodological, terminological and biological arsenal that made up the doctrinal *corpus* of medieval Arabic natural philosophy was required. The summary that we have provided of the *K. al-tibb al-qastali* demonstrates in sufficient detail that both the author and his public were familiar with this *corpus*.[87] Above

---

86 Musa ibn Sasun (or Susan), probably a member of the Banu Susan, a family of physicians of Toledo to whom belong some of the medical manuscripts which have been preserved. The first of them was written in 1182 in Toledo. The last famous member of this family associated with medical manuscripts was Mayir b. Ishaq b. Susan, physician and financial adviser of Alfonso X, King of Castile (1252–84): see van Koningsveld, 'Andalusian-Arabic manuscripts in Christian Spain', Appendix, no. 72.

87 A good summary of Arabic medicine and its relationship with the natural philosophy used by physicians is given in the long introduction written by M. W. Dols, *Medieval Islamic medicine. Ibn Ridwan's treatise 'On the prevention of bodily ills in Egypt'* (Berkeley, 1984), pp. 1–42.

all else, the work reveals the existence of an intellectual atmosphere in which medical problems were of interest and discussed, a process for which the Arabic language was used.

The work which is being described adopts as its starting point a clinical problem that was apparent to any medieval physician who approached his medical career with a minimum of rigorousness. What were the causes of the clinical peculiarities of the sick in the various parts of Castile, whose diseases were on occasions different from the descriptions to be found in classical medical works, and how could they be explained? What could be done when the intellectual tools which were available to the physician (i.e. the works of the great physicians) were of no use in finding effective advice that enabled him to solve the particular cases that occurred in his everyday medical practice? The author provides an answer by resorting to two tools: rational analysis by means of the intellectual resources that contemporary natural philosophy and Galenism made available to him, and personal clinical experience, extraordinarily rich in his own case. For all these reasons, the *K. al-tibb al-qastali* cannot be considered to have been an isolated phenomenon, a matter of chance. It is evident that its existence and contents place before our eyes a chink that enables us to peek into a medical intellectual world that has been lost. Our image of this world is strengthened if we bear in mind the eminently educational nature of the text:

Many times, on reflecting upon the works that the great authors composed concerning medical science, I found that their approach was limited, especially as regards the particular aspects of medicine that are connected with the maintenance of health and the cure of diseases in specific regions never alluded to by them in their books of medicine (fol. 1r).

All the medical treatises that circulate nowadays among us – both the most famous and the more ordinary – were composed in regions and countries with very different customs to those of this region of Castile. Thus none of the peculiarities described in them can be applied in Castile. For this reason I have seen fit to draw up this work, which deals with the practical norms to take into account in the treatment of the diseases of this region. These norms differ from those listed in the treatises, especially with regard to the two kingdoms [he is referring to Leon and Castile] of this region (fols. 7r–v).

The author took great care to indicate directly or indirectly (through the references he used) which were the authors and works that normally circulated among the Jews of Castile. The most frequently cited author, both as regards the number of references and the number of works, is Galen. The following works are directly referred to: *De methodo medendi, Quod animi mores corporis temperamenta sequantur, De flebotomia, De compositione medicamentorum secundum locos, De sanitate tuenda.* The Galenic commentary to the Hippocratic treatise *Airs, waters, places*, which was translated from the Arabic into the Hebrew in the year 1299 by Solomon ha-Me'ati, is not explicitly quoted.[88] The texts of Hippocrates cited are the *Aphorismi* and *Epidemiarum libri*. As for Arabic authors, at the end of the first introductory part, the author says:

The most famous treatises of medicine existing today and known unto us [the Jews] are: the *Kitab al-Hawi fi-l-tibb* [*Continens*] of al-Razi, the *Kitab al-Qanun fi-l-tibb* [*Canon*] by ibn Sina, which follows in its particularities [the clinical part] the instructions of *al-Hawi*, the book of al-Mayusi [*Pantegni*] and that of Julaf al-Zahrawi [*Kitab al-Tasrif*], in addition to other habitual treatises (fol. 7r).[89]

Among these are mentioned *On the pains of the joints* and *On blood-letting* by Rhazes and the *Book of Foodstuffs* by Isaac Israeli.[90] He also includes works of natural philosophy, such as *al-Tahafut* (*The refutation*) by Abu Hamid al-Gazzali, and he summarizes the cosmological opinions of Al-Zarqali (Azarquiel), whom he describes as 'modern' (fol. 21v).[91] He also seems to make allusion to Ibn al-Kammad (fol. 21v).[92] He has a wide knowledge of Galen's works, which is especially evident when he demonstrates the authenticity of the Galenic text *De flebotomia* – probably based on the authority of Rhazes – the authorship of which had been placed in doubt by Abu Harun b. al-Lawi, the Jewish physician of Seville with whom he maintained a dispute (fols. 20v–21r).[93] Galen was for him the unquestionable medical authority. It is his work which is always chosen to settle conflicting views. This Jewish physician held the following opinion of him:

Galen displaced all other physicians both of Antiquity and those of modern times, like Asclepiades, Thessalus and others, in such a way that his teachings have remained beyond any doubt down to our days (fol. 15r).

Of Avicenna he states that:

It is he who consolidates the art of medicine with the book *al-Qanun*, something which no other author has managed to achieve until now ... His Agrabadin [*Antidotarium*, Book v of the *Canon*] contains marvellous texts which are the fruit of his experience (fol. 20v).

---

[88] A. Wasserstein (ed.), *Galen's Commentary on the Hippocratic treatise* Airs, waters, places, *in the Hebrew translation of Solomon ha-Me'ati* (Jerusalem, 1982).

[89] The *Kitab al-Tasrif*, as is known, consists of thirty books; only four were translated into Latin, and have the following names: *Liber theoricae necnon practicae* (Books 1 and 2: generalities and description of diseases *a capite ad calcem*), *Liber servitoris* (Book 28: in fact a treatise on pharmacy), and *Chirurgia* (Book 30: the most famous and influential Arabic treatise on surgery).

[90] F. Sezgin, *Geschichte des arabischen Schrifttums*, vol. III (Leiden, 1970), pp. 287–8 (al-Razi), and p. 296 (Ishaq al-Isra'ili).

[91] *DSB*, vol. XIV, pp. 592–5.

[92] On Ibn al-Kammad (d. 1195), an astronomer who lived in Al-Andalus, see J. Vernet, 'Un tractat d'obstetricia astrológica', in *Estudios sobre historia de la ciencia medieval* (Barcelona and Bellaterra, 1979), pp. 273–300. I am grateful to Julio Samsó (University of Barcelona) for his help in acquiring this information.

[93] The authorship of this work has been questioned by scholars of medieval Arabic writings: see Sezgin, *Geschichte*, pp. 115–16. On al-Razzi's references, see ibid.

This did not prevent him from disagreeing with him on those points that he considered to be unsuitable for application to patients in Castile, and even on matters of natural philosophy, as in the case of his disagreement about the components of the 'efficient natural causes' cited by Avicenna.

It is worth considering briefly the attitude that this Jewish physician adopted towards the Christian physicians that he had contact with during his medical career, and to whom he makes allusion on several occasions. Throughout the work, it is possible to detect a climate of constant critical contrast with what his Christian colleagues did and wrote. On one occasion, he explicitly refers to a Christian surgical treatise with the title in Arabic of *Balagtu-hu al-yabr al-yadid* (*On the new art of surgery*). He does so in connection with a debate on the therapeutic use of wine in the case of patients with wounds, 'according to the nature of each injured individual and the part of the body where the wound is to be found' (fol. 15r). In opposition to the attitude of those who took into account both sets of circumstances (which is the position defended by the author), there existed that of

[some] Christian surgeons in favour of giving wine instead of water to those who are injured whether by blows or by wounds. They base their argument on what was written by a great Christian friar, who composed a book on the subject some sixty years ago, to which he gave the title *On the new art of surgery*. He believed that he had invented something new and different from what Galen had already put forward on this art of surgery. As a consequence of this book, two groups were formed among Christians surgeons: the ones who professed the new surgery; and those others who supported the ancient view, which is none other than Galen's medicine (fol. 15r).

He appears to be referring to the *Cyrurgia* of Teodorico Borgognoni, who was a Dominican friar (*c.* 1205–98).[94] From the evidence of Henri de Mondeville (1316), a disciple and fervent supporter of the new surgery, we know that the therapeutic procedures explained by this Dominican caused great debate among the Christian surgeons of Italy, Montpellier and Paris, and his supporters were described as 'modern'.[95]

Putting aside the dispute, and the version of it that is provided by this Castilian Jew, what is important to point out at this stage is his opinion of

[94] The date ('sixty years ago'), the debate (the giving of wine 'to those who are injured whether by blows or by wounds'), the social condition of the Christian author ('a great friar'), and the controversies following the spreading of the work are coincident with the circumstances surrounding Teodorico Borgognoni and his treatise on surgery. This treatise was translated twice into Catalan in the first decade of the fourteenth century, and it was very well known both by Jewish and Christian Catalonian physicians and surgeons of the time. I suspect that the treatise was also translated into Spanish at the end of the thirteenth or beginning of the fourteenth century. On Teodorico's opinion on the use of wine, see his *Chirurgia* (Venice, 1499), vol. I, p. 25. He based his therapy on the authority both of his teacher Ugo da Lucca and Galen himself (*De methodo medendi*, 8,3).

[95] Henri de Mondeville agreed with Teodorico. See E. Nicaise (ed. and trans.), *Chirurgie de maître Henri de Mondeville ... composée de 1306 à 1320* (Paris, 1893), pp. 187–8 and 284.

the new Christian medical literature. He was not full of admiration for the writings of the medical scholasticism of Montpellier, unlike his brothers in religion who were physicians in Provence or Catalonia in the second half of the fourteenth century.[96] On the contrary, the Jewish physician of Toledo, living in the last third of the thirteenth and first decades of the fourteenth centuries, disputed, on an equal footing, certain specific opinions sustained by Christian physicians, calling upon his training in natural philosophy and his knowledge of the Galenic *corpus* to which he had access in Arabic, something which his brothers in religion in Provence and Catalonia were unable to do as they had forgotten this language and because manuscripts in Arabic were scarce amongst them. On the other hand, neither is there any feeling of respect in the passages in which the author of the *K. al-tibb al-qastali* mentions his relationship with Christian colleagues in the case of specific patients. It was a relationship of professional equality, and even endowed with a certain superiority on his part. Expressions such as 'his opinion is erroneous' (fol. 32r), 'it is easy to refute them' (fol. 31v), 'do not pay attention to what is mentioned by non-Arabic-speaking practitioners' (fol. 31r) are not unusual when he mentions Christian physicians. He clashed with them, not only on clinical matters (differences of opinion in the case of a course of treatment, as in the above-mentioned situation), but also on others of a theoretical character, in which both parties put forward 'logical arguments taken from natural philosophy' (fol. 31r) to settle the questions raised (all of clinical origin), as, for instance, the suitability or unsuitability of using cold water on patients suffering from certain fevers.

The author was aware of the differences and even contradictions existing between the various authors mentioned (both ancient and modern) when it came to deciding upon a form of treatment. In a way similar to what happened in the already sophisticated Galenism of Latin scholasticism, he made an effort to find arguments that harmonized the conflicting opinions and endeavoured to explain the differences rationally. As regards the question of the amount of blood that should be let on each occasion, a subject that was widely debated in Jewish medical circles in Toledo, as we know from this work, the author was faced with serious differences between what was stated to be usual by Galen (six pounds!), what was practised by Rhazes (three pounds), and what his own common sense imposed on his practice of medicine (not more than a pound and a half). The reasoning used by this author allows us, to a certain extent, to come close to the type of arguments put forward in these discussions among Jewish rationalist physicians, about which we otherwise know hardly anything. It was in these discussions that the greater or lesser degree of training in natural philosophy of the participants was made evident. At the core of the argument was the cosmological question of whether the created

---

[96] See García-Ballester, Ferre and Feliu, 'Jewish appreciation'.

world was or was not variable. The author himself states: 'on reflecting upon this problem, I saw that it had to be considered in the context of natural philosophy [*'ilm al-falsafa*]' (fol. 21r). He adduces arguments from al-Gazzali, Ptolemy and Al-Zarqali (Azarquiel), among others, against 'those who maintain the theory that both the world and all that there is in it have suffered no changes from their original state' (fol. 21v). When he discovered that the above-mentioned quantities of blood were in the proportion of 1:2, he concluded as follows:

If we accept our arguments as valid, the question for which we could not find an answer is resolved. I refer to the quantity of blood to extract indicated by Galen and by al-Razi. According to our suppositions, in the time of Galen – let us remember that more than one thousand two hundred years have elapsed until the present time – people used to bleed the quantity of six pounds, in view of the size of their bodies and the vigorousness of their faculties or virtues. In contrast in the time of al-Razi – let us not forget that more than six hundred years have passed down to our days – the quantity of three pounds was bled. That is to say, half the amount that was let in Galen's time. However, since the time of al-Razi to our days exactly half the length of time from the period of Galen to that of al-Razi has gone by. For this reason, at present, the maximum quantity of blood that is let is exactly half that extracted in the time of al-Razi, approximately a pound and a half, a quantity similar to that which I have just mentioned that I let from a heavily built woman [22 ounces] (fol. 22r).

This reasoning indicates a certain concern for quantifying biological processes, but unfortunately, the author does not offer us any more data to enable us to develop such conjectures any further. The work is planned in a context of a debate – if I might say so – of a very academic nature, the structural framework for which makes use of the scheme of the 'six natural efficient causes' mentioned earlier, together with the elements that make up the other three causes (material, formal and final), all in an intimate functional relationship. These are of course the same as the scheme of the *res naturales*, *non naturales* and *praeter naturam*, so familiar to Latin medieval Galenism. The *K. al-tibb al-qastali* is in no way a rough, direct, word-by-word commentary on a text of a medical authority. It is an authentic systematic medical treatise which integrates the reality of the author's own clinical experience with this Aristotelian-Galenic scheme. The author introduces his clinical experience as a problematic factor – the different forms of behaviour of the sick and the healthy according to whether they live in the high, cold lands of Leon and Castile (Burgos, Avila, Segovia) or in the warmer, lower areas of Toledo and Seville. Together with this factor, the author puts forward the Galenic doctrine of the relative nature of the individual and climatic constitution as the key to the intellectual problem of the divergence between experiential knowledge and what is stated by medical authorities, who not only lived in other climates, but also – like Galen, Rhazes or Avicenna – several hundred years beforehand.

For example, the inhabitants of the region of Toledo forbid youths to drink wine until they reach the age of twenty; and neither do those with fever consume wine for several days. This is due to the fact that the air of the region of Toledo is very warm in comparison with that of the area of Burgos, apart from the fact that its wines are thicker and warmer than those of Burgos. In contrast, the inhabitants of Burgos agree with their children drinking wine, and some even give it to those who are suffering from fevers – provided they are not continuous or burning fevers. And this is because the air of Burgos is softer in comparison with that of Toledo, and as a result the wine is also thin and acid-tasting, so much so that it may be compared with the juice of the bitter pomegranate, as is easy to prove. If this is the difference existing in medical treatment caused by the different air of the two cities mentioned, between which there is only a difference in latitude of two degrees, how much greater will be the variation in treatment [between cities] whose difference in latitude is of five or ten degrees (fol. 7r).

The author of the *K. al-tibb al-qastali* did not aim to write an abstract treatise, but a work addressed to the practising physician – a 'useful' work – but without renouncing the intellectual equipment without which medicine is reduced to a simple handbook of prescriptions or to a catalogue of clinical casuistry. He placed great emphasis on this last point. All the steps that he mentions directed towards the maintenance of health or towards explaining the application of specific treatments are preceded by a brief physiological summary which gives a natural basis for the particular medical approach that he is considering. Recommendations like the following, with a touch of medical ethics, are not unusual:

The practising physician will apply this treatment [one associated with wine in the case of special patients] only after having acquired solid knowledge and when able to diagnose the disease well. He should not use it to challenge the merits of other physicians, and for this reason neither will he pretend to establish a precise diagnosis to gain fame (fol. 14r).

We have already mentioned the complex doctrinal background that the author presupposes in his potential readers, and the authors and medical works recommended. We are now going to turn to a discipline that has not yet been mentioned, but is present in the medical activity of this author: astrology. We have already alluded to the knowledge that he demonstrates of the works of Ptolemy and Al-Zarqali (Algazel). He also seems to have known the astrological work of Ibn al-Kammad. The clearest allusion to astrology appears in a digression in which he considers one of the questions that most concerned Castilian Jewish physicians: the amount of medicine necessary to achieve a certain measurable effect. This is closely connected with the concern for measuring biological phenomena mentioned before. The author resorts to a minor therapeutic experiment for this purpose. His account helps us to recognize the central role that astrology played in the practical medicine of his time.

As for the relation existing between the amount of medicine needed in this region [Castile] and what has to be given in warm regions, I can explain what I obtained in the course of my lengthy experience. I have frequently seen that the quantity of medicine required to evacuate any quantity of humour in this region has to be double what needs to be taken in Al-Andalus [Toledo] in order to evacuate the same amount of humour. In fact, a single drachm of finely powdered agaric evacuates five depositions of humour from any body in Toledo. The same quantity in Burgos does not produce this effect in a body of similar nature and build ... What I have just said does not rule out any individual from Burgos responding favourably, and the person from Toledo unfavourably. This is due to the fact that the natural disposition and complexion of people differ considerably and that is decisive. This is the norm in this matter. For this reason I pointed out that the following requirements should be met to check the strength of one or two grains of agaric: that the two individuals who are the object of study in both these regions should be similar in nature, complexion and in the abundance of humours. However, if we wish to be more demanding in this matter, we also have to make the position of the moon at the moment when the purgative is consumed a condition in order to be able to compare both individuals in the two regions. This is a natural circumstance that may or may not facilitate the action of the medicine. In effect, if, at the moment when the laxative is taken by the man in Toledo, looking towards the planets the moon is to be found in the astrological houses of earth and fire – in other words with all the circumstances required to diminish the strength of the medicine – its efficacy will be reduced. The humours even though they naturally tend towards it, will not respond to evacuation easily. In contrast, we will assist the response of the humours – even though the humours are not disposed [towards evacuation] – if the man from Burgos should consume the purgative when the moon is in a watery sign of the zodiac, other than Cancer, and with aspects towards Venus or Mercury, and both are also placed in the same sign of the zodiac (fol. 26r–v).

The *K. al-tibb al-qastali* had a clear didactic intention. The work is aimed at a hypothetical pupil to whom instructions and recommendations are given. As a result it provides us with the means to reconstruct the most personal parts of the system of medical instruction practised within Jewish quarters, the general lines of which are already known. We refer to what has been called the 'open' model, in contrast to the closed institutional model practised by the Christian university institutions, to which the Jews were forbidden access. According to the open model, he who possessed medical learning transmitted it or imparted it, following his own personal criteria and without being protected by any institution. Teaching activity in the open system reflected the master's interests and abilities rather than the university system.[97] This is apparent in the case of this author, who made an effort to place the pupil who was to practise in the lands of Castile face to face with continual practical examples and specific situations. As we have already seen, the work is not just a set of specific cases hurriedly put

[97] Ibid.

together, but is endowed with a logical structure and a certain standard of abstraction. This latter aspect was to enable the author to pass on his personal experience in a more efficient manner since it was set within the framework of the underlying doctrinal Galenism of his medical practice. He endeavoured to focus the pupil's attention, using the starting point of a specific problem which is likely to arise when the student comes to practise medicine. On other occasions, the pupil's attention is attracted by discussion of questions that were the subject of debate among the practitioners of his time. In this case, the teacher immediately follows with examples from his own experience. He then moves towards an ever-increasing level of abstraction. For example, when dealing with the therapeutic use of cold water with patients suffering from fever in Castile, once he has encouraged the pupil to consult Galen's works on the matter, he explains the seven conditions necessary to establish the individual treatment (this was the abstract level):

First, that the humour causing the fever should not be either phlegm nor black bile. If it were yellow bile, this would have to be subtle and mature. Secondly, that the functions of the stomach should not be weakened nor should they be cold; this last circumstance rarely comes to pass in this region [i.e. Castile]. Thirdly, that the liver should perform its functions perfectly and should not be cold, which also rarely happens in this region since the internal organs of the inhabitants are usually found to be, in the majority of cases, healthy and they are warm, as we have already explained. Fourthly, that there should exist no inflammation nor pain in any intestine, nor subtle yellow bile, something that has to be taken into account in this land. Fifthly, that the patient should possess plenty of innate warmth and blood. Among the inhabitants of this region, those who belong to the nobility and royalty usually fulfil this condition, as we have already explained in the first chapter of this book. Sixthly, notice whether the feverish patient, when in a state of good health, was or was not in the habit of drinking cold water; this point may affect the consumption of cold water in this region. Seventhly, that the person affected by fever should not be an extremely thin person. When you know that these conditions are fulfilled, or are dominant, in the person suffering from fever, then you may let him drink cold water (fols. 31r–v and 32r).

After a series of theoretical considerations, he goes on to explain an individual case history (the case of an old man of seventy who was suffering from fever and severe back pains); the aim of this was to capture the attention of the pupil and lead him towards the specific field of medical practice: 'I mention this example so that you take it into account during treatment, and so that you know the norms of medicine as regards the consumption of cold water during sickness' (fol. 32v).

One aspect of the medical practice of the author of the *K. al-tibb al-qastali* that has been mentioned and which we should not omit is his relationship with noble and royal circles. The biological justification for the 'different' character of the physiology of those belonging to such high ranks was the basis on which rested the whole literary genre of what Christian physicians called *regimina sanitatis*. This genre reached its peak in such circles in the early fourteenth century. By means of these texts, physicians aspired to order the whole life of the addressee, both when he enjoyed good health and when he was sick, thereby hoping to convert medicine into a way of life for the individual in question.[98] These biological characteristics came into existence at the very moment of conception and were hereditary – hence the individual way in which patients had to be treated both in health and in sickness. They could only be detected by a physician, and they differentiated those who belonged by birth to the rank of the nobility from those who did not. The latter all shared a common nature. Thus, their treatment or the norms for preserving their health did not require the same degree of individual attention as demanded by the nobility and the royal family. These arguments, from the point of view of bio-medicine, stressed the social differences of Christian feudal society, which was served by the Jewish author of the work being described. These social characteristics were clearly reflected in the medical treatment provided (fols. 10r–11r). Such arguments were also developed by his Christian contemporary, the royal physician and surgeon Henri de Mondeville, when he describes the social and bio-medical elements that the practitioner has to bear in mind when starting to establish a relationship with his patient.[99]

CONCLUSIONS

Medieval medical Galenism found in the Arabic language an adequate and rigorous vehicle of scientific communication, which survived in south Europe during the late medieval centuries and the Renaissance; people trained in this language could have access to medical texts of scientific and practical value. Between the twelfth and the fifteenth centuries Arabic medical manuscripts circulated in the Christian Kingdoms of Castile and the Crown of Aragon. Although the majority have been lost, nevertheless a total of eighty-one medical works by Greek and Arabic authors, written in Arabic, that circulated in this period and in these regions, are available for study today, surviving in various repositories. The users were members of the three religious communities that co-existed in the Christian kingdoms of the Iberian peninsula during these centuries – Christians, Muslims and Jews. Within the Christian group we have to distinguish between those of Arabic culture (*Mozarabs*) and those of Latin culture. The former would appear to have ceased to make use of Arabic in the early thirteenth century,

[98] L. García-Ballester, 'Changes in the *regimina sanitatis*: the role of the Jewish practitioners', in S. Campbell (ed.), *Health, disease and healing in medieval culture* (Toronto, 1992).
[99] The biological and social characteristics on which medieval physicians, both Jews or Christians, grounded their socially differentiated treatment were systematized and described by Henri de Mondeville in the long introduction to the second book of his treatise on surgery: see Nicaise's edition of the *Chirurgie*, pp. 121–81.

whereas the latter continued to demonstrate interest in medical writings in Arabic down to the transition from the thirteenth to the fourteenth centuries. There is direct evidence that this is actually what happened in the Crown of Aragon and in Murcia. Interest in the employment of Arabic on the part of Latin Christians can again be detected at very localized centres in Valencia in the second half of the fifteenth century.

The only geographical areas where intellectual medical activity on the part of members of the Muslim minority requiring the use of Arabic medical manuscripts can be identified were in the south of Valencia (Crevillente) and Murcia (late thirteenth to early fourteenth centuries), together with Aragon and Valencia once again (last third of the fifteenth century). The evidence is scanty and that from the fifteenth century is particularly difficult to interpret. It is of interest to note that the latter information is derived from Muslim sources, which would appear to indicate that the culture of the Muslim communities was not as poorly integrated as might be suggested by the use of Christian documentary sources alone.

As far as the Jewish minority is concerned, both their own and Christian sources are unanimous in confirming the intense activity of Jewish practitioners – both in Castile and in the Crown of Aragon – which also involved the treatment of members of the Christian community. There is no available information as regards them practising their profession among the Muslim minority. Diachronic analysis of the surviving medical manuscripts in Arabic, as well as the study of the medical sources mentioned in the only surviving fourteenth-century medical work, written in Arabic by a Castilian Jewish physician (probably from Toledo) – the *K. al-tibb al-qastali al-maluki* (*c.* 1312) – demonstrate that the level of medical culture of certain Castilian Jewish rationalist physicians in the first third of the fourteenth century was equal to that of their contemporary Christian colleagues in universities. This learning was nourished by the *corpus* of Galen's medical works, by certain works of Hippocrates, and by the medical writings of Arabic and Jewish authors, written in Arabic. Works of natural philosophy of Aristotelian inspiration and of astrology are to be added to these. All this circulated among the Jewish communities of Castile during the whole period under study here, although the pace of movement declined substantially in the late fourteenth century. The survival of Arabic among the minority of Jewish medical scholars seems to have acted as a limiting factor for their level of scientific knowledge and their intellectual independence as regards Latin scholastic science and medicine.

Internal analysis of *K. al-tibb al-qastali* allows us to draw further conclusions. This work illustrates the author's concern for the application of doctrinal considerations to particular problems and, on urgent occasions, to everyday medical practice. Throughout the work, the author presents himself as a physician who practised for the greater part of his life in the area of Castile now known as the autonomous region of Castile-Leon (see map). There is a predominance of clinical problems and others concerning the maintenance of health of the highest ranking members of society (the nobility and royalty), circles which were well known to the author. He took particular care to emphasize prudence in the application of remedies (e.g. blood-letting) and also to point out the need to study the clients belonging to such ranks of society individually.

Although the author made use of surgery, and had no reservations about employing medicines, of both simple and compound nature, the text reveals that he is also convinced of the benefits that the physician's use of the natural agents that regulate the functions of the body, ranging from the air to the movements of the soul, can have for the client – whether he be sick or healthy. He considered that the physician's study of these external agents (among which astrological factors are also included) should be accompanied by knowledge of the individual 'complexion' of each patient. Thus the physician must be in possession of detailed knowledge of both the region in which he works and of the natural resources of the region. The patient is not an abstract entity disconnected from his environment, but a part of a microcosm incorporating a complex series of natural factors (the word 'natural' should be emphasized) that must be familiar to the physician for him to evaluate them correctly. The diagnosis-prognosis will effectively consist of this. The physician's actions – both in order to maintain health, and also to recover it if lost – will make sense only after this process of evaluation; this process tries to integrate the microcosm–macrocosm relationship at an individual level, by resorting to astrological techniques. This relationship is a consistent factor in the work under study and makes up the core of the natural factors mentioned above.

The author does not reject the study of the great treatises, nor the constant consultation of medical authorities. Three stand out among these: in the first place, Galen, to whose writings he resorted in order to settle conflicting points in medical disputes, whether of a practical or a theoretical nature; in the second place, Rhazes' *Hawi*; in the third place, Avicenna's *Canon*. The intellectual leadership of the last author was for him indisputable, in spite of minor points of disagreement. Avicenna thus appears as the most suitable and lucid interpreter of the Galenic *corpus*. Concerning this point, we can point to the earlier and more direct evidence for Avicenna's prestige among the rationalist Jewish physicians of Castile (first third of the fourteenth century). The version of the *Canon* that was used among the Jewish physicians of Catalonia by the 1350s was in Hebrew.[100] However, the author did not tire of repeating that his work was addressed to the practising physician, and he insisted that the practising doctor had to be mindful of the peculiarities of what might be called the 'regional path-

---

[100] ACA, C., reg. 686, fol. 69r–v, 2 December 1355; reproduced by Rubio y Lluch, *Documents*, vol. II, p. 111, no. 117.

ology', in other words, the set of illnesses dominant in a given region, shaped by physical and psychical factors and in which astral factors were also significant.

The author strongly criticizes the lack of similar works which take as their starting point the clinical problems particular to any geographical area. In this respect, there is constant veiled criticism of the abuse of speculative medicine which relegates the specific patient to the background. The author clearly prefers medicine to be a practical activity based on biological knowledge given by a living Galenism. The physician should have a wide range in his practice; a range which is directly proportional to his knowledge and his clinical experience. The knowledge is acquired through study and reading – in this respect there are constant allusions to consulting and studying medical works and authors. The clinical experience is a matter of time, but it may also be transmitted – and thus learnt – by means of writings. Knowing how to communicate one's own clinical experience through the written word is considered to be the greatest expression of the physician's maturity. This communication should adopt a direct and specific style. Arnau de Vilanova – a Latin contemporary of this author – exemplified this by his aphoristic writing.[101] In this way it was intended to make the conceptual and intellectual complexities achieved by Galenism in the early fourteenth century, in the Latin as well as the Arabic and Jewish worlds, accessible to the practising physician.

The Jewish author of the *K. al-tibb al-qastali* therefore adopted a direct style. His text lacks conceptual solemnity, even though all the sophisticated conceptual complexity of early fourteenth-century developed Galenism underlies it. The Galenism is not presented as a uniform and immutable doctrinal block, but offers different options for interpretation, both at a doctrinal level and in the application of particular forms of treatment. In this work there is not the slightest trace of elements alien to Galenic rationalism. We believe it to be a good example of the Galenism practised by the Jewish rationalist minority in Castile.

The text exhibits a form of Galenism resulting from total intellectual tools and resources of its own, totally separate from the intellectual resources and doctrinal means that were being produced in the nearby world of Latin medical scholasticism in Montpellier or Italy. The author exhibits evidence of knowing some of the intellectual products of this Latin scholasticism, although he does not appear to have been aware (or at least he does not show it) of the intellectual products of the most recent medical scholasticism of these medical centres; neither does he show any interest in the scholastic technique of reasoning, nor in the background (the liberal arts) required by Latin university medicine, which converted medicine into a *scientia* with consequent practical repercussions. The sources of

---

[101] *Repetitio Arnaldi de Villanova s. canonem 'Vita brevis'*, ed. by M. R. McVaugh in AVOMO (Barcelona, in progress).

information were the same as those that the most demanding Christian university physician of the first third of the fourteenth century had access to, with the additional advantage of access to them directly through Arabic. During this period Jewish rationalists do not yet seem to be very attracted by Latin scholastic medicine, although this was to happen to Jewish rationalist physicians at the end of the fourteenth century in western Mediterranean countries.

The information that we possess on the state of the intellectual atmosphere of the Muslim and Jewish minorities in Castile at the turn of the thirteenth and fourteenth centuries indicates that only those scholars who were members of the Jewish minority used the Arabic medical sources in existence in Castile. These manuscripts circulated in Castile with sufficient freedom for Jewish physicians to have access to them without difficulty. The text also clearly reveals the existence of intellectual freedom, at least in those Jewish circles that the author moved in, together with a certain climate of intellectual exchange between Christian surgeons and physicians and their Jewish counterparts. All these points may be deduced from the repeated allusions of the author to problems that were the subject of debate both among Jewish physicians and between the latter and individual Christian surgeons and physicians, whom he refers to, though unfortunately not by name. This indicates a degree of communication between the practitioners of the two communities characteristic of the fourteenth century.[102] Nowhere in the text does there appear any reference to contact with contemporary Muslim professionals practising in Castile. From other sources we know that a relationship with Muslim colleagues living in the Kingdom of Granada, however, did occur.[103]

[102] There is much clear evidence in fourteenth-century Catalonia and Majorca of professional collaboration between Jewish and Christian medical practitioners in the treatment of the same patient: see, for example, Regional Archive of Puigcerdá, notarial records, Joan Torrelles, *Lib. extraneorum*, 1361–2, fol. 45v, 18 March 1362. The collaboration was between the Christian Magister Anthonius de Capeyll, *physicus*, and Samuel Adday, *judeus physicus*, both living in Puigcerdá. See note 51 above.
[103] See note 64 above.

Index